THE GREEN CITY WITCH

THE GREEN CITY WITCH
Weaving a Magical Life in Urban Spaces

Lynn Shore

AEON

First published in 2025 by
Aeon Books

Copyright © 2025 by Lynn Shore

The right of Lynn Shore to be identified as the author of this work has been asserted in accordance with §§77 and 78 of the Copyright Design and Patents Act 1988.

All rights reserved. No part of this publication may be reproduced, stored in a retrieval system, or transmitted, in any form or by any means, electronic, mechanical, photocopying, recording, or otherwise, without the prior written permission of the publisher.

British Cataloguing in Publication Data

A C.I.P. for this book is available from the British Library

ISBN-13: 978-1-80152-188-8

Typeset by Medlar Publishing Solutions Pvt Ltd, India
Cover design and illustrations by Hannah McDonald,
https://www.hannahmcdonald.co/

www.aeonbooks.co.uk

DISCLAIMER

The information in this book has been compiled to provide general guidance, including insights into spells, charms, meditations, and herbal remedies. It is not intended to replace the advice and treatment of qualified health professionals. Please do not attempt to self-diagnose or self-prescribe for serious or long-term issues. When exploring spells, charms, meditations, or herbal remedies, always heed the cautions provided. If you are pregnant, nursing, or taking medication, consult a professional before using herbal remedies or engaging in any magical practices that use herbs.

By choosing to use any information in this book for personal use, you acknowledge your constitutional right to do so. However, the author and publisher cannot assume responsibility for your actions or outcomes.

To the best of the author's knowledge, all information presented here is accurate and up-to-date at the time of publishing. As with all matters of health and wellness, whether physical, spiritual, or magical, exercise caution and proceed with care.

CONTENTS

ACKNOWLEDGMENTS ix

INTRODUCTION xi

LIFESTYLE

Belonging 3
Reconnecting with urban nature 7
Green living for urban witches 19
Covens and community 29
Wheel of the Year 33
    Samhain 36
    Winter solstice 41
    Imbolc 46
    Spring equinox 51
    Beltane 56
    Summer solstice 61
    Lughnasadh 66
    Autumn equinox 71

Urban foraging 77
    Ethical foraging 78
    Urban foraging calendar 80

NATURE LORE

Plant lore directory 88
Animal lore directory 261

TOOLS AND TECHNIQUES

Tools 288
Techniques 303
Symbolism 319
Rituals 329
Nature spirits 337
Divination and special senses 341
Prayer 351
Sound 355
Protection techniques 357
Spells and charms 367
    Charm directory 379
    Spell directory 388
Moon Magic 401
Blood Magic 409
Shapeshifting 413
Conclusion 419

BIBLIOGRAPHY 423

INDEX 435

ACKNOWLEDGMENTS

I would like to thank Livvy and Frank de Graaf for their love and patience, Peter Sweers and Ranju Roy for their encouragement at much-needed times. And, not least, Hannah McDonald for her beautiful illustrations.

Special thanks:
While researching this book, many others were consulted. Their experience spans eight decades, all seven continents, and a wide range of practices.

Andy Hamilton – Author, forager, and thinker.
theotherandyhamilton.com

Ash – Crystal Keeper, Alchemist of culinary and botanical delights.
aether-obscura.com

Bobby – Revivalist craftsman, forager, and fleece tamer

Brian – Thank you for sprinkling extra charms into these pages

Diana Zuican – Exploring human complexities through the lens.
didoaska.com

Esther Heidr Rheintochter – Priestess of Freya, Daughter of the Rivers

Jules – Equity advocate and creative catalyst

Louise Hawkins – Rose and Passionflower charmer

Mahaut Vidal – Enchantress of Paris, Citrus, and gelée

Marisa Conde – Protector and blender of nature's gifts. @primalessencecosmetics

Melissa Love – Transatlantic hedgewitch and shadow dancer

Michael – Warm-hearted world traveller with very green thumbs

Mana Sundari – Yoga Witch, animal lover; of many homes & hobbies. @mana.sundari

Mara – Researcher, doula, creative. Rewilder of hearts
@mara.mamamagick

Nastya – Rewilder of smooth cityscapes

Sam Webster – Forager, North UK
@ForagingForAges

Sian and Cathy – Diolch am eich cymorth

And, to the wonderful team at Aeon Books, for bringing this book to life.

INTRODUCTION

Welcome to *The Green City Witch*, a guide to bringing magic and nature into city life. With most of us living in small or shared apartments, often without gardens, in bustling cities, it can feel as though nature is far away. Yet even the smoothest urban landscapes teem with life and offer countless opportunities to engage with nature. Whether you were born and bred in your current town or have been highly mobile throughout your life, there are always ways to nurture a connection with nature and your surroundings.

Plants and animals are not constrained by the languages and beliefs that divide humans. Governed by nature's laws, they have much to teach us. By observing and connecting with urban wildlife, we can elevate ourselves above the stress and pain that often accompany modern living.

Magic is here too, waiting for anyone seeking a deeper connection with the spiritual world. It is what sets magical practitioners apart, but you don't need to identify as a witch, shaman, or wise wo/man to use it. Magic is the art of engaging with the energy, or spirit, that connects all things. It offers a means to bring change or disruption to the natural course of events. All magic requires is clear intention and passion;

no religious affiliation, no props, no tools—just hyperfocus and drive. And it works.

The field of quantum physics gives scientific validation to what magical practitioners have understood forever: all aspects of the universe are intricately connected. By manipulating one part, we can create change elsewhere. Through these subtle changes, magic offers ways to improve the world. In these times of climate crisis, social polarisation, and work–life imbalance, magic lights up the parts of our brains that make our souls sing. It helps us see connections where others see separation and trains our minds to remain open to possibilities and growth.

Humans are amazing creatures, capable of incredible good. But the lives we create can stifle our brains' potential if we allow them to. When the left and right hemispheres of our brains aren't given opportunities to work in harmony, we limit what we can achieve and enjoy. The analytical, detail-focused left hemisphere is essential for making decisions like "yes/no" or "safe food/poison", while the holistic, context-aware right hemisphere excels in imagining blue-sky possibilities. There should be a dynamic balance between the two.

Yet many of us suppress our creative and magical side. To reawaken it, we must push algorithms and schedules aside, immerse ourselves in nature, write poems and spells, listen to the wind, find stories in the clouds, watch Beetles at work, and feel Moss beneath our feet! This is the inspiration behind the offerings in this book.

You may like to think of *The Green City Witch* as a woodland retreat for your soul. It contains practices to help you cultivate a life that embraces your surroundings, values, and dreams. What unfolds for you might include foraging on side streets, connecting with Crows, or learning about local heroes. It could also involve rituals, spells, divination, and befriending nature spirits.

The book is divided into three parts:

Lifestyle: Explore ways to live sustainably, grow roots in new cities, align with seasonal changes, and develop a sense of belonging through connection with urban nature. This section also provides guidance on urban foraging as a means to source magical natural materials and supplement your food supply.

Nature Lore: A plant lore directory of wild and feral plants that thrive in urban spaces, along with their magical symbolism, folklore, and practical uses. An animal lore directory introduces the creatures that share our city spaces; their symbolism, special characteristics, and ways to engage with them spiritually.

Tools and Techniques: Guidance on working magic, from grounding and self-protection to rituals, charms, divination, and shapeshifting. These techniques are offered in a sustainable context, using local, ethically sourced natural materials.

City living is full of contradictions, offering chaos and calm, challenges and opportunities in every neighbourhood. This book helps you engage with these contradictions and bring about positive change. Its practices are designed to be accessible, sustainable, and safe. Some come with reminders to approach with care, particularly when working with potent herbs or exploring altered states of consciousness. Their goal is to help you craft a magical life that feels connected, authentic, and uniquely yours.

This book celebrates the hidden opportunities in what are often seen as the challenges of city living; embracing compact homes, limited time, and shared resources. Green city witchcraft offers a way of being that is open to everyone and brimming with potential. This is an invitation to engage with the diverse lifeforms of our towns and cities, regardless of your experience with nature or magic. The aim is to inspire creativity, connection, and transformation. Urban life holds immense possibilities for those ready to nurture both the practical and imaginative sides of their mind.

LIFESTYLE

What does the life of a witch really look like? Is it cloaked in mystery and bound by rituals? Or is their magic seamlessly woven into daily life? For witches practicing in cities, magic can't be confined to quiet woods or ancient ruins; it thrives in bustling neighbourhoods, verdant parks, and graffiti-tagged streets. These cunning folk blend spells into their routines and form deep connections with urban nature. They work with the rhythms of local wildlife, street trees, and spirits of place. Each cityscape carries its own energy, and Green City Witches move through them with awareness, drawing strength from energetic shifts. Wherever they go, they blend with nature to feel at home; from putting down roots in a new town to shaking off jetlag on trips abroad.

Some practise alone, quietly crafting their magic, while others join loose-knit or closely bonded groups. What unites them is their eco-conscious approach: a reverence for the natural world, even in smooth, grey urban settings. Their magic uses locally sourced materials, often foraged or crafted by hand. Their choices deepen their bond with the environment. These men and women hail from all walks of life and are frequently drawn to careers that honour the earth. Above all, sustainability and simplicity guide their practice and strive to bring respect and balance to all around. This section of the book explores how to live this way, developing renewed nature-connection and a sense of belonging in the urban world.

Belonging

City life offers a vibrant mix of cultures, new experiences, and the potential to flourish. But it can also feel overwhelming. The fast pace, ever-changing surroundings, and sheer scale of urban environments often lead to loneliness, detachment, and a lack of belonging. Those feelings make it difficult to thrive, but there are practical ways to help grow roots through rituals and exploration. They can help whether you're moving home, travelling, or simply want to deepen your roots in a familiar town.

Local energy

Every city and neighbourhood has its unique rhythm and spirit. So take time to walk, pause, and observe the contrast in energy from one area to the next. Walking or biking through your neighbourhood will connect you to its layers of history, culture, and nature, better than travelling by car. Seek out lesser-known greenscapes like cemeteries, school gardens, and arboretums, but also visit landmarks and historical sites, to discover stories of the land and its people. To help your search for interesting places, seek out maps of street trees, community gardens, or heritage trails.

As you settle into the flow of a town, you'll more quickly be able to sense where you feel nourished or drained. Some areas may feel chaotic and draining, while others will bring you calm and inspiration. Don't rush, take time to explore, as this will help the experiences to sink in and strengthen your inner compass.

Take time to observe what goes on there, use all your senses and notice how the feel of the environment depends on the time of day or week that you visit. On a city map, mark places you have visited that feel nourishing or interesting. These might include parks, markets, historic sites, cafés, and secret courtyards. Then use the map as a personal guide to pull out and lead journeys on days when you need to recharge.

Local food

Very local food, especially plants native to the region, can quickly connect us with local surroundings. Try foraging familiar herbs, like Dandelion flowers or Stinging Nettles, and experiment with incorporating them into your meals. Visit a farmers' market to sample some local produce and support organic businesses. Do this regularly and reflect on how this "taste of place" influences your sense of belonging. Eating local edible *weeds* can align our internal rhythms with the place almost immediately, so you may like to try it when feeling jet lagged.

Green connection

Urban environments can feel detached from nature, but opportunities for connection exist everywhere: Nurture plants indoors, on a doorstep or balcony. Plant a window box, adopt a small green space, and perhaps explore guerrilla gardening in your area. Connect with urban wildlife, from birds to bugs; observe how they adapt and thrive. You may like to look for opportunities to support local greening and rewilding. Your local council may keep a directory of this kind of project. Indoors, set up a nature display with found objects—stones, leaves, or feathers—and change it with the seasons. And, try developing small, personal rituals, to deepen this bond; the Wheel of the Year section contains plenty of ideas. You may also find plants that grow almost exclusively in your area, such as Bristol Rock Cress (*Arabis scabra*), or Cornish Heath (*Erica vagans*).

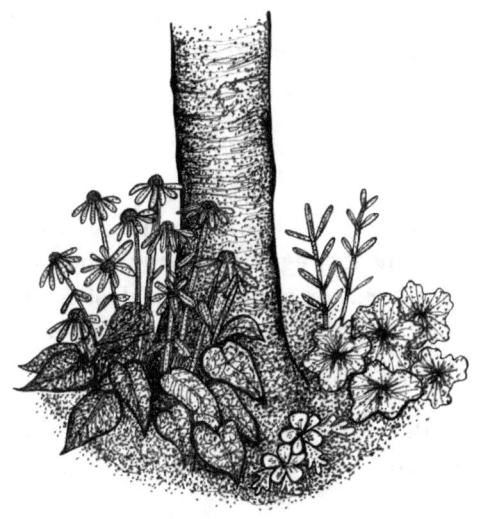

History and folklore

Understanding the history and mythology of a place can increase our sense of belonging, so research the origins of your neighbourhood. Find out how it was built, its cultural influences, and local legends. Folklore often holds clues about the environment, like plants and animals of significance, and may offer a sense of connection with those who came before. Learn the names of some plants and animals in the local language, which can often reveal traditional uses or symbolic meanings. Your city may have a local history museum or offer heritage walking tours, too. Explore regional tales and consider honouring these by blending symbols of them into your spiritual practices.

Pilgrimage

Getting out of the city, even briefly, can refresh your perspective on life and help you to understand the culture that created the town where you live. Find out about ancient landmarks, nearby forests, or coastlines and how to reach them. Spend some time tuning into the energies there, and leave simple natural offerings to honour the place and ancestors.

You may also like to go on short pilgrimages to the resting places of key figures from your community. This could involve marking the graves of well-known poets, community leaders, activists, writers, artists, etc., on a map of your local cemetery, then visiting and researching what they added to the world during their lifetime.

Immersion

To feel at home in an environment, you will need to immerse yourself in its rhythms. This means regularly taking time to engage with the people, plants, and creatures around you. Listen to the "language" of your place, from the sounds of the wind in trees, the movements of wildlife, and the hum of your neighbourhood. Belonging is both a practice and a feeling, so take time to connect with your neighbours, learn the language they speak, join in local activities, talk to people, and expect to fit in. In no time you will feel connected to the place.

Reconnecting with urban nature

In the rush of city life, it's easy to overlook the magic of daily encounters with nature. Yet small moments like pausing to admire a tree, listening to birdsong, or tending a plant, can improve your wellbeing and enrich your magical practice. Connecting with the natural world brings peace into your life and awakens your awareness, helping you weave its details into your spells and rituals.

This chapter invites you to see urban nature from a fresh perspective, and rekindle some of the awe you felt as a child exploring the outdoors. By opening your heart to the plants and creatures sharing your city, you'll form a deeper bond with them, one that strengthens your magic and reminds you that even in a bustling city, nature is never far away.

Biophilia

Why is connection with nature so vital? Biophilia, a term coined by biologist Edward O. Wilson, describes a bond shaped by evolution to ensure our survival. We are attracted to green spaces filled with living plants. Studies confirm what has long been realised, that being in nature, or even just imagining being in it, can lift our spirits, ease stress, and boost our creativity.[1] This need for nature connection reminds us that we're not separate from nature—we are a part of it. And by embracing this bond, we nourish both ourselves and the planet.

There are many ways to benefit from engaging with nature. One is simply being near soil. That can be deeply healing. Studies show that the tiny microorganisms in soil release volatile organic chemicals (VOCs) into the air that help reduce inflammation and improve emotional well-being. So, whether through gardening or simply touching the earth, working with soil and inhaling its volatile chemicals can be incredibly grounding and restorative.

Our eyes are particularly drawn to the colour green. We are able to detect its infinite shades with remarkable precision, a skill that once helped us identify nourishing plants. Many cultures have special words for life force, such as *prana*, *viriditas*, or *nwyfre*. With a little practice it is possible to appreciate which plants are rich in this vitality, by observing the hues of green.

In cities, whether we are wandering in a park, gazing at fresh Moss, or simply caring for a houseplant, even small interactions with the green world can renew our energy. These moments ground us, calm our racing thoughts, and anchor us in the present. Our relationship with nature goes beyond convenience; it's about recognising that the same forces nurturing the Earth sustain us, too.

Although the colour and form of plastic plants and wallpaper trees can improve our mood, they mimic the aesthetic of life, lack its essence, and indeed may harm us.[2] To gain the most benefit from nature connection, we need to interact with real living soil, plants, animals, microbes, and the weather.

Three simple ways to cultivate a real, living relationship with nature are to regularly observe, communicate, and meditate on aspects of it. For example, when you next walk by a beautiful flowering Rose, pause for a moment to take in its details. Breathe softly yet deeply, and let its fragrance fill you. Notice how the Rose makes you feel, and silently thank it for its gifts. Later in the day, find a quiet moment to revisit this sensory experience in your mind. Through these three simple steps

---

[1] M. Cordoza et al. Impact of nurses taking daily work breaks in a hospital garden on burnout. *Am J Crit Care* (2018) 27(6): 508–12.

[2] The 2018 article by K. Kelleher, Scheele's Green: The color of fake foliage and death. *The Paris Review* (2 May), is both fascinating and disturbing, especially given that some French florists are suffering from contemporary work-related disease.

of observing, communicating, and meditating, you'll open yourself to a deeper connection with and appreciation for the natural world.

Observation

One of the simplest and most rewarding skills, observation requires no special tools and causes little disruption to nature. All it takes is a calm, patient approach and an open mind. Find a spot, busy or quiet, and tune into everything around you. Use whichever senses you have available to pick up on the scents, sounds, textures, light, and even the feel of the air on your skin. With regular practice, this mindful awareness creates a sensory memory bank unique to every place and time. For instance, you might recognise your hometown from the sound of birdsong in a recording, or sense that a storm is brewing by a particular scent in the air.

This sensory connection links to your emotions, teaching how environments affect your mood. For example, a walk on a windy day might stir your thoughts if you're feeling stuck, while a calm green setting could ease anxiety. By observing regularly, you'll learn to recognise how nature influences your state of mind and use that knowledge for balance and wellbeing.

Move gently when observing, this helps urban wildlife and plants feel at ease around you and gives you time to process what your senses are picking up. Observe whatever catches your attention, from vibrations in the soil to the textures of grass and stones. Trace a Daisy's stem to its roots with your fingers and eyes, observe the tiny hairs, and see how each petal is unique. Feel the autumn mist on your face as you cycle. Immerse yourself fully in the small wonders of the natural world and be open to the messages that other living beings send to you. This can quickly build appreciation for nature's wisdom. Here are some more observation activities to try:

Weather watching

Watching clouds drift and imagining their shapes is a calming meditative practice and a traditional form of divination. Whether you read patterns in the sky or reflect on how the weather shapes cloud formations, weather watching sharpens your observational skills and helps you tune into nature.

Over time, you may notice how your body senses weather changes. For example, your hair might stand on end before snow, or you might feel the dampness of approaching rain on your skin. And, standing outside as the first storm of a heat wave breaks is exhilarating—just remember to be cautious of lightning and take cover if needed! The subtle cues that our body detects, along with spending more time outdoors, improves our ability to anticipate changes in the weather. Even opening windows to air your home each day, year round, can help you live more in sync with the natural climate and build a stronger connection to the world.

Learning about clouds and air pressure can also build your weather watching skills. In simple terms, high pressure creates clear, dry weather by keeping moisture grounded, while low pressure allows moisture to rise, forming clouds and often leads to rain or storms. Sudden shifts in pressure bring strong winds, while smaller changes produce subtler effects. Cloud formations show what is happening; Cirrus clouds (the high, wispy ones) signal fair weather; Cumulus clouds (fluffy, lumpy and grey) often predict rain; Nimbus clouds are thick and dark, bringing rain, snow, or hail, while Stratus clouds form gloomy blankets across the sky. They predict rain.

Also watch out for special light effects at twilight. You may see crepuscular rays, sunbeams that radiate from a point, or the Green Flash, which is a fleeting green spot at the top of the Sun as it sets or rises. Both are special sights to observe.

Moss watching

Moss watching, or *koke kansatsu* in Japanese, is a soothing way to reconnect with nature. By observing the tiny world of Moss (and also liverworts, and lichens) you can gain a deep appreciation for life's details. Whether you investigate Moss in the wild or bring a small piece home, this is a quiet and rewarding activity that sharpens observation skills and invites us to notice often overlooked aspects of nature.

Stretching your fingers and gently resting them on a soft patch of Moss is very grounding. Moss has a distinctive scent and grows in countless shades of green, which keep our biophilia superpower sharp. Some enthusiasts create small Moss gardens in shallow trays or pots, others prefer to observe the wild.

Start Moss watching by finding a nice specimen. Then with or without a hand lens, simply sit quietly and examine its textures, colours, and patterns. Look closely at the delicate structures, tiny water droplets, and the subtle beauty of these simple plants. Over time, you'll notice their growth patterns and how they change with the seasons. If you want to go further, squeeze a few drops of Moss water onto a slide and examine it under a microscope or hand lens. You might spot tiny creatures like Tardigrades (Water Bears), Nematodes, or Amoebae moving within this miniature ecosystem. If you don't have a lens, simply imagining the unseen life within Moss can be a deeply meditative experience.

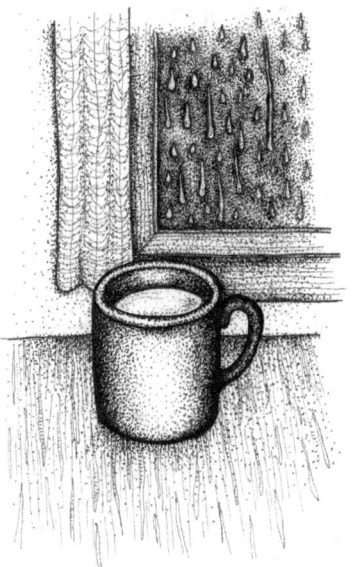

Rain watching

Rain offers countless opportunities to pause, observe, and connect with the natural world. Whether walking through a spring shower or watching droplets slide down a window, there is so much to notice. On a Sun-cloud sort of day, you might spot raindrops clinging to leaves or railings. If the light catches them just right, you may see them sparkling like tiny jewels. If you shift your head slightly, you may be able to see the droplets refract the sunlight into rainbows.

Then there's petrichor, the fresh, earthy scent made when rain mixes with soil and plant oils. It helps to ground us, so try taking a deep breath during or after a rain shower to tune into your environment.

Observing how rain feels on the skin is another simple and underappreciated thing to do. When it next rains, notice how the raindrops falling from leaves differ from those falling straight from the sky; each carries the unique essence of what it has touched. And how does it feel on your skin? How does it differ from tap water?

Rain also reminds us of nature's cycles: travelling constantly from river to sea, then to clouds and droplets, and finally back to the earth. Rain brings life and balance, so rather than rushing to avoid it, take a moment to observe, or even enjoy. You may find yourself connecting more deeply with the rhythms of the world around you.

Animal watching

Observing animals in the city offers a chance to connect with nature in unexpected ways. Every creature has unique talents and adaptations, with some that thrive in urban environments while others struggle. Watching city animals closely can reveal their intelligence and survival strategies, and even inspire your shapeshifting work.

Start with the animals you see around you. Pay attention to birds like Magpies, Crows, and Blackbirds: observe their calls, movements, and behaviours to learn to distinguish between species. Sitting quietly in a park, you might notice Rats scavenging near benches or bins. Stay still and calm, and you'll begin to see their natural behaviour.

Companion animals also have much to teach. Cats, for instance, communicate their feelings in subtle ways that we often overlook. A slow blink can indicate trust and affection, and learning their body language can help us keep them healthy and deepen our connection.

Water watching

Water offers a wonderful opportunity to enhance your observational skills, whether you're by the sea, near a river, a canal, or simply beside a garden water feature. Observe how water moves, the reflections it creates, and the life it supports. The pebbles and flints lining a path, perhaps washed down from distant mountains or rivers, each hold a story of their journey. Even gravel in a driveway or seaweed along the shoreline can offer moments of wonder and insight.

If you can't reach a natural waterway, sit with gravel or pebbles, which often come from riverbeds. Notice their smoothness, imagine their origins, and reflect on the journeys they've made. Simply being near water, listening to its sound or noticing its scent, can bring a peaceful awareness of the world's cycles and rhythms.

Tree watching

Tree watching is a wonderful way to sharpen your nature observation skills. Trees hold countless stories and offer a calming presence to those who spend time with them. Begin by finding a tree that calls to you, perhaps in a local park or cemetery. Spend time observing its leaves, bark, branches, and the way it interacts with the surrounding environment. Notice how it sways with the wind or changes with the seasons. Return to visit it regularly and watch how it adapts over time.

Seek out unusual trees in green spaces, or use online tree maps to locate different species nearby. Tree watching also introduces you to the animals and fungi living on or within these majestic plants, so take your time and notice the details you may have missed before. This practice cultivates mindfulness, connects you to urban nature, and enhances your ability to observe and appreciate the natural world.

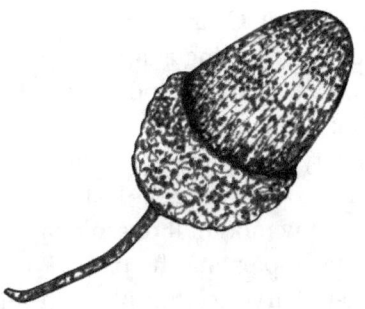

Communication with nature

There are endless ways to explore and practice communication with nature. Every living being has unique methods for exchanging information. Animals use calls, body language, eye contact, proximity, and even subtle changes in breath rate. Plants release chemical signals, fungi emit scents, and the weather *speaks* through its changes. Observing these interactions can deepen our connection to the natural world and sharpen our communication skills.

Wildlife provides many opportunities to practise: calming a stranded Frog or gently helping a rain-soaked Bee relies on communicating trust, calm, and care through our tone and body language. Animals often sense intent, responding more positively when approached with respect. These principles apply when a bird strays indoors or a Grasshopper hops into your home, when staying calm helps them feel safe and find their way out without harm.

Developing nature-communication skills also involves developing your instincts. Foragers often know a plant or mushroom is nearby before they see it, which suggests an intuitive connection and well-developed senses. By tuning into the cues of other living beings, we can start a dialogue with them and encourage harmony.

Plant communication

Plants communicate in fascinating ways. Damaged Acacia trees, for example, produce chemicals to warn of grazing animals. This prompts nearby trees to produce defensive compounds that deter the grazers. Mimosa trees do the same, while underground fungal hyphae are known to communicate using electrical messages and altering the flow of their protoplasm.[3] The VOCs that fungi emit also communicate the ripeness of mushrooms to foraging animals.

A personal experience with Ground Elder (*Aegopodium podagraria*) shows how plants may communicate with human forgers. This fast-spreading plant has tasty leaves and grows in colonies. I've noticed that as it begins to bloom in early summer, the leaf scent changes, and nibbling them causes a tingle in my mouth. It doesn't happen at other times but seems a clear signal to stop eating the plant. Further experimentation showed that the longer I harvested this plant, the more intense the reaction became. I now avoid the problem by picking only small amounts at a time, and avoiding it completely around seed-setting time.

Ground Elder colonies grow from a shallow root network, and I suspect these may be used to quickly communicate and ramp up the production of defensive chemicals. Another forager, Sam Webster, noted a similar effect on her skin; the longer she spent harvesting the plant, the more intensely her skin reacted. Ground Elder isn't thought

---

[3] A. Adamatzky, Language of fungi derived from their electrical spiking activity. *Royal Society, Open Science* (2022) 9(4).

to contain the harmful furanocoumarins of its Apiaceae relatives like Giant Hogweed (*Heracleum mantegazzianum*), but it does contain potent phytochemicals. Whatever the cause, Sam and I have listened to Ground Elder, and learned to be extra cautious around it.

Here are some less irritating ways to develop your powers of communication with nature:

Talk with trees

It is possible to engage with trees by speaking to them aloud or silently. Some trees seem to welcome attention, while others prefer solitude, so respect the feelings they evoke when you attempt to connect. As you walk among trees, notice how different species or individuals affect your emotions. Try quietly leaning against one or sit nearby, to tune into its energy.

When city trees fall during storms, you might like to honour them by gathering keepsake leaves, seeds, or cuttings to create offspring. Reflect on their history, the creatures they supported, and their contributions to the ecosystem. We can learn much about resilience and renewal from grand old street and park trees.

Show respect by clearing litter from their surroundings or offering gifts like water, herb tea, or flowers. Be mindful not to stunt their growth by raising the soil level around their roots, or tying objects to them. Simple acts of care are enough to show your appreciation of these incredible beings.

Autumn leaf art

Celebrate the changing seasons by creating ephemeral designs with colourful fallen leaves. Dab a little honey on each leaf and arrange on tree trunks or pavements. As trees save resources by pulling nutrients back into their trunks, the autumn leaf colours may indicate the remaining chemicals such as yellow xanthophylls, orange carotenoids, and brown tannins. Autumn is when these are naked and possible for us to see. If Liquidambar trees grow near you, their balsam-scented autumn leaves are well worth including in such ephemeral art.

Deepen your connection with nature through art at any opportunity. Use whatever medium attracts you and let your creations inspire your spells and rituals.

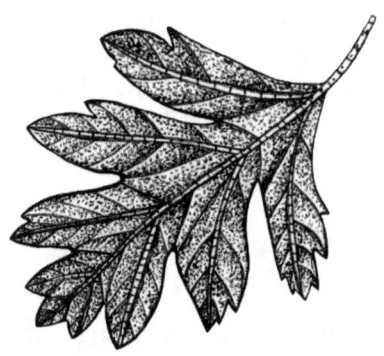

Talk with birds

Birds offer many opportunities for interaction if you take the time to observe and respond to them. Notice their body language, such as head movements, and mimic them respectfully. If a Robin visits you while gardening, tilt your head to acknowledge it, and avoid direct eye contact or sudden movements (often interpreted as a threat). Over many days, build trust through gentle communication. Eventually, it may choose to land on your hat or shoulder.

Listening to the patterns of bird songs and calls, try to interpret their meaning, and perhaps mimic them to encourage a response. Patience and a non-threatening presence are key to communicating with urban birds.

Calm communication

Approach wild creatures and plants calmly, using gentle words and gestures. Be open to subtle messages they may send out, perhaps expressing the need to be left alone, or how they can be helped. For instance, you might dry a rain-drenched Bee with the warmth of your hand, or keep hazards away from a bird, fallen from a nest. Some foragers ask herbs to prepare for their harvest, believing it increases their potency. Whatever your intention, be calm near wildlife, and listen to their messages.

Baring skin

We tend to spend most of our time with almost completely covered skin and a great separation from the elements. Regularly exposing even small areas of flesh to fresh air and sunlight can boost vitamin D production, build resilience to the Sun's rays, and help us pick up on information from nature.

Gardening outside with bare hands and feet takes this a step further. Bare skin on soil is grounding, and channels any worries into the earth. It also lets us feel the Earth's energy and soak up beneficial VOCs from soil microbes. Try it year round, if you can.

Dew bathing

Walking barefoot on dewy grass in the morning or using dew to refresh your skin is a great way to engage with nature. Try collecting dew from clean plants like Lady's Mantle or Hawthorn, and notice the invigorating tingle it brings, an experience unmatched by expensive skincare routines.

Meditation and contemplation

Tree meditation

Try sitting at the base of a tree, leaning gently against its trunk, or simply placing your hands on its bark. Let your breath settle at a natural pace. You may feel the energy within the tree; does it feel fast or slow, throbbing or still? Imagine the deep network of roots below, intertwined with fungi and other plants, creating a vast, unseen web of life. Visualise yourself moving into the tree trunk, exploring the tree's great skeleton of branches, twigs, and leaves.

Take time to appreciate the tree's shape, the creatures it shelters, and how it responds to its environment. Extend your attention to the Ivy climbing its trunk or the birds and insects resting in its branches. See the world through the tree and its ecosystem. Be open to any messages it has for you. Then gradually withdraw from the tree, return to your own body, and thank the tree for its teachings.

Skull meditation

This meditation invites us to reflect on the interconnectedness of life and death. Sit comfortably and trace the gentle contours of your skull with your fingertips, feeling its strength and shape. Visualise your skull glowing with golden light, a sacred vessel holding your consciousness and the memories of your spiralling journey. Reflect on how your skull supports and protects you. Release any tension by softening your facial muscles, neck, and scalp. When ready, gently return to the present moment.

Contemplations on found objects

Take time to explore the origins of the materials around you, whether made from wood, metal, plastic, or glass. Consider the journey it has made, from its source. If a wooden object, contemplate how it grew from seed to sapling, to tree, supporting wildlife, standing in all weathers, through many seasons. How it was transformed into something new. Consider what will happen to the object, when its useful days are through. This practice can build an appreciation for the interconnectedness of all things, from the natural world to the human-made.

Alternatively, contemplate natural found objects like feathers, stones, or shells. These small treasures have been shaped by nature, by elements. How did they arise, and how will they be recycled and transformed anew?

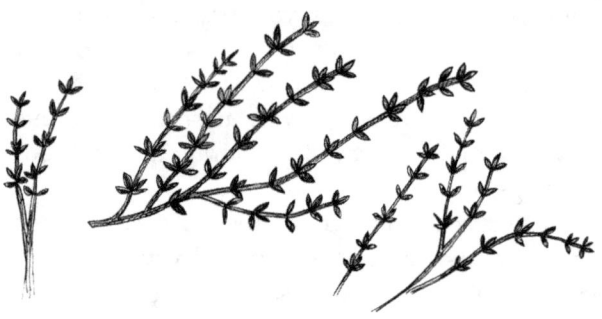

Elemental meditations

Sit by a tree, hold a stone, feel the wind on your skin, dip your toes in a canal, or gaze into a flickering candle flame. Each element carries unique energy, offering a chance to connect with the spirits of nature and the place around you. Hugging a tree, or simply touching its bark, can connect you with all elements at once, as trees reach from earth to sky, water courses through them, and the chemical processes inside each leaf resemble tiny controlled fires. Consider how other living beings encapsulate the elements in similar ways.

Green living for urban witches

Living sustainably and authentically as an urban witch involves cultivating habits that nurture the Earth and yourself, from reducing consumption, minimising waste, and forging intuitive connections with the natural world. The key is to make your lifestyle intentional and circular. Choices regarding your home, work, craft and play all make this possible.

When it comes to your home, choose décor and furnishings that align with your values. Opt for natural, ethical, non-toxic, and durable materials. Many furnishings, decorating supplies, and cleaning products contain synthetic and toxic chemicals such as formaldehyde, benzene, and phthalates, which can seriously harm your health. To minimise exposure, focus on reducing consumption, using natural products, and maintaining good ventilation in your space. Additionally, minimise reliance on energy-intensive climate control systems by adjusting your clothing and acclimating to seasonal rhythms; this can also improve your health.

Growing plants can improve the quality of your indoor environment, and reduce the need for air conditioning. If you want to fill your home with plants, find organically grown options that suit your usual indoor climate (think temperature fluctuations, air humidity, and light intensity). Water and mulch green housemates with leftover herb tea or rainwater, and take good care of them, to let their personalities and talents shine.

Choose your possessions wisely also. Opt for energy-efficient appliances, natural cleaning products, and support businesses that use recycled materials or locally sourced, sustainable materials. Be cautious of greenwashing, where businesses claim to be environmentally friendly without genuinely practising sustainability, and look at the long-term effects of your purchases. Installing solar panels, for instance, can seem a great way to reduce fossil fuel use, but their production requires the mining and transportation of quartz, heavy metals, and other issues of significant environmental and social impact.

Rather than buying more solutions to our problems, it is better to scale up efforts to reduce consumption, energy use, and to question the wider effects of our decisions. One way is to extend the life and usefulness of appliances and tools, by considering *Tsukumogami*, a Japanese belief that items with a strong connection to people acquire power over many years of use. Rather than replacing items, develop a sustainable mindset by maintaining, repurposing, and repairing them.

One of the benefits of city living is the proximity to resources and networks. Cities offer the ability to share tools, space, skills, and knowledge, which can reduce your dependence on traditional, resource-draining systems. Developing self-sufficiency by learning how to fix clothes, bake, or grow your own food can relieve financial and emotional stress. Your local community may have repair cafés, where items are mended and reused rather than discarded, or networks where people with occasional-use items register and lend them out. There may also be local skill share groups, to learn alongside each other. Networks like this reduce waste and reliance on consumerism, building stronger, more resilient communities. If there is nothing similar happening near you, why not start a group? You may quickly find that life becomes less stressful and more fulfilling, when you are part of such a community.

A cluttered home can mirror a cluttered mind or spirit. So, regularly declutter, and ensure that your possessions serve you both practically and energetically. Each season, you may find that ritually cleansing your space and stuff helps keep you feeling fresh.

Living sustainably also means being mindful of your energy consumption. Rising costs and planetary crises make this essential for everyone. So alongside turning the thermostat down, cycle around town, prepare low-energy meals, and phase plastics out of your life.

Buy seasonal, local and organic fruit and vegetables to nurture the ecosystem around you. Support the local businesses, restaurants, and community-supported agriculture that take sustainability seriously. This can help sustain the local economy and reduce the need for long-distance transportation. But remember that "local" doesn't necessarily mean sustainable. Consider the wider environmental impact of your choices and know that consumers hold immense power. So shop wisely to guide the market towards planet-friendly practices.

Sustainability touches all areas of life, whether cleaning, clothing, cooking, or travel. At times, our actions may seem futile against the size of global crises but small steps, repeated many times, can make a huge difference.

Seasonal city living

Living in harmony with the seasons is an aim of most Green Witches, but we each interpret seasonal living differently, and have unique circumstances to contend with. For most, the ideal scenario involves flexible and fulfilling work, where we can adjust our working hours according to our needs and the seasons. With some planning and effort, you can adjust your lifestyle to align more closely with the natural rhythms of the days, months, years, and phases of your life. Adapting the foods we eat, the herbs we use, and our daily routines to reflect seasonal needs can make a huge difference.

During summer, energy levels often run high, and we may use some of that energy to harvest and process local plants for magical and medicinal purposes. Autumn tends to be a time of winding down, leading into winter, when many of us feel the need for more sleep, grounding foods, and a focus on quieter, introspective activities. Spring, often seen as a season of awakening, can be energising but also quite overwhelming because the initial excitement of spring sometimes leads to overexertion.

Of course, we are all unique, even from one day to the next. Some of us concentrate best around midday, while others thrive in the early or late hours. Learning when to rest, work, and play, and listening to our changing internal needs during each season, can enhance our wellbeing. But we often seem to lack the ability to act on these feelings.

Work and careers

Adopting a holistic approach to work that aligns with natural rhythms and spiritual beliefs can transform how you navigate life and your career. Whether you're transitioning to a new path or adjusting your current role, the key is to stay aligned with your values and nurture your connection to nature.

Some employers now offer menstrual leave and menopause support, recognising that energy levels and priorities can fluctuate throughout the menstrual cycle and different stages of life. And within more traditional work structures, it may be possible to incorporate spiritual practices into your routine. For instance, one practitioner books a holiday at each Pagan festival, like Samhain, and shares her blessings with colleagues through out-of-office reply messages.

One way to achieve a healthy work–life–nature–magic balance seems to lie in having multiple strings to our career bows, so if one path falters, the others can support. Many Green Witches also see *currency* in the widest sense, and exchange energy, skills, and resources through bartering or local trade.

Building a strong network of people with complementary skills is essential if we are to thrive. Networking should not be about self-interest, but about creating mutually beneficial relationships that help everyone grow. Strengthening these connections, whether for emergencies or collaboration, increases your resilience and allows you to contribute more positively to your community.

Achieving financial independence is another component of a fulfilling life. Working towards noble ecological causes cannot be sustainable if it doesn't also maintain your lifestyle. Debt, in any form, limits the potential for growth and freedom, so clearing debts, reducing expenses, and prioritising saving and investments, can create more flexibility in our lives. Financial independence is not selfish either, it's empowering and helps us to help others. It also allows ethical choices to be made and gives the power to leave situations that are unhealthy.[4]

There are ways to bring green magic to anyone's working life. From initiating sustainability audits, or requesting holidays and work hours in line with seasonal needs, we can all make a difference.

---

[4] For a toolkit on how to achieve this, see J.L. Collins, *The Simple Path to Wealth* (2021).

In researching this book, I spoke with many magical practitioners. Each found ways to align their careers with nature-centric values and many enjoy some seasonal flexibility in their work. Some had gradually transitioned into these roles, while others specialised from the start. Careers in green, magical, and sustainable sectors are not only achievable but can be deeply rewarding. It may take some time to arrange but aligning work with your values is possible, and can result in a life that is both spiritually and financially rich.

Of course, other options are possible, but those interviewed work in urban gardening, herbalism, yoga, teaching sustainable skills, woodworking or soap making, while others are community leaders, professors, NGO consultants, artists, writers, translators, and landscape architects. These nature lovers align their careers with their spiritual beliefs and ecological values, creating lives that are both meaningful and financially sustainable.

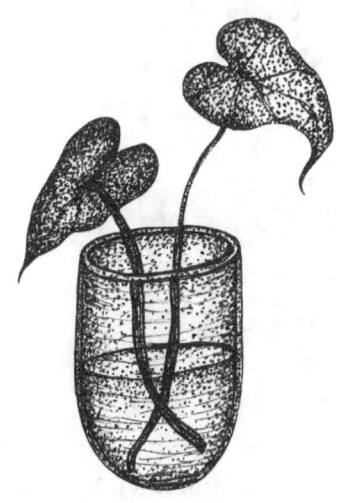

Routines

We have the greatest impact on the world around us when we are strong; emotionally, spiritually, and physically. So it is important to take care of ourselves.

Eat wholesome food and be mindful of what you expose yourself to. Move your body regularly, breathe deeply, and appreciate beauty in all its forms. Take time to recharge with practices like ritual baths, herbal teas, and getting daily fresh air, and develop a gratitude or prayer practice. Surround yourself with supportive people and places that inspire you, so you can learn together and grow.

Of course, it helps to know which direction you would like to grow in. Creating a personal manifesto can help with this: Take some time to jot down your long-term emotional, social, financial, and physical goals. Sketch out what your ideal life looks like. Within your manifesto, ensure that your basic needs are met, such as clean air, nourishing food, good health, and a peaceful, caring environment. Spend time sharpening your goals; meditate on how it feels when you get there, and think about the steps you need to take to make it happen. Then take those steps, small and large, as often as you can. Check in with your manifesto occasionally, to help stay on track. Choose spells and rituals from the Techniques section to boost your success.

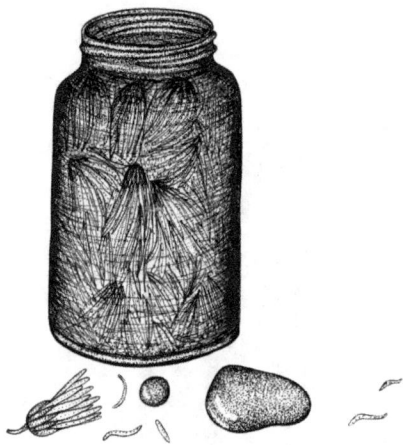

Incorporating nature-based routines into your life can increase connection with nature, and increase your ability to work magic. Here are some ideas to consider incorporating into your daily routine:

Waking

Rise early to enjoy some quiet before the world stirs. Let fresh air into your home while you brew tea, and sweep yesterday's energy out of your space. Greet and water your houseplants. Tend to companion animals and refresh your altar. Watch the sky brighten. Notice weather signs, and the first bird you hear. Morning sky-stretch: seated or standing, inhale, swing your arms out and over your head. Press your palms together above you, then exhale as you draw them down to your solar plexus. Repeat several times to welcome the day.

Hydrate & nourish

Start with warm water or herbal tea, and eat a nourishing breakfast as late in the morning as possible. Make your first meal of the day seasonal and grounding. Eat at regular times, as far as possible. Listen to beautiful music, or practise a meditative instrument.

Psychic hygiene

Use a tongue scraper in the morning, to clear the way for today. Skin brush before showering, rinse with a gentle herbal infusion, and apply herbal oil. This keeps your physical boundary with the outside world strong. Ground, centre, and shield before leaving your home, upon return, and as often as needed through the day. Use natural incense and candles, and ventilate rooms well. Bury pocket stones in soil regularly, to discharge held energy. Maintain your tools, cleanse and recharge them at each seasonal festival.

Movement & breath

Incorporate gentle stretches, yoga, or breathing exercises into your day. Keep it simple and aligned with your energy level and the season. Spend time outside before 10am to help align yourself with your local environment. Walk barefoot.

Record & reflect

Make time for meditation, gratitude, and journaling. Notice what inspires you in nature each day. Record dreams, synchronicities, and any magical symbols that you may encounter.

Wind down

Enjoy moments of relaxation between activities. Avoid news and external distractions in the period before bed. Encourage restful sleep with soft lighting, soothing sounds, and Chamomile tea.

Clear your mind

Before bed, take some time to prepare for the next day. Record any pressing concerns and gather anything needed for the coming day. Pray to the spirits that support your spiritual work; tell them your concerns, ask for guidance or help, and send gratitude to them.

Witch book of hours

Not everyone thrives on routine, but if you would like to try, the following ideas may be interesting. The Catholic Book of Hours was very popular in medieval times. It divides daylight hours into eight segments, known as canonical hours. These books offered spiritual activities to try during different hours, days, and seasons. They were often personalised with beautiful nature illustrations.

You might like to create your own Book of Hours, based on what nourishes your life. It could contain activities and rituals to build intuition and connect you with nature. Favourite meditations, poetry, and songs, could be included, to read at certain hours. And nourishing food and drink recipes to help recharge you. Meditative crafts, spells, and charms would also fit well. On days where you want to recharge, simply choose options to suit your needs.

If you have the luxury of a whole free day to try this, start by checking when sunrise and sunset are due. Choose a selection of spiritually nourishing activities from your Book of Hours and plan your day. An example could be:

First Light:	Meditation by candlelight
Dawn:	Watch the sunrise, with herb tea
Morning Task:	Recharge the protective boundaries of your home
Walking Outside:	Enjoy nature in a local park and take something home to craft with
Creative Task:	Write a poem, craft or paint
Lunch:	Enjoy nourishing food
Social/Outside Time:	Street gardening or foraging
Evening:	Share a communal meal or read something inspiring
Dusk:	Practise using divination tools, before meditating as the Sun sets.

Creating a personal Book or Hours, or simply planning days to intentionally nourish yourself can be a real treat. You may also like to mark Wheel of the Year Festival days, in this way.

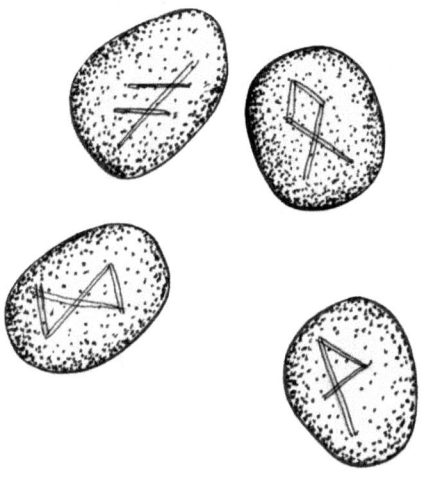

Covens and community

You might wonder if witches really need to connect with one another, especially since many enjoy practising alone. While they certainly don't have to, many urban witches find that building relationships with other like-minded folk enhances their lives and leads to greater success.

Connection

City life can sometimes feel isolating and overwhelming, making it harder to grow spiritually. Some alone time is essential but true loneliness can take a toll on your health. We are social beings who need meaningful connections. Many witches find personal and magical support through joining a coven or circle. These groups are designed to be safe, shared environments where wisdom is exchanged, problems are shared, and growth occurs collectively. Joining a group doesn't mean sacrificing independence; it's about balancing solo practice, companionship, and learning.

A coven is a group of witches who meet regularly, formally or informally. They share practices and collaborate on magical projects. The stronger the relationships within the group, the better the dynamics tend to become. Connections may grow naturally through shared interests, and urban witches may find kindred spirits in street gardening groups, crafting circles, or local Pagan events.

Patience, mutual respect, and trust are key, and there's no need to rush forging these friendships. If you're struggling to find others who share your interests, try casting a spell to invite meaningful connections into your life. Cities offer endless opportunities to meet new people, and when we set clear intentions, we become more attuned to the right people and moments when they arise.

Working in a group can amplify the potency of our magical work, especially when group members share the same intentions. Covens often unite to solve problems or support environmental and social causes. They use collective magic to achieve shared goals. Coven members often come to see each other as family and meet regularly. Some covens have monthly attendance requirements, initiation processes, or specific training, while others have a more relaxed structure.

Coven size varies; usually there are fewer than twelve members, allowing for closer connections and collaboration. Whatever the format and size, covens thrive when their magic is fuelled by intention and passion. When the focus is strong, the results are powerful.

Activities

Covens have different values and strengths, but their activities usually blend magical and mundane. They may perform group rituals at the New or Full Moon, celebrate seasonal festivals, set collective intentions, craft spells, learn new techniques together, or enjoy shared feasts. Some mark life transitions, such as with croning ceremonies and handfastings. Coven gatherings aim to strengthen bonds and positive outcomes.

Covens sometimes meet to craft together, such as making spell bottles, herbal remedies, sacred tools, or even quilts. Gatherings may include singing, storytelling,[5] and learning nature skills together. Taking walks to find special trees, or learning bird song can help build

---

[5] Storytelling has many positive effects on wellbeing. See G. Brockington et al. (2021) Storytelling increases oxytocin and positive emotions and decreases cortisol and pain in hospitalized children. *Proc Natl Acad Sci USA* 118(22): e2018409118; and T.K. Houston et al. (2011) Culturally appropriate storytelling to improve blood pressure: A randomized trial. *Ann Intern Med.* 154(2).

knowledge, care for the environment and strengthen the group. Coven activities tend to be dynamic and rooted in earth or community care.

Meetings often take place in homes, garden houses, outdoors, or even in cafés. They may happen spontaneously such as after storms to gather wood from fallen street trees. Most involve ritual, feasting, and sharing conversation.

Following group rituals, coven members often continue the work at home, solo, perhaps at agreed times, between meetings. This certainly intensifies the effects.

Many covens are involved in ecological and community efforts. They might transform derelict ground into wildlife sanctuaries, care for street trees or help at soup kitchens. Some maintain gardens for elderly neighbours. Others choose a different local project to support each year. Most find many ways to support nature.

Some covens plant groves at their regular meeting places. Over time these can grow into powerful reservoirs of spiritual energy, and beautiful places for the community to enjoy.

Safety and trust

If you are interested in joining or starting a coven, pay attention to the physical and emotional safety of all involved; It helps to have clear guidelines to encourage mutual respect. Some covens have appointed leaders, while others share responsibilities according to the strengths of members. Alongside fairly sharing tasks, shared leadership also helps ensure that members are equally valued.

Some covens appear to be exclusive, giving the impression that they are better than others. But magic is as powerful as the intention behind it. Exclusivity is usually an illusion to protect the group from unwanted energies.

A coven should not become a therapy group. It is useful for coven leaders to have a basic understanding of mental health, but members with deeper needs should be encouraged to seek professional help, rather than relying on the group. Coven members need to be able to trust each other, and that comes gradually through spending time together. Successful covens enjoy a balance of openness, respect, privacy, and respect.

There's no single right way to build a magical community, but successful covens find approaches that suit their locality and members.

For those needing more guidance on how to lead groups safely, or who may like to benefit from the advice of large organisations, OBOD (Order of Bards, Ovates, and Druids) and the Pagan Federation may be worth exploring.

At the heart of any coven is trust, belonging, and collective growth. By balancing private and group practice with social connection, both your magical abilities and overall wellbeing are sure to grow.

Wheel of the Year

Many NeoPagans divide the year into eight parts, often known as the Wheel of the Year, with festivals happening about every six weeks. Some of these are known as quarter days and others as cross-quarter days. The quarter days are related to the Sun; the longest and shortest day of the year (the solstices), and the days of equal dark and light hours (equinoxes). Previously, quarter days were times to settle rent, legal and social matters in Celtic Britain. Cross-quarter days fall between the quarter days and are seen as more important, or by some, less. Some of the festivals (Samhain, Imbolc, Beltane, and Lughnasadh) were celebrated with great fires and merriment. Many NeoPagans celebrate all eight festivals, although some choose only the quarter days or the cross-quarter festivals.

You may notice alternative names for each festival and reference to deities. A mix of Celtic, Nordic and astrological are common but there are many others. All ancient cultures observed the seasons in some way, and most associated different spirits and deities with specific seasons. Use the names and traditions to which you feel most akin, and avoid being restricted by ideas of how to celebrate the seasons and festivals; embrace what feels right to you.

The dates below show when the festivals occur. The cross-quarter dates are a guide, as these festivals are linked to the energy of the land rather than solar events.

Samhain—All Saints
Northern Hemisphere: October 31
Southern Hemisphere: May 1

Yule—Winter Solstice
Northern Hemisphere: December 20 to 23
Southern Hemisphere: June 20 to 23

Imbolc—Early Spring
Northern Hemisphere: February 1
Southern Hemisphere: August 1

Ostara—Spring Equinox
Northern Hemisphere: March 19 to 22
Southern Hemisphere: September 20 to 23

Beltane—Late Spring
Northern Hemisphere: May 1
Southern Hemisphere: October 31

Midsummer—Summer Solstice
Northern Hemisphere: June 20 to 23
Southern Hemisphere: December 20 to 23

Lughnasadh—First Harvest
Northern Hemisphere: August 1
Southern Hemisphere: February 1

Herfest—Autumn Equinox
Northern Hemisphere: September 20 to 23
Southern Hemisphere: March 19 to 22

You may want to take time off work to mark the festivals, to give opportunities to do things that nourish you. Some city witches plan technology-free time, or spend days without artificial lighting, to help them wake and sleep with the Sun. These are also good reminders to declutter and reorganise, to cleanse space and tend to houseplants, boundaries, and magical tools.

The following chapters offer ways to align with the changing energies of the year through crafts, rituals, foraging, and meditation. Choose those that attract you and enjoy following the turning year.

Samhain

Northern Hemisphere: October 31
Southern Hemisphere: May 1

This cross-quarter day, between autumn equinox and winter solstice, is seen as the start and end of the Pagan year. It is a liminal time for divination and ancestor worship, and is related in focus to All Saints Day, Hallowe'en (All Hallows' Eve), Diwali, and Día de los Muertos.

By Samhain, autumn weather is usually here, leaves swirl, and the nights are long. Wild animals prepare food stores and hibernation nests. We also begin to turn inward: eating hearty food, layering warm clothes, and looking forward to quieter months. The darkness makes it easier to slip unnoticed through the streets; and so it becomes easier to work magic outdoors. This is the ultimate witching season and, like Beltane, Samhain offers an easier connection with the spirit world.

Traditions

At Samhain the Wild Hunt, of Celtic folklore, is said to rip through the land gathering up the souls of the recently deceased. It symbolically makes space for new beginnings and can be a useful way to let go of those we have loved and lost. Many Samhain traditions honour the dead, such as the custom of Dumb Suppers where an extra place is set at the table to invite ancestral spirits to join the meal. Jack o' lanterns, initially carved from swedes rather than pumpkins, light up homes and gardens to ward off ill spirits. Apples, symbolic of wisdom and insight, are buried to guide and nourish spirits as they journey to the Isle of Apples (the Celtic dream land of eternal spring). Bobbing Apples is an old divination game used to predict love matches at Samhain. Trick or treating is a far cry from the Souling and Guising of previous times. Then, the souls of the dead were prayed for and appeased with tasty offerings.

Foraging

This is the time of nuts, seeds, late fruits, and fungi. Leave plenty for local wildlife and avoid those that have lost their glow. Semi-evergreens catch the eye as falling tree leaves let more sunlight reach the ground. Now is the time to go on mushroom walks, with experts and, if you have landowner permission, time to dig edible roots. Harvest what you need before the first frosts arrive but forage lightly, as many creatures depend on this last harvest to survive winter.

Altar

Natural autumn items in shades of orange, red, and brown capture the spirit of Samhain, as do nuts and Apples. A simple altar arrangement, symbolising ancestors and the Isle of Apples, can be made with a circle of apples on a plate, surrounding a simple beeswax tealight.

You may like to add mementos of ancestors, which can be anyone who has contributed to your life, whether blood relatives, spiritual figures, or someone else dear to you. Display photos or items that remind you of them, perhaps their favourite drink or game. You may also like to display some stones, cleaned bones, and seeds, to symbolise clarity and new beginnings. The blood red of Hawthorn and Rosehips also works well.

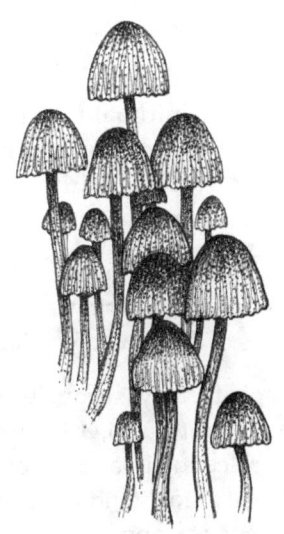

Activities

Support wildlife by creating piles of leaves and sticks in garden corners, postponing deadheading plants until spring. Plant winter nectar plants, like Ivy and Mahonia, to help animals prepare for winter.

Prepare for winter by setting up tasty herbal infusions and ferments, to be ready at Yuletide. Learn or develop a craft to keep you warm through the colder months; perhaps knitting, carving, or making a cloak.

Walk in parks to observe how plants and animals respond to the shorter cooler days. Notice autumn scents, colours, and wildlife activity. Gather natural items for your journal or altar, and plant flowering bulbs, like Daffodils, to enjoy in spring.

Weave soul nests, palm-sized nests from twigs, stems, and an Apple leaf. Line them with Moss, then place in a tree, to give passing spirits a rest, as they travel to the Isle of Apples.

Candle gaze to develop concentration and mindfulness. Sit about a metre from a lit candle. Get comfortable and turn down the lights. Softly gaze at the flame, keeping a wide, relaxed focus. If your thoughts wander, guide them back to the flame. After a few minutes, close and cover your eyes with your palms. Observe how long the flame's image remains in your mind's eye. Repeat the gazing and palming several times before safely extinguishing the flame.

Divination is often easier at Samhain, as it is a liminal period when the veil between the physical and spiritual realms is most thin. Try using Yarrow sticks and love charms, and play Bobbing Apples with friends. Gaze through hag stones, interpret ink drops in water, read tea leaves, or try another divination technique.

Cemeteries are especially interesting to visit at Samhain. Visit green and pleasant cemeteries. Just be there and enjoy the quiet. If appropriate place a small pebble at the graves of those who you have some affinity with.

Communication with spirits may seem attractive at Samhain. We can only invite them to attend to us. Let them visit naturally through dreams, familiar scents, or fleeting images. Show gratitude and respect, rather than commanding them to attend to your needs. So offer shelter or food, perhaps a dumb supper, apple, Bread of the Dead, or lanterns in carved Swedes. Help souls pass onward and rest; if they chose to somehow speak, thank them, and let them go on their way.

Reflect on the gifts of your ancestors. What legacy have they left you? How have they shaped your life? Light a candle in their honour and perhaps do an activity, or eat foods that they enjoyed. Reflecting in this way is sometimes difficult, especially when ancestors have caused harm, and of course everyone has shadowy and bright sides. The following contemplation could be triggering to some, yet for others, it can be healing and beneficial. It can be used to think about any ancestors, as well as elders in your community who are still alive.

Hold an item that is symbolic of the ancestor(s) who you would like to focus on. Sit in a safe and familiar space; perhaps by your altar. Light a candle and call upon the nature spirits to guide you towards positive thoughts about this ancestor. Gaze softly or with eyes closed, allow your thoughts to drift. Do any positive memories or thoughts bubble up? How has your ancestor added to who you are today? Do this for as long as you feel comfortable. When ready, thank the spirits for supporting you, extinguish the candle, and note any insights in your journal.

Samhain tree meditation

Don't try the following meditation, if you have yet to recover from psychiatric difficulties. It involves spiritual journeying.

You will need an anchor stone (details in the Tools section), and a little food, to help ground yourself at the end. Begin by visiting a local tree, perhaps one that is overlooked by most people. Spend some time observing its shape, bark texture, and how it coexists with animals and other plants. Consider how it reacts to other life forms. Does it show signs of human intervention, like pruning?

Hold your small anchor stone in the palm of one hand and sit at the base of the tree. Lean your back against it, if possible. Ideally, remove your footwear and sit barefoot, allowing your skin to contact the ground beneath the tree. Let your gaze soften and look downwards, or close your eyes. Allow your breathing to flow smoothly without any control; simply let it come and go.

Ask the spirits of this place to protect you as you spend time communicating with the tree. Feel the anchor stone in your hand. Visualise roots growing from your tailbone into the soil. Just as the tree has roots, envision your roots spreading throughout the ground beneath you. Your roots seek out the roots of the tree, and perhaps those of other trees and plants as well. You might sense the shallower roots of grass and weeds nearby or small creatures moving through the soil. Imagine your roots growing gently around them all. Inviting the roots of the tree to interact with yours.

Keep your focus on the roots of the tree that you are leaning against. Use this exploration to learn more about the tree. What do the tree roots tell you? Are they different from the other roots in the soil? Be open to sensing any information it may wish to share with you. This may come to you through light, sound, scents, images, or other sensations. Stay open to whatever comes; do not be disappointed if you sense nothing. Enjoy your time in close relation to the tree and its roots, for a while.

When you are ready, begin to retract your roots. Bring them back into your body. Sense them being neatly reabsorbed. Consider something you would like to remember as you completely dissociate from the tree roots and return your attention to the physical plane. Hold or rub your anchor stone to remind you of the way home.

As you become more aware of the physical plane, take deeper breaths to ground yourself, fully sensing where you are sitting on the ground and ensuring your roots are completely retracted. Sense your body as an intact form, and recognise the tree behind you as a close but separate entity. You are you, and the tree is the tree.

Inwardly thank the tree and your guides for their protection and for the communion you experienced today. When you feel ready, slowly bring your attention fully to the present, becoming more aware of the sounds around you, and how your skin feels. Gently open your eyes, stretch, and take a few deep, nourishing breaths. If needed, eat something to ground yourself further. Finally, record any notes about the experience in your journal before continuing with your day.

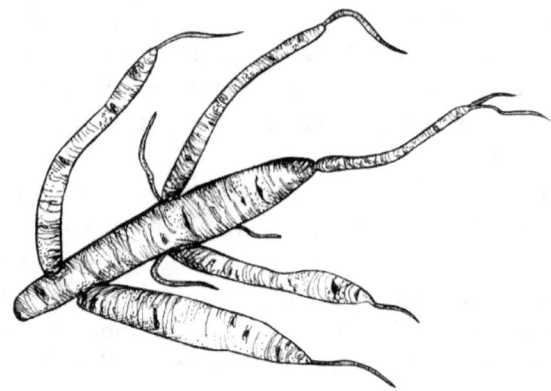

Winter solstice

Northern Hemisphere: December 20 to 23
Southern Hemisphere: June 20 to 23

This quarter day occurs at the winter solstice, the shortest day of the year. Yuletide lasts fourteen days from the solstice. This is a time of returning light. The Sun's path has reached its lowest point in the sky, leading to short days and long nights, but from now until midsummer, daylight hours will steadily lengthen. This festival honours the return of the Sun. It is a chance to show gratitude to those who support us. Yuletide shares this focus with Soyal, Dongzhi, and other festivals.

Midwinter is often dark, brittle, and cold. Many wild animals hibernate, flowers are scarce, and plants lie dormant or static. Birds who did not migrate to warmer lands may struggle to access food and water in the cold. It's easy to feel dark or isolated from nature at this time, but spring is near and we must trust in the power of the long winter nights.

Traditions

Yuletide traditions are rich with practices that bring light and warmth to dark midwinter days. Evergreen Holly, Ivy, and Fir are used to brighten homes, and Yule logs are kept burning. A clairvoyance-enhancing Elderberry wine is made from the last gathered berries and fruit trees are blessed by Wassailing; cider is poured onto cake in branch hollows, while lots of noise is made to drive away evil spirits. Ancient Romans celebrated Saturnalia at this time; laws were relaxed, slaves enjoyed some freedoms, Bay leaf crowns and simple gifts were exchanged. Yuletide traditions blend those from many cultures.

Foraging

The ground is often barren at Yuletide, but urban foraging can yield small winter salads. Many plants struggle to recover, if foraged in midwinter. It is best to watch and wait until spring, and use preserved foraged foods instead of harvesting fresh. Leave wildlife refuges, like leaf piles, undisturbed for hibernating creatures, and tread lightly as others may sleep beneath your feet.

Altar

Include evergreen foliage, red berries, small stones, bones, and nuts, if you can. A circle of Holly, Ivy, or Bay leaves, placed around a tealight, with some Mistletoe hanging above, is very suited to Yule. You may like to burn a large Yule candle, which can be lit each day through Yuletide.

Evergreens represent resilience through winter. Their presence encourages nature spirits into our homes. Holly and Ivy are used to symbolise longevity, renewal, and protection. Mistletoe, associated with love and fidelity, has poisonous berries, so beware of those.

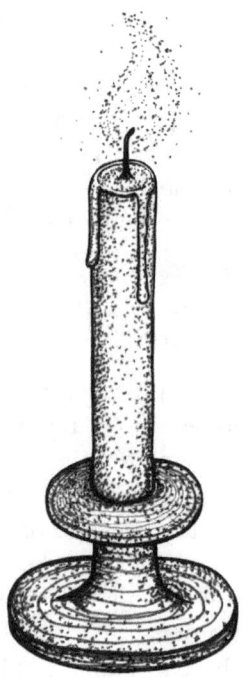

Activities

Holly and Ivy create beautiful evergreen decorations. Circular wreaths, hung on doors, encourage the Sun's return. Less prickly Ivy crowns, threaded with tiny rechargeable lights, and Mistletoe can be worn at gatherings. Use Ivy in winter binding spells, and Holly for protective charms. Holly, Ivy, and Mistletoe can be added to charm bags. If travelling during Yule, carry a protective amulet, like a vial of ground

Holly leaf. Alternatively, visualise Holly and Ivy growing around your home and possessions, keeping them safe while you are away.

Support wild birds by packing a mixture of birdseed, chopped Chickweed, and unsalted peanut butter or animal fat into Pine cones. Hang them in bird-friendly spots. Also consider filling shallow bowls of water for them on frosty days.

Moss watch in damp, shaded areas. Use a hand lens to study mossy details, touch it, draw or photograph it. Take off your shoes and walk on Moss. As you do, visualise your worries being absorbed by the Moss, passed to the earth, and transformed into fertile soil.

Welcome the returning Sun by checking the local sunrise time for the Winter Solstice and visiting a nearby natural space to wait and watch it happen. Or observe the sky brightening from a window. Spend time quietly reflecting on which aspects of your life could benefit from fresh light. Set simple intentions for the coming weeks until Imbolc. If you can't be with loved ones at Yule, consider sharing this ritual, despite the distance. Perhaps watch the sunrise together-apart, while sipping Rosemary tea, which helps to align minds.

Ritual root harvesting at Yule can yield great results, especially if the ground is soft (and you have the landowner's permission). Wood Avens (*Geum urbanum*) roots release a wintery, Clove-like scent when chewed. Harvest sustainably, taking only a small portion of the roots. Afterwards, replant the Wood Avens carefully. Clean, dry, and use the roots in rituals.

Walk with friends, at night carrying lanterns, torches, or wearing sparkling crowns. Enjoy walking on crunchy frost, notice nocturnal wildlife and feel fresh air on your face. Sip hot drinks, share stories, and reflect on the past year. Make fun plans for the year ahead. Enjoy the light and warmth of decorations as you pass by homes and shops. If you wander by day, look for leaf buds on Lime and Magnolia trees. Find the small leaves of the Elder and notice how nature is resting. Pay attention to wildlife and where birds are looking for food. Try to identify a winter tree.

Yule logs are possible in small spaces: Carve indentations in a log to fit small candles, and line them with metal foil. Burn and replace the candles throughout Yuletide. Ash from Yule logs is very protective so burn the wood shavings made when carving the indents. Use the resulting ash in protection rituals throughout the coming year. After Yuletide, burn the log or branch outdoors or let it decompose back into the land.

Candle making is easy. Try rolling beeswax sheets around a wick, or melt and pour wax into moulds. Use sustainably sourced wax and dress them with crumbled dry Pine needles, Rose petals, Cinnamon, and Orange peel. You can personalise further by etching sigils, or decorating with coloured threads.

A light meditation

This visualisation-based meditation requires a candle and lighter, and a little food, to help ground you at the end.

Sit comfortably, indoors or out. Remove your footwear and allow your skin to contact the floor. Light the candle and place it safely in front of you. Gaze softly at a flame. Feel the light and warmth of the candle slowly filling you. As you breathe, visualise the light growing, until it fills every part of your body. Then expand the brightness and warmth into the space around you. This light, symbolising the returning warmth of the Sun, grows ever wider, touching the earth, the trees, the creatures beneath you, and eventually the whole world. Imagine this ever-expanding, beautiful, and life-giving light. Breathe into this feeling for a little while. Feel yourself and the world filled with warmth and light.

When you are ready, let the image fade. Take deeper breaths to ground yourself, and move your gaze away from the flame. Become more aware of where you are sitting. Think about the ground beneath you and the feel of your feet on the floor. Thank the light of the universe for its warmth.

Extinguish the flame, then stretch, and take a few deep breaths. If possible, eat something to ground yourself further. Record any thoughts in your journal before continuing with your day.

Midwinter spell for light

Gather a small handful of evergreen leaves, a natural wax candle to symbolise the returning light, a leaf to write on (Bay or Holly), and a pen or pencil.

Arrange the leaves in a circle, around the candle. Light the candle and take a moment to centre yourself. Feel the warm glow of the candle and take a few relaxing breaths. Write an intention, on Bay or Holly, linked to returning light, clarity of mind, or something else.

Read your intention, aloud or inwardly. Then, place the leaf under the candle or herbs. Breathe smoothly, visualising the candle light filling your body and illuminating your spirit. Imagine this energy pushing aside darkness and cobwebs; see it manifesting your wishes. Imagine the evergreen leaf circle growing upward, like a column around the candle. It shoots up into the sky, directing your intention up into the atmosphere to find all it needs to manifest your will. See your intention complete, as if it is completely achieved, here and now.

Enjoy this meditative state for a few minutes, then visualise the column of evergreen leaves reducing back to the ring around the candle. Breathe smoothly and become more aware of your surroundings and the floor beneath you. Extinguish the flame with a little herb-infused water and take more time to ground yourself. Eat something to further ground yourself, if needed.

Leave the spell candle and evergreen foliage undisturbed, if possible, and return each day during Yule, to relight the candle and repeat the practice. After fourteen days, use the candle flame to burn your intention leaf. Dispose of the ashes outside, in the earth.

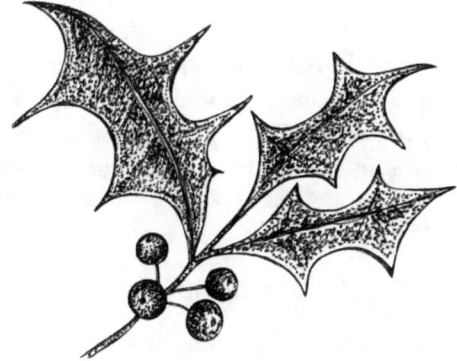

Imbolc

Northern Hemisphere: February 1
Southern Hemisphere: August 1

This cross-quarter day, between Yule and the spring equinox, is the earliest spring festival. Imbolc occurs when the very first stirrings of life are seen, and is rich in traditions about purification and fresh starts.

Many subtle signs indicate the arrival of Imbolc, and these often appear earlier in towns and cities owing to metropolitan microclimates. Sunlight strengthens, sap rises in trees, and hints of green appear on the ground. Imbolc air has a specific essence: the pure, rejuvenating scent of wintergreen, released by stretching leaf buds. Flower bulbs also push through the earth, and many animals leave hibernation. Mixed with the anticipation of warmer days to come is slight regret at losing winter's peace. This festival is about renewal, cleansing, and preparing from the verdant times to come.

Traditions

Imbolc marks the start of the lambing season and is traditionally celebrated with milk. Blackthorn flowers are white, and early seedlings start to show. Foraged spring greens, like Stinging Nettle, Chickweed, and Cleavers, are eaten or enjoyed as tea daily until the spring equinox. Water features in Imbolc rituals, with pilgrimages to springs, rivers, and wells to cleanse and renew. Brigid's crosses are woven from Ribwort stems, to honour the Celtic goddess of poetry, healing, smithcraft, fertility, and the hearth. Imbolc is an ideal time to start or bless new projects.

Foraging

Many wild edibles start to build strength at this often cold time but overharvesting them will reduce their health and size in the coming months. If you choose to forage at Imbolc, pick lightly, leave plenty to grow and flourish, and focus on strong mature plants. Learn to recognise the Birch trees, and follow your nose to Wild Garlic, pushing its way up through woodland soil.

Altar

Green and white altars symbolise the pure, fresh life of Imbolc. A circle of variegated green–white Ivy, placed around a tealight, with damp pieces of Moss, will welcome spring indoors. Alongside you might include a pot of flowering Snowdrops, or some fallen Birch bark; these plants symbolise rebirth, purity, and hope. Brigid is often honoured, with symbols of metalwork, spring water, young animals, poetry, and dairy produce.

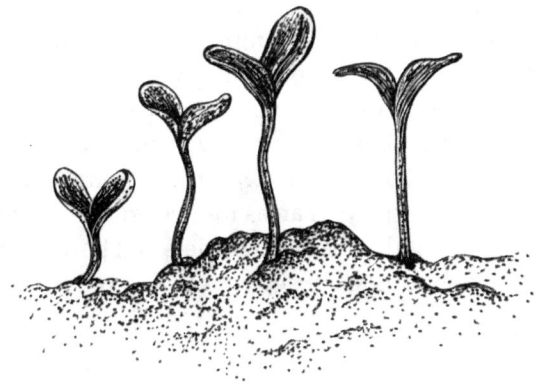

Activities

Birch bark paper. Find naturally shed pieces of bark near mature Birch trees. Clean gently under running water, then pat dry. Carefully peel apart the bark layers; some will be tissue paper-thin, so handle with care. Once separated, lay the pieces on a clean tea towel, and flatten by pressing between books. Spells, poems, intentions, and symbols can be easily written on the bark sheets. This burns well but composts slowly, as Birch bark is filled with protective substances.

Walk in nature, paying attention to bare trees and shrubs as they start to hint at green. Look out for the lamb's tail catkins of Hazel, Birch, and Alder. Snowdrops may be flowering in shady places, and Blackthorn flowers in wilder hedgerows. In mild weather, you might see Bumblebees on their first flights of the year. Try to find the flowers that they are seeking, such as Lungwort, Lesser Celandine, and the earliest Daffodils. If your surroundings are looking barren, seek out quieter signs of life such as Lichen and Moss, on trees and walls.

Scatter wildflower seeds though early spring. Seeds naturally lie dormant through winter, waiting for the right conditions to germinate. Sprinkle seeds where flowers are welcome, trusting that some will grow while others will compost or feed wildlife.

Barefoot time at Imbolc is likely to be fresh and invigorating. Find a clean spot near trees to place your feet on the ground. Feel the earth on your skin and try to detect the gentle throb of rising sap through your soles. Enjoy the sensations that this brings.

Refresh your home and body. Try simple self-care routines such as skin brushing before showers and nourishing your skin with infused oil. Freshen your surroundings by reorganising your wardrobe, donating unneeded items, and letting fresh air flow through your home to invite renewal and growth. Craft a ritual broom from Birch twigs (see Tools chapter). Gently prepare garden areas for new growth, plant Pansies or Primroses, and thoroughly clean bird feeders and bowls before topping them up. Gently rinse dusty houseplants with tepid water and top up their soil.

Ritual bath or shower

Release the old and welcome the new by bringing ice and candlelight into your bathroom. Arrange ice cubes, and perhaps Ivy, around a candle, in a bowl. Place this safely and within sight as you take your bath or shower. Light the candle and enjoy your shower or bath. Visualise the water carrying away any worries and obstacles from your life. For a final rinse, pour a soothing herbal tea or decoction over your body; ideally from Chickweed or Ivy (*Hedera helix*) leaf. When dry, apply Olive oil or Birch infused oil, to nourish and protect your skin.

Snowdrop meditation

This meditation involves meeting the spirit of a Snowdrop through visualisation and journeying. Those with psychiatric difficulties should wait until they are recovered to try this. You'll need an anchor stone (see the Tools section for details), Snowdrops (an image or plant), and some food for grounding at the end.

Sit comfortably near the chosen Snowdrops, or image. Observe the plant's shape, colours, scent, and texture. Breathe naturally, hold your anchor stone in one palm, and let your gaze soften on the Snowdrop. Ask your spirit helpers for protection. Visualise the Snowdrop bulb, hidden beneath the soil. Gently touch the stem of the Snowdrop and ask permission to merge your spirit with it. If the answer is yes, feel yourself enter the plant.

Visualise yourself exploring within the stem, the leaves and the flower. Notice its delicate scent and the complexity of its structures. Then, descend into the bulb. Just beneath the soil is a place of warmth, activity, and transformation. Move into the roots, feeling them draw nourishment from the soil. Explore the plant for a while. Enjoy absorbing some of the Snowdrop's viriditas. When ready, rise up through the stem and into the flower again. This time, prepare to leave the plant. Visualise yourself being birthed from the Snowdrop flower, and flowing back into your body; fully formed, securely within each cell of the physical body.

Thank the plant and become aware of all parts of your body, especially those touching the floor. Ground yourself by rubbing the anchor stone, and take deeper breaths. When ready, open your eyes, stretch, and breathe deeply. If needed, eat something to further ground. Reflect on your experience in your journal.

Spell for renewal

This is best performed in the morning, after a ritual shower or bath.

Gather a natural candle, a few seasonal leaves and flowers, a heatproof container, lighter, Birch spell paper or a Bay leaf, pen or pencil, and a cup of warm milk (or plant-based alternative), sweetened with honey or syrup.

In a quiet place without distractions, arrange your materials in front of you. Light the candle to symbolise the renewing power of Imbolc. Hold the Birch paper or Bay leaf and close your eyes. Take a few smooth, deep breaths. Then focus on what you want to release from your life, and what you wish to invite into your life.

Choose one word, or a symbol, to represent what you wish to release. Write this on one side of the paper or leaf. Choose another word or symbol to represent what you wish to attract. Write this on the other side of the Birch paper or leaf. Allow the ink to dry and dab a little milk and honey onto the side of the leaf that shows what you want to attract.

Whisper the following incantation as you hold the leaf or Birch paper and visualise the changes you desire, as if they are real now. Repeat three times:

From winter's hold, I break away,
With light and love, I greet the day.
As sap does rise, in Birch and Bay,
I embrace renewal—Come what may.

Burn the Birch paper or Bay leaf in the heatproof container. As it burns, visualise your worries and obstacles being consumed by the flame. Let the smoke carry your intentions away. Once the burning has finished, drink the warm milk and honey while reflecting on the nourishment that it brings. When you feel ready, extinguish the candle, perhaps with the last drop of milk and honey, and take a few moments to reflect on the experience.

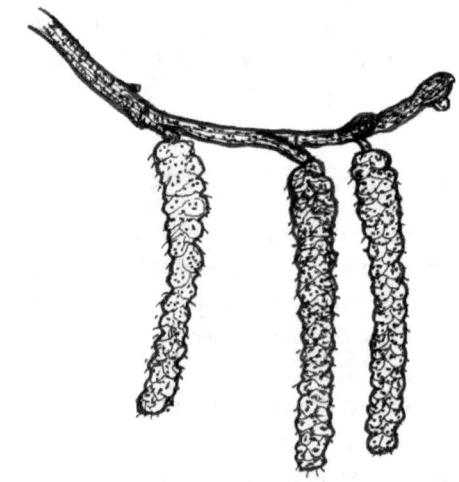

Spring equinox

Northern Hemisphere: March 19 to 22
Southern Hemisphere: September 20 to 23

This quarter day occurs when the Earth's equator is directly in line with the Sun; the hours of light and darkness are equal. This is the second festival of spring, and is strongly associated with rebirth and fertility. Also known as Alban Eilir or Ostara, this festival has links with Easter, Nowruz, and Holi.

Spring fever is in the air at spring equinox; birds nest and wild animals mate, leaf buds open, Daisies bloom and the world slowly strengthens in the extra sunlight. Nature is full of promise. This is a time of rapid growth, which should be balanced with plenty of rest.

Traditions

Eggs and Hares, symbols of fertility and renewal, feature in many spring equinox rituals. Hares were sacred to the ancient Celts. They symbolise fertility, abundance, and rebirth. They are also messengers from the spirit world. In cities, Rabbits are more often seen and they have similar traits. Seeds are often sown at this time. The Green Man, depicted with a leafy face, is often used to represent spring's regenerative energy. He is closely associated with the Cernunnos, the Celtic horned god of fertility and nature.

Foraging

This is the end of the hungry gap, where many wild edibles start to emerge, so there is usually plenty to forage. As always, harvest sparingly and with intention, knowing how you'll use the herbs, in food or rituals, before picking them. Spring flowers are particularly appealing—just remember how much pollinating wildlife needs them. Focus more on rapidly growing leafy herbs, such as Stinging Nettle, Dead Nettles, and Cleavers.

Altar

Ostara altars often include bright yellow spring flowers or leaves. A circle of Willow, surrounding a beeswax tealight, with yellow Forsythia flowers sprinkled around works very well—Forsythia is a common garden shrub.

A small handmade nest, lined with Moss, containing a stained egg, or a broken shell (they often fall from street trees), can add further symbolism.

Wild Garlic, budding Willow stems, and Hazel with dangling catkins, all symbolise fertility and rapid growth. Objects representing Hares or the Green Man could also be added. Potted flowering bulbs, like Narcissi, Wild Garlic, and Grape Hyacinth can be nurtured at your altar and, later, planted outside.

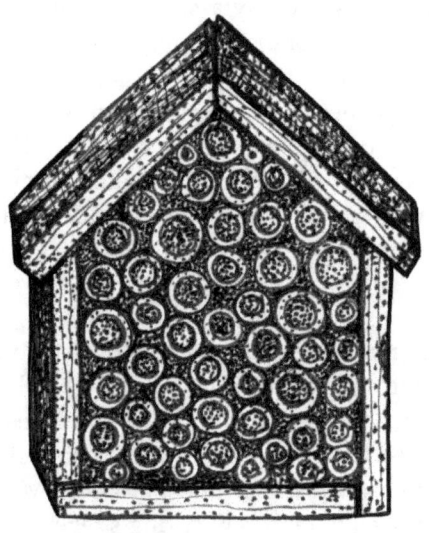

Activities

Egg staining is possible with common plant materials. Try using Onion skins, Beetroot, Red Cabbage, Spinach, Coffee grinds or Avocado skins from the kitchen. Or, from local nature, acorns, Gypsywort, Dock root, Black Walnut hulls or Chamomile flowers.

Hard boil six eggs. Remove from the cooking water and allow to cool. Separately, simmer a handful (about 3 heaped tablespoons) of your chosen chopped dye material in about 500 ml of water. Keep the lid on for 20–30 minutes. Strain the dye material from the liquid into another bowl or pan, then add 1 tablespoon of vinegar for every 250 ml of dye infusion you have made. Repeat with as many dyes as you like. Submerge the cooled eggs in the dye water for 1 to 12 hours, depending on the desired depth of colour. Then remove the eggs and dry them off. If you'd like a glossy finish, rub a little vegetable oil on the eggs. Use in Ostara decorations and egg hunts.

Walk with seeds to plant intentions in the ground and your heart at Ostara. The life of a seed can reflect the life of our goals: germinating, rooting, shooting, and blossoming. Primrose, Hawthorn, Wild Rose, and Mallow can be mixed in your pocket, to sprinkle and press into soil near hedges and neglected edges. As you walk, look for traditional signs of spring such as the yellow flowers of Lesser Celandine (*Ficaria verna*), Forsythia, and Daisy. Find Moss, dropped by nesting birds, and notice tiny plant seedlings. The first true leaves of Cleavers are always fun to find.

Egg magic

This spell requires a fresh egg, pen, small piece of spell paper, a bowl, a fine marker pen, candle, and lighter.

Cleanse the egg by rinsing with Rosemary or Lavender water, or pass it through incense smoke. Write your intention for spring growth, as a sentence or sigil, on a small piece of paper. This needs to be small enough to fit inside the eggshell.

Then blow out the egg: Use a pin or needle to carefully poke two small holes, one at each end of the egg. Gently enlarge one hole with the pin. Hold the egg over a bowl, then blow through the smaller hole, so that the egg white and yolk flow out through the larger hole. You can help the process by gently shaking or tapping the egg. Rinse the shell thoroughly with water and leave to dry completely. Use the egg contents in cooking; as you eat, think about your spring intention.

Now roll up your spell paper and push it inside of the shell. Decorate the eggshell with symbols or patterns, using the marker pen. You may like to write a prayer or poem on the shell.

To activate the egg magic, light the candle and whisper your intentions to the egg. Then place it on your altar. If you have a small nest, or Moss, place it there to symbolise the incubation and growth of your intention. Leave the egg there, or another safe place, until Beltane. Then bury it in the ground.

The spell is done.

Journey with the Spring Hare

Shapeshift with the agile Hare, a traditional symbol of spring. Anyone with psychiatric issues should wait until they have recovered before trying this practice.

If you have never encountered a Hare, you may prefer to use a more familiar animal for this journey, perhaps a Squirrel, Fox or Rat. Choose one that is resourceful and agile. You will need an anchor stone, a symbol of your animal (such as a nut, feather, or photo), and some food for grounding at the end.

Sit comfortably, with your anchor stone in one hand and the symbol of your chosen animal in the other. Relax with a few smooth, deep breaths. Visualise energy rising from the earth through your body, connecting you to the sky with a silver thread. Imagine walking into a beautiful garden and sitting by a stream. Let the scent of spring surround you. Explore the garden, looking between plants and shrubs.

If an animal spirit appears, ask if you could engage with it for a while. It may be the animal you pictured at the start, it could be another. If the creature's response is positive, spend time moving around with it. If you and the animal welcome it, become closer by breathing together. As you breathe in, take some of their breath and energy within you. As they breathe in, they take in some of yours. Get to know each other in this way for a few breaths.

Then, if it feels good, ask if your spirit can merge with that of the animal. If the response is positive, let your spirit pass into the animal. Feel yourself sensing the world from within its form. Move around the garden as it would; run, leap, dig as you will. Sense through the eyes, ears, nose, and skin of the animal. Fully engage with it—learn what it has to show.

Notice the anchor stone in your palm. It calls you to return to your human form. Thank the animal for this experience. Make a mental note of the knowledge you obtained and then shift from the animal's body straight back into your own. You and the animal are now separate. Become more aware of your physical body, squeeze or rub your anchor stone and sense the weight of your body. Hear the sounds around you, feel the air in your nostrils and notice your body move as you breathe. Rub your hands together and place them over your eyes. Open your eyes, lower your hands, and stretch. Clap, stamp, or eat nourishing food to further ground yourself. Reflect on your experience, and note any insights.

Seed spell for balance and growth

This is best performed at dawn or dusk, when light and dark are in balance.

Gather a candle, lighter, a few spring flowers, a small handful of Sunflower or Pumpkin seeds in their shells, and a heatproof bowl.

Sit comfortably in a quiet place, where you won't be disturbed. Arrange the flowers and seeds around the candle. Light the candle, then take a few deep breaths. Think about how we are constantly trying to maintain balance. Allow yourself to consider areas in your life where that is difficult. Pick up one of the seeds and imagine that challenge as the outer seed shell. Feel how the shell is tough to protect the dynamic, living kernel within. Whisper the following words onto the seed:

Perfect balance, strong and true,
I crack the shell, good things come through.

Slowly eat the seed. Crunch through the shell and enjoy the inner edible seed kernel. Spit out the tough shell and save near the candle. As you eat the tasty kernel, visualise its nourishing energy merging with yourself.

Repeat with a few more seeds; each representing a different obstacle in your life. Afterwards burn the collected seed shells, in the candle flame (or compost them later) to completely remove the obstacles. Extinguish the flame.

It is done.

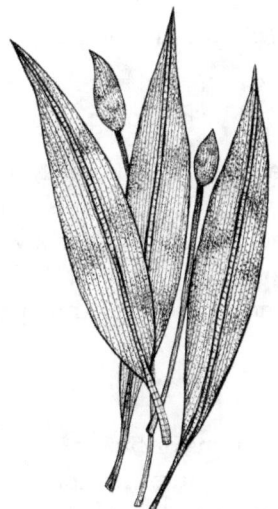

Beltane

Northern Hemisphere: May 1
Southern Hemisphere: October 31

This is a cross-quarter festival, between the spring equinox and the summer solstice. Beltane marks the end of spring and the start of summer. It is associated with warmth, creativity, fertility rites, and abundance. Also known as May Day, Beltane occurs around the same time as Walpurgis Night, Japanese Greenery Day, Akshaya Tritiya, and the ancient Roman festival of Floralia.

Beltane energy is invigorating and empowering. By now plants are growing well, many trees are in blossom. Butterflies have begun to emerge and most herbs are in their prime. This is the time that viriditas spills over the land. As with Samhain, this is a liminal time when contact with the spirit world is easier.

Traditions

Beltane festivities often include merry gatherings, hilltop fires, and ritual herb gatherings. In parts of Britain, the May Queen, Green Man, and Maypole dances still symbolise Beltane's fertile spirit. Several towns in Somerset and Cornwall still enact Hobby Horse processions, which stem from ancient fertility rites. Those seeking to preserve their beauty, wash their face with the morning dew of Hawthorn.

Foraging

At Beltane wild edibles are usually abundant, and the foraging season is at its peak. If developing your foraging skills, it may help to focus on just a few local edibles and get to know those really well during this season. Yarrow is at its most potent and magical at this time, and Hawthorn blossom needs to be found, but there are many plants to choose from.

Altar

At Beltane, bring fresh herbs inside but not Hawthorn branches, as they can lead to bad luck if taken into the home. A simple altar arrangement could include a crown of fresh Oak foliage woven with a few seasonal flowers. Oak leaves and acorns symbolise the verdancy and fertility of Beltane, and the Green Man.

Primrose, Daisy, and Wild Garlic are often in flower now, and can bring Beltane energy to the altar. Images of the Green Man, found bird feathers, and Moss are also very appropriate at this time. Small pots of organic Bluebells may be available in your area and can be nurtured at your altar while they flower, and later planted outside.

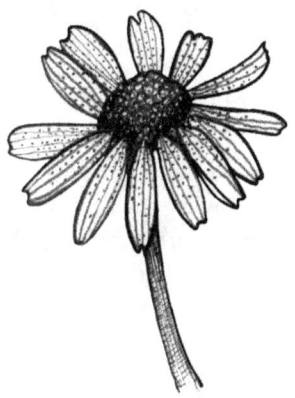

Activities

Willow drying frames can be woven from the long flexible branches of Willow. Find them in public spaces during the pruning season. Take two pliable stems, of about the same length. Cross the wider cut ends, then create a rough heart shape. Weave shorter, thinner Willow stems across that frame for support. Keep weaving until the rack can hold itself together. Thread foraged herbs and flowers through the frame, to dry them. Hang on a wall to store between uses.

May Bowl is a traditional German drink, made by infusing Sweet Woodruff (*Gallium odoratum*) in white wine. Sweet Woodruff has pretty white flowers and a fresh-cut hay scent in May. It grows in shady areas and looks quite similar to Cleavers, but it doesn't stick to clothing or climb up other plants. Cleavers can be used as a substitute in May Bowl, although Sweet Woodruff tastes better. The toxic look-alike Madder (*Rubia tinctorum*) should not be used in foods.

To prepare May Bowl, mix one bottle of white wine (Riesling works well) with 2 handfuls of lightly chopped Sweet Woodruff foliage and flowers. Let it infuse, chilled overnight in a sealed glass container. After straining the mixture, add a good pinch of grated Citrus zest and perhaps honey or sugar to taste. The result is a pale green drink with the distinctive fragrance of Sweet Woodruff.

Beltane tea blends are easy to make. Harvest small quantities of edible herbs from clean local areas. Dry each in a separate paper bag. When they are tinder dry, combine and store in a clean glass jar. A tasty Beltane blend might include Willow leaves, Mint, Chamomile, Ribwort, and a few Rose petals.

Visit sacred wells. Wells are often considered to be entrances to the underworld and are visited at Beltane by those seeking healing and inspiration. Seek out a local well, bubbling spring, or some other natural body of water. Spend time enjoying the area and make an offering to the water spirits. In lowlands, without springs and wells, you could visit natural water filtration systems, where purification takes place through sand dunes.

Daisy chains capture the playful spirit of Beltane. To start, pick Daisies with long stems from a lawn, snapping them off close to the ground. Use your thumbnail or a pin to make a small slit near the flower end of each stem. Thread another Daisy stem through the slit, gently pulling it until the flowerhead rests snugly against the stem. Repeat this process to create a chain of your desired length, then link the last Daisy to the first to close the loop. Wear your chain as a garland, bracelet, or crown, and keep it fresh by misting with water every few hours.

Go a-Maying. This tradition combines foraging, socialising, and celebrating the fertility of Beltane. Visit a beautiful green space with friends, to admire local herbs. Take a picnic to share, and look for Cleavers to shape into small foraging baskets. Forage lightly and focus on plentiful perennial herbs. Craft a Beltane crown from Willow or Ivy, and thread it with edible flowers like Dandelion and Daisy. After your excursion toss it into flowing water with a wish, or take it home to dry. Maying was historically a chance to collect flowers and enjoy a roll in the hay, on sunny Beltane days.

Dew bathe. Greet the Beltane sunrise by walking barefoot to a Hawthorn or Oak tree and washing your face with the dew. This ritual may enhance beauty, and radiance, and attract good fortune for the coming year. Beltane dew from Hawthorn leaves or blossoms is thought to connect us with the Fae and bring blessings of vitality and strength.

Yarrow divination is common at Beltane, which is the best time to harvest this powerful herb. Yarrow sticks are used with the I Ching, but can be interpreted without an oracle (see the Divination chapter). Cut some tall, flowering Yarrow stems; make tea from one and use it to cleanse and charge your divination tools. Place a sprig of Yarrow under your pillow to foretell the future. Or simply try looking around as you harvest Yarrow: the first person you see may well be your next romantic partner.

Maypole ceremonies can be recreated in city parks. Gather friends and choose a sturdy tree, perhaps a Hawthorn. Tie colourful cotton or paper ribbons around the trunk, as high up as possible. Each friend holds the end of a different ribbon. Dance around the tree, some of you moving clockwise, the others anticlockwise, weaving in and out to wrap the ribbons around the trunk. As you dance, focus on visualising your dreams coming to fruition. Afterwards, remove the ribbons, leaving the tree unharmed. Sprinkle protective herbs, such as Bay leaves, around the tree base, in thanks.

Spell for abundance and creativity

This is best done outdoors, or indoors with a soil-filled plant pot.

Gather a natural candle, lighter, pencil or knife (to mark the candle), some fresh seasonal flowers, a few seeds (and pot of soil), natural items linked to fertility (such as Hawthorn flowers or acorns), a little honey or rosewater, Bay leaf or Birch paperbark, a pen/pencil, and a heatproof bowl.

In a quiet space where you won't be disturbed, place the fresh flowers and symbolic items around your candle. Clarify your intention then, with a sharp point, mark your candle with a symbol to represent it (perhaps a heart, flower, or something to represent creativity or abundance). Anoint the candle with honey or rosewater, to attract growth sweetly. Light the candle and watch the flame; with each movement of the flame, feel the creativity and abundance stirring in the air.

Take a few smooth, deep breaths to centre your energy. As you breathe in, envision the abundance or creativity you desire flowing into your life. See it growing like the plants at Beltane. Hold the seeds and imagine them absorbing your wishes for abundance and creativity. Say:

Creative sparks, come to me,
Fertile seeds, in earth I see.
Let the blooms of Beltane grow,
And bring forth gifts, let them flow.

Carefully plant the seeds in the earth. As you plant, visualise the seeds sprouting and growing, to help manifest your intentions. Then sit quietly for a few moments. Extinguish the candle or stay with it until it burns down. Gather up the remaining natural items from the spell and bury them or compost them.

So mote it be.

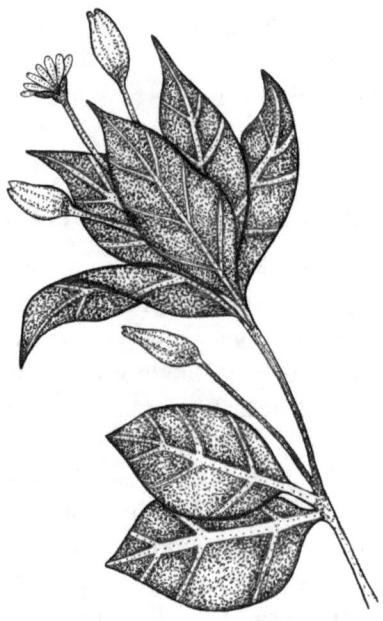

Summer solstice

Northern Hemisphere: June 20 to 23
Southern Hemisphere: December 20 to 23

This quarter day festival marks the longest day and the shortest night of the year in the Northern Hemisphere. Also known as Litha, Alban Hefin, or Midsummer. This is the pinnacle of the year, associated with bright light, and peak energy.

Midsummer is full of nectar-rich flowers, Bees, Butterflies, and sunbeams. Wild animals enjoy plentiful food, and we spend more time outdoors, soaking up the long daylight hours. This is a time to let the Sun uplift our hearts while the Moon cools our minds.

Traditions

Midsummer traditions celebrate the power of the Sun, and appreciate that until midwinter, the hours of daylight will fade. The sunrise is welcomed at first light, and the mighty Oak is honoured. Bonfires are lit at gatherings, their flames honouring the Sun. Midsummer's Eve is considered the best time to harvest many medicinal and magical herbs. This is a popular time for love divination. Perambulations, circular walks, are another long-held tradition.

Foraging

Many herbs and plants reach their peak, and seeds start to form at this time. Midsummer is the best time to harvest many herbs because they are potent, and drying is made easy by warm days. Some seeds are already ripe and can be gathered sparingly.

Altar

You may like to include Willow or Oak foliage, with Lime blossom, Roses and St John's Wort flowers. These midsummer flowers symbolise happiness, love, and health. The Green Man or Oak King is said to rule the land at this time. Willow symbolises fertility and health, and Lime blossoms are now as sweet as honey.

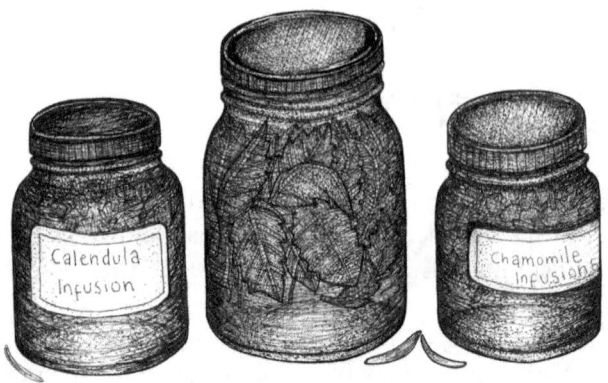

Activities

Flower crowns are simple to make using supple Oak or Willow branches. Thread with edible flowers like Lime blossom, Dandelions, and Daisies. Wear to gatherings, then either float the crown on water, as an offering, or take home to dry.

Charge houseplants, stones and crystals in sunlight. Midsummer is often a good time to move houseplants outdoors, if you have space. This will charge them with solar energy, to keep them healthy during the rest of the year. The same is true for crystals and stones. Rinse them in clean running water before placing them outside, or in a sunny windowsill. As they soak up the Sun from dawn till dusk, you may also like to set intentions for how each stone will be used.

Midsummer fires are a great way to build community. In the city open fires are rarely an option but a BBQ with friends could be a good alternative. Otherwise you can use candles to symbolise the cleansing qualities of traditional midsummer fires.

Perambulations are circular walks around an area. They were often used to assert the right to live in a district. If you enjoy walking, perambulations can be a great way to connect with your local landscape. Plan and walk a route around your local park, estate, town, or national park. As you wander, take in the sights, sounds, scents, and energy around you. If you have a map of local trees, you could even plan a halfway picnic under Lime trees, to enjoy the uplifting scent of their blossom. On sunny days, these trees will be filled with Bees.

Midsummer's Eve harvests are traditional for medicinal herbs like St John's Wort, Meadowsweet, Mugwort, Yarrow, Elderflower, Chamomile, and Lime blossom. Make it a ritual harvest by offering your gratitude to the earth and seeking permission to harvest from the plant spirits. Cleanse your harvesting blade or scissors with Yarrow or Bay-infused water. Cut the herbs cleanly and harvest lightly.

Stay up with the Sun

Celebrate the longest day of the year by staying awake all night. Begin your day with meditation at sunrise, breakfast with friends and be somewhere that you can forage sacred herbs. Take your tools for creating a tincture: small jars, vodka, scissors, and a chopstick. Once you've harvested your herbs, clean and chop them, then place them in the jars, before filling with vodka. As the Sun sets, gather around a fire (or candle, brazier, or BBQ). As you enjoy the glow, set your intentions for the season ahead. Use your midsummer tincture later in the year, on days when the Sun's energy seems far away.

Mugwort divination. Mugwort flowers are most useful for this, but the leaves can also be used. Try making Mugwort Moon water, by infusing Mugwort in a jar of water, which is exposed overnight to the Full Moon. Use to cleanse and charge your magical workspace, tools, or altar.

For dream work, place a Mugwort dream pillow or a sprig of fresh Mugwort inside your pillowcase. This invites prophetic dreams and can deepen your connection to the spirit realm. To make a dream pillow, sew a small pouch from natural fabric. Fill it with dried Mugwort and relaxing herbs like Lavender or Chamomile, and stitch it closed. Place it under your pillow or beside your bed to enhance dream work and spiritual connection.

If you are experienced with herbal teas and know that Mugwort is safe for you, brew a light infusion. Drinking this tea before meditation or a midsummer ritual can enhance spiritual journeys and deepen intuition.

Saining bundles are traditional Celtic cleansing tools used to purify spaces, objects, or individuals. Saining involves wafting the smoke of herbal bundles during rituals. Midsummer is an excellent time to craft saining bundles, particularly from herbs such as Mugwort, St John's Wort, or Lavender, which flower at this time and are associated with purification, protection, and spiritual awareness.

To make a saining bundle, gather small bunches of fresh or dried herbs. Bundle them so the cut ends of the herbs are all together. Bind the herbs together with natural twine. Ensure they are snug but not overly tight to allow proper airflow for burning. Hang the bundle to dry for a few weeks. To use them in rituals, light the leafy end and blow out the flame once it has caught. Then blow on the smouldering end so that it glows and smoulders. Place it on a heatproof dish, or stone, to prevent hot embers causing damage. Then allow the smoke to flow over the desired area, object, or person. Carry it around for this, if needed. Sain using non-toxic herbs and ensure proper ventilation.

Midsummer spell for abundance

To invite new opportunities, we must first release blockages. Begin by gathering some pieces of paper, Birch bark, or Bay leaves, a few Lime flowers, a few Sage leaves, a candle, pen, and a heatproof bowl.

Onto each small piece of paper, write something that you want to release, or be free from, such as old habits, doubts, and fears. On another larger piece, write the word Abundance, and surround it with symbols that represent abundance to you. Rub one of the Lime flowers onto this piece of paper, until it is scented by the nectar. The nectar attracts positive energy, just as it attracts Bees. It will amplify your intentions. Next, rub a Sage leaf over each of the small papers. Sage will help to banish the things you wish to be free from.

Once the notes are ready, light the small ones, one by one. As the papers burn say the following, then eat a Sage leaf.

> *With the Sun's light and fire's might,*
> *I release the old and welcome the bright.*
> *Abundance flows, my heart is free,*
> *I call forth joy, prosperity, and glee.*
> *As these words burn, so it shall be,*
> *Wishes drawn near, my obstacles flee.*

Focus on the flame consuming the things you wish to be free from. Then repeat the incantation while burning the larger paper, with what you wish to attract. Visualise the qualities you seek growing clearer and stronger in your life. Then eat the rest of the Lime flowers.

When you are finished, extinguish the candle.

It is done.

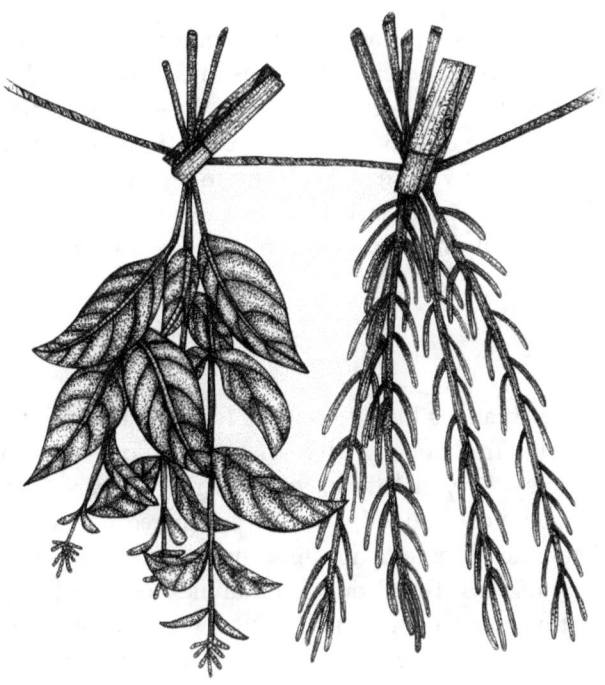

Lughnasadh

Northern Hemisphere: August 1
Southern Hemisphere: February 1

This cross-quarter festival falls between midsummer's day and the autumn equinox. Also known as Lammas (meaning Loaf Mass), this is traditionally when the first grain harvest of the year takes place.

Lughnasadh is the time when nature turns from green to gold, and plants become heavy with seed. We begin to reap what we have sown. Lughnasadh is the time to harvest, preserve, and share food. It reminds us that achievement and abundance happen best through teamwork and unity.

Traditions

Lughnasadh celebrations blend gratitude for the harvest with preparation for the future. Traditionally, harvest knots or favours were made from sheaves of Barley, Rye, or Wheat, to give to sweethearts. Grain-based foods, like elaborately braided loaves, were shared at festivities. Fairs, feasts, and strenuous contests are still common at this time of the year, in agricultural regions; They bring communities together but once were a chance for tribal leadership contests. There was a great sense of camaraderie and resilience at Lughnasadh, which often lasted for six weeks.

Foraging

There are plenty of wild edibles to choose from at Lughnasadh, but some herbs are starting to fade. Fruits are ripening, many street trees are sticky with Aphids, and some leaves are past their best. Look out for apples, haws, Lavender seed stems, grapes, blackberries, and soft Japanese Rosehips. Focus your harvest on the vigorous plants, and shift your attention towards seeds.

Altar

Add symbols of harvest and ripening seed. You might include Oak foliage, green acorns, rosehips, and Lavender stems. A handmade Ribwort seed dolly could serve as a herbal harvest knot. Plants that are partly in flower, and partly in seed, such as Meadowsweet, and Lavender, can be added to symbolise this festival of gratitude and hope.

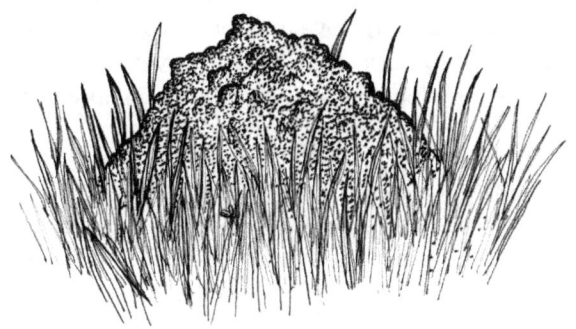

Activities

Grow Elder babies by planting forearm-length cuttings from healthy Elder trees. Gently push them halfway into pots of molehill soil, gaps in hedgerows, or barren spaces near your home. Remove most of the foliage from these cuttings, to help them to set root. By spring, they should burst into leaf. The world can never have too many Elder shrubs, with their edible and medicinal gifts. Be sure to mark where you plant them so you can visit in spring and summer. Within a few years they will flower and fruit in sunny locations; within months there will be leaves to harvest for skin balms.

Harvest seeds from local plants. When foraging, carry a paper bag to harvest ripe seeds. Shake them into the bag, but leave plenty on the plants to disperse naturally. Some tiny seeds, like Poppy and Garlic Mustard, can be difficult to collect individually, so remove whole seedheads and let them open at home in dry warmth. As with many leaves and flowers, the best way to dry seeds is simply to leave them in the paper bag. Label and place somewhere that dry air can circulate. Some other seeds to harvest at this time of year are Pot Marigold, Hollyhock, and Burdock.

As you travel around town, carry a pocketful of these seeds to push into soil-filled cracks near buildings and street poles. Eventually, your travel routes will be lined with Hollyhocks, Poppies, and Marigold flowers.

Garlic can be grown from organic bulbs from grocery stores. They grow tall and thin, so they don't need much space and can be planted in pots of molehill soil. Carefully crack the bulb open to separate the cloves. Discard any that look unhealthy or feel soft. Leave the papery skin on and push the flat end of each clove into the soil, leaving just the pointed end visible above the soil. Space individual cloves about a thumb length apart. Place in a sunny location and water occasionally through winter.

Natural Ink can be made by mashing a handful of juicy Blackberries or Elderberries. Strain the juice to remove any seeds or pulp. To thicken slightly, simmer in a small pan over a candle, and dissolve a pinch of powdered Pine tree resin. Use the ink with a dipping pen, or sharp twig, to write intentions, symbols, and spells. Many berries can be used to make ink, but if using poisonous ones, be sure to avoid inhaling the fumes while simmering to thicken.

Plan quiet time. Lughnasadh is a good time to reflect on how you wish to spend the months ahead. To avoid overextending yourself, consider slowing down on promised engagements and resist the urge to over-commit as autumn and winter approach. Plan quiet time to rest and recharge. Give yourself space to reflect on your practice, and preserve your energy during the darker months.

Ribwort knots are simple corn dollies, or favours, made by plaiting together Ribwort seed stems. This is a crafty way to connect with the harvest and save a few seeds from this valuable city plant. They can be given to friends or placed on the altar as a symbol of Lughnasadh gratitude and hope. As you weave, reflect on the progress of your inner projects since spring. There's still time to align your efforts with your goals, so try to weave a plan of action.

Start by gathering four tall, fresh Ribwort spikes. Cut them as close to the base as possible; you may like to do this with a special tool that you reserve for ritual harvests. Secure the seed ends of the stems together (with string or an elastic band) then open the four stems into a cross shape. Arrange them so one points to you, one points away and the other two point right and left. Weave them together by folding the top stem down, then the bottom stem up, left to the right, then right to the left. Keep folding the stems this way until you reach the end of the stems and a simple, sturdy braid is formed. Secure this (with another elastic or string) into a simple loop shape.

Seed planting charm

This charm can be used as you plant seeds at Lughnasadh. It helps to focus intentions for growth and prosperity. You will need a handful of seeds.

At your chosen planting site, ground and centre yourself. Then hold the seeds. Close your hands around them and feel your energy flowing into them. Let it activate them and make them ready to germinate when the conditions are right. Whisper these words onto the seeds:

> *Seed by seed, I plant with grace,*
> *Abundance blooms in Earth's embrace.*

Now start to plant them, and repeat the charm as often as you like while doing so.

Harvest protection spell

As the harvest season settles in, this simple spell can be used to protect what has been gathered and preserved, helping it remain safe and potent through the coming months. You will need a candle, lighter, small bowl of grain or seed, some fresh or preserved foraged herbs or fruits, and a length of Ivy.

Arrange the seeds and herbs around the candle. Light it to symbolise the Sun's warmth and protection. Hold your hands over the seeds and herbs—these symbolise the harvest that you wish to protect. The harvest can be anything that you have worked for. Say aloud:

> *By earth and fire, by sky so wide,*
> *Protect this harvest, with love as guide.*
> *Frost and pests, from here alight,*
> *What's gathered, safe through winter nights.*

Now place the Ivy around the seeds and herbs, to form a ring of protection.

> *Shield the bounty, keep it whole,*
> *Fill with strength and make it gold.*
> *Bless these gifts, may they endure,*
> *Through cold months, their power pure.*

If possible, sit with the candle as it burns down completely and spend time visualising your harvest safe and whole.

The spell is complete when the candle is extinguished or burns out.

It is so.

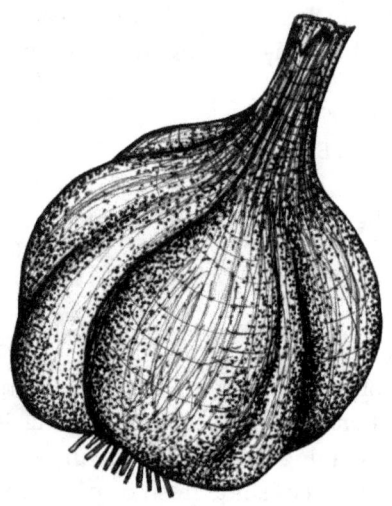

Autumn equinox

Northern Hemisphere: September 20 to 23
Southern Hemisphere: March 19 to 22

This quarter day occurs when Earth's equator is directly in line with the Sun, causing the hours of light and darkness to be equal. This is the second harvest festival; a time associated with balance, completion, and movement into darkness. This festival is also known as Alban Elfed, Herfest, or Mabon.

In nature, all stages of life can be seen at once; there is fresh growth on some plants with flowers, fruits, leaves, and seed spikes but also plants that have completely faded and are returning to the soil. Animals are beginning to prepare for winter, and in green spaces, the scent of autumn creeps through the air. Tap roots thicken and the days shorten. Nature is about to start its steady retreat into winter.

Traditions

The late grain harvests were previously big community affairs in country regions. These were followed by nourishing meals, sometimes the best of the year, and social gatherings for all concerned. In cities, flower-cutting days and group harvests at community gardens offer locals a chance to gather herbs and vegetables, before frosts or soil cultivation clear them away. At Herfest, the Holly King is said to dethrone the Oak King. The Ivy Queen also comes into her own.

Foraging

Most plants have started to direct nutrients from their leaves into their roots by this time; it is a way to conserve their resources for winter. Frosts will soon change the landscape and limit wild-foraged foods, so preserve what you'll need for the months ahead. Light harvesting will be possible through winter, but the main foraging season returns in April, so now is the time to prepare. Evergreens like Rosemary, as well as brambles, hips, haws, and nuts, are abundant now but harvest lightly, taking only what you can use or preserve. Leave plenty for wildlife.

Altar

You may like to add to your altar some fresh Holly or Ivy foliage, a tealight candle and some Marigolds, and seasonal fruit. Turkish Hazel nutcases and Michaelmas Daisies can look especially good too. Orange-coloured flowers, nuts, and evergreen branches, all symbolise nourishment, plenty, and resilience. Small pots of organic Basil or Mint, which will soon fade if outdoors, can be grown on your altar in pots—very useful for money spells.

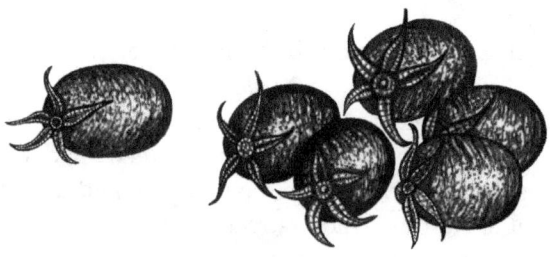

Activities

Balancing the breath involves matching the length of your inhalation and exhalation. It calms the mind and eases stress. To practise, sit comfortably but upright, and allow your body to relax. Gently close your eyes and take a few natural breaths. Then count in your mind, as you inhale. Without force, match the same count as you exhale. When ready, repeat. Let the breath flow smoothly, without force, and add short pauses before inhaling, if it feels comfortable. Keep your focus on the steady rise and fall of your breathing for a few minutes, then relax and breathe normally again.

Walk in nature, paying attention to fading leaves, the last berries, nuts, and signs of animals storing food. If you have one, take a pocket mirror, and look up at the tree canopies while viewing their reflection below. This gives a different perspective on the world. Let your many senses guide you to what's ripe or ready to eat, whether edible herbs, seeds, or fruits. Even if you don't harvest, notice which signs show you that these things are ripe. Where do you sense this knowledge?

Michaelmas Daisies (*Aster amellus*) are resilient plants, often grown alongside city streets. They are overlooked before flowering time, when they erupt into a mass of starry flowers. The purple flowers and young leaves, when clean, are edible and taste like Chrysanthemum. The plant has medicinal and magical qualities, and is associated with purification and love. You may like to add a few flowers to incense blends, place them on your altar, or float them in a bowl of water before adding ink drops for autumn divination.

Plant trees at the autumn equinox, to give them a chance to settle before winter. Rehome or repot any that you may have been nurturing from seeds. Move tiny seedlings from large trees, such as Oak, Ash, and Sycamore, to locations where they can flourish.

Oxymels are a simple way to make bitter or pungent herbs more palatable. Made with vinegar and honey, they represent the sweet and sour balance of the equinox. To make an oxymel base, combine 5 parts honey and 1 part apple cider vinegar in a small jug. Stir well to mix. Then, half-fill a glass preserving jar with your chosen herb (perhaps Sage, Black Horehound (*Ballota nigra*), or Garlic). Pour the oxymel base over the herbs, until the jar is completely full. Close the jar, after prodding the mixture with a chopstick, to release any air bubbles. Let it sit for several days to weeks, before straining. Store the oxymel in a glass jar with a non-metallic lid. Take a teaspoonful in water to soothe sore throats or to remind of the need for balance.

Ritual harvesting of the last grain plants of the year is an ancient British practice. In agricultural regions, the spirit of the corn had to be captured, to ensure future harvests. To do this, harvesters would circle the crop, cutting the field in ever-decreasing circles. This was to trap the Corn spirit at the centre of the field. When the final stalks were left standing, harvesters would cut them, by throwing sharp sickles, from a safe distance. The last crop stalks were then woven into a Corn dolly.

This ritual can be recreated using a plentiful urban *crop*, such as Stinging Nettle. If a dense patch of Nettles needs to be cut down for some reason, begin harvesting from the outer edges and move inward in ever-decreasing circles. The final stems can be woven into a Corn dolly using the Lughnasadh Ribwort knot activity, or can be saved until next spring, to retain the spirit of the plants.

Consult the Ivy Queen Oracle. The spirit of Ivy can be a powerful guide through the autumn and winter. To begin, go outside and find a healthy patch of Ivy. Take time to observe closely, notice how it climbs and twists; how it holds trees and walls. Ivy cloaks and protects, symbolising the invisible power of the witch, moving through the darker months.

Sit near the Ivy, close your eyes and breathe smoothly and deeply. Feel the energy of the plant around you and ask it for guidance. Hold an Ivy leaf in your hand and ask:

What wisdom do you have for me in this quiet time?

Pay attention to any impressions, thoughts, or feelings that come to you; these could be symbols or messages related to your inner journey, as you prepare for the winter months. Thank the plant and note any insights. This simple practice can be done with any plant that you feel drawn to.

Spell for Herfest

This spell is a nod to the Harvest Lords of ancient agricultural communities in Britain. These leaders of the agricultural workers wore Red Poppies and Bindweed around their hats. They were the first to be served at feasts, because they were the ones that negotiated pay and conditions for the harvest workers.

Gather a candle, a length of Bindweed, a length of Ivy, some Poppies (or other bright flowers), and some food. Shape the Ivy and Bindweed into a circle or crown and weave the Poppies into it. Place this around the candle.

Light the candle and take a moment to centre yourself. Imagine the Harvest Lord's spirit coming into the room. Satisfied at a good harvest, and care for the workers, the Harvest Lord is ready to feast before enjoying a period of rest. Say aloud:

> *Harvest Lord, shining bright,*
> *With Poppies red and bindweed tight,*
> *You walk the fields, your work is done,*
> *Now give thanks for the bounty won.*
> *Guide the harvest, make it right,*
> *Bring peace and balance, with your might.*

Hold your hands near the candle and feel the energy of the Harvest Lord, balancing the work and the rewards of the season. Eat the food as you consider the labourers and harvest workers, past and present, who have helped bring food to your table.

Sit quietly for a moment, then blow out the candle to close the spell.

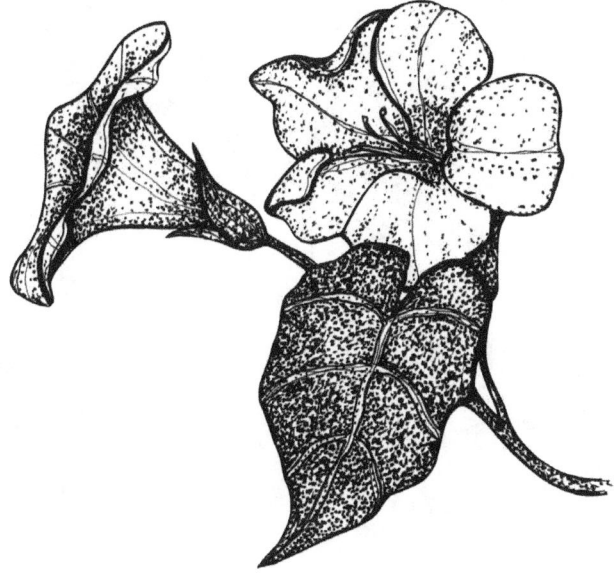

Urban foraging

Towns and cities are home to an astonishing range of plants. Many of them are edible and/or medicinal, and can be used in spells, and rituals. Foraging is more than just gathering food; it is a chance to tune into the landscape, and get to know local plants. These plants face constant challenges—pollution, foot traffic, and poor soil—and yet they thrive. They can teach us a great deal, but to learn we must listen to them.

There are concerns about the safety of food plucked from polluted urban spaces but it has been found that, when properly washed, they can be as healthy as plants from agricultural land. Urban foraging gets us outside, in the green, which we know improves wellbeing. When practised responsibly, foraging benefits us and the environment.

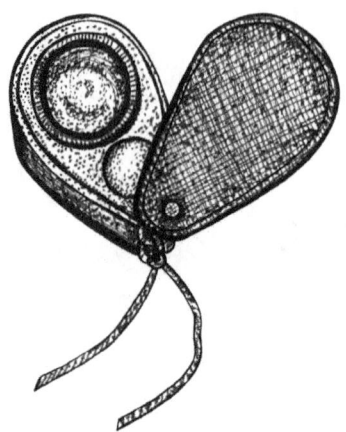

Ethical foraging

Foraging is a partnership with nature that requires respect and thoughtfulness. Try to find plants that have chosen where to grow, and thrive; these are usually more potent than those intentionally planted by gardeners. Keep the following guidelines in mind, using the acronym *CALLES* (Spanish for streets):

Clean: Avoid heavily polluted areas, and spots where animals might have left their mark, and always wash your finds thoroughly before use.

Accurate: Be absolutely sure of a plant's identity, using trusted identification tools, and understand this plant's role in the ecosystem.[6]

Light: Harvest only what you need; aim for 10% of any plant that you find growing in large numbers. Some plants, like Japanese Knotweed, are invasive and can be harvested in greater quantities, but avoid heavy harvesting of any plant from one location, in case of unseen pollution. Leave enough for wildlife and the plant's regrowth. Gather fallen bark, Pine or Fir cones and excess resin from tree wounds. These materials are gifts that allow you to connect with the plant without causing harm.

---

[6] Clearly illustrated field guides, such as *Collins' Wildflower Guide* (2nd edn) by David Streeter, and *Collins' Tree Guide* by David Johnson, are extremely useful, and worth regularly consulting to check finds and build knowledge. Don't rely on apps or foraging books for plant identification.

Legal: Follow local foraging laws, respect private property, and avoid picking protected species.

Enriching: Leave the space better than you found it. Scatter seeds, plant native herbs, and remove litter.

Safe: Ensure plants are edible or safe for their intended use, avoid contamination, label your harvests, and store them properly away from children.

Ritual harvests

For many city witches, foraging is a sacred act. Before harvesting they seek out wild edible plants that are brimming with energy. They ask them to prepare to be harvested, knowing that this intensifies the plants' potency. Then, using their hands or clean tools, they are guided by the plants and take gently what they need. They thank the plants and ensure they are left unharmed.

Every plant has its own personality and talents. The Green City Witch taps into these. Making a ritual from foraging connects us to ancestors who realised that we are the land, we rely on its gifts, and must treat it as well as we would our own child.

Urban foraging intimately connects us to our local environment and encourages us to take care of it. Rather than depleting the landscape, ethical foraging makes cities greener, healthier, and more vibrant.

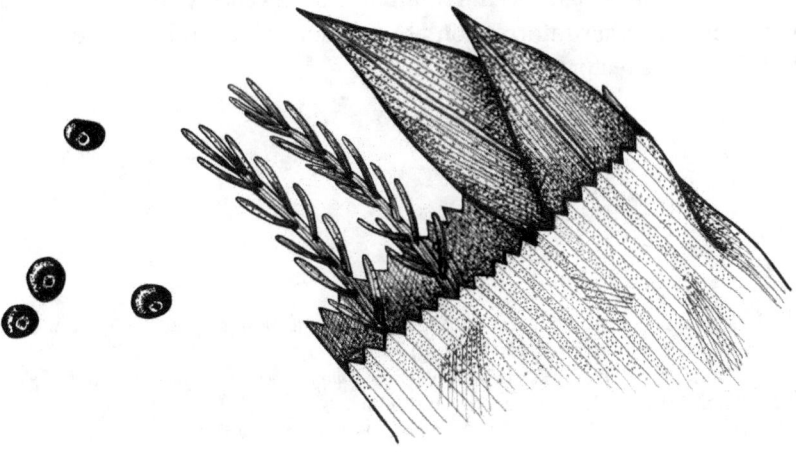

Learning the plants

If you're just beginning your foraging journey, start slowly.[7] Focus on one plant at a time, observing its uses, growth habits, and seasonal availability. Keeping a foraging journal can be a useful way to track your discoveries; simply noting the date, plant names and those growing close by will help build a picture of the ecosystem.

Start by focusing on familiar plants like Stinging Nettle or Bramble; follow them through the year to observe how they change and which animals they support. Find out more from experienced foragers.[8] And try to learn the characteristics of plant families, as this can reveal connections between related species, and help build your knowledge more quickly.[9] Joining The Herb Society UK can also provide access to a wealth of information about growing and using herbs. With patience and care, you will develop a rich relationship with the plants around you.

Urban foraging calendar

Each season offers urban foragers a wide range of edibles and medicinals. Some are possible to harvest year round but most have seasons when they really shine. You will notice these extra potent times by the vibrant colour of individual plants.

This calendar indicates when you are most likely to find favourite wild and feral plants. This doesn't necessarily mean that you should harvest them then, but you should be able to find them, and build your understanding of them. As the weather changes each year, use the dates as a guide. Further information about each plant can be found in the Nature Lore directory.

---

[7] And seek out an expert guide from professional organisations such as the Association of Foragers (https://foragers-association.org).
[8] Andy Hamilton's book *The First Time Forager: A complete beginner's guide to Britain's edible plants* (National Trust 2024) is a good place to start.
[9] Thomas Elpel, *Botany in a Day* (2013) is particularly useful for this.

Key: bd = leaf bud, lf = leaf, fl = flower, fr = fruit, nt = nut, sd = seed, sp = sap, st = stem

Late Autumn/Early Winter — Samhain

Bay	Hawthorn fr	Rue
Bramble bd	Hazelnuts	Sage
Burdock lf/sd	Ivy	Self-heal
Chameleon Plant rt	Japanese Plum lf	Shepherd's Purse
Chickweed	Lady's Mantle	Stinging Nettle
Comfrey lf/rt	Lime bd	Sweet Chestnut
Daisy lf	Mahonia fl	Thyme
Dandelon lf/rt	Mallow	Violet
Dead Nettle lf	Mint sd	Wild Rocket
Feverfew	Mugwort sd	Willow st
Gallant Soldiers	Nasturtium	Winter Purslane
Geranium	Oak sd	Wood Avens
Ginkgo fr/lf	Parsley	Yarrow
Ground Elder rt	Pot Marigold	Yellow Dead Nettle
Ground Ivy	Rose fr	
Hairy Bittercress	Rosemary	

Winter Solstice — Yule

Bay	Japanese Plum lf	Shepherd's Purse
Bramble bd	Lime bd	Stinging Nettle
Chickweed	Mahonia fl	Violet
Geranium	Parsley	Wild Rocket
gingko fr	Pot Marigold	Willow st
Ground Ivy	Rose fr	Winter Purslane
Hairy Bittercress	Rosemary	Wood Avens
Holly	Rue	Yarrow
Ivy	Sage	Yellow Dead Nettle

Late Winter/Early Spring — Imbolc

Bay, Birch sp	Cleavers	Dandelion rt
Bramble bd/lf	Cranesbill lf	Garlic Mustard
Chickweed	Daisy	Geranium

Ground Ivy
Hairy Bittercress
Hawthorn bd
Holly
Hollyhock lf
Ivy
Japanese Quince fr
Lime bd
Moss
Parsley Pine

Poplar bd
Pot Marigold
Primrose lf/fl
Rosemary
Rue
Sage
Shepherd's Purse
Stinging Nettle
Sweet Cicely lf
Sycamore sp

Violet
Wild Garlic lf
Wild Rocket
Willow st
Witch Hazel fl
Winter Purslane
Wood Avens
Yarrow
Yellow Dead Nettle

Spring Equinox—Ostara

Apple lf
Ash lf
Bay
Beech lf
Birch lf/sp
Bramble bd/lf
Burdock lf
Catnip
Chameleon Plant
Chickweed
Cleavers
Coltsfoot fl
Comfrey
Daisy
Dandelion
Dead Nettle
Dock
Primrose lf/fl
Fennel
Garlic Mustard
Geranium
Grape Hyacinth fl

Ground Elder lf
Ground Ivy
Hairy Bittercress
Hawthorn lf
Hazel lf
Herb Robert
Holly
Hollyhock lf
Ivy
Japanese Knotweed
Lady's Mantle
Lavender lf
Lilac fl
Lemon Balm
Lime lf
Magnolia fl
Mallow
Moss
Mugwort
Oak lf
Parsley
Pine

Plantain
Poplar bd/lf
Pot Marigold
Ribwort
Rose lf
Rosemary
Rue
Sage
Self-Heal
Shepherd's Purse
Stinging Nettle
Sweet Cicely lf
Thyme
Violet
Wild Garlic lf/fl
Wild Rocket
Willow fl
Winter Purslane
Wood Avens
Yarrow
Yellow Dead Nettle

Late Spring/Early Summer—Beltane

Apple lf
Agrimony lf

Ash lf
Bay

Bramble lf
Burdock lf

Catnip
Chameleon Plant
Chamomile
Chickweed
Cleavers
Clover
Comfrey
Daisy fl
Dandelion
Daylily fl
Dead Nettle
Dock
Elder fl
Elm sd
Enchanter's
   Nightshade lf
Fennel
Feverfew
Garlic Mustard
Geranium
Grapevine lf
Ground Elder lf
Ground Ivy
Hairy Bittercress

Hawthorn lf/fl
Hazel lf
Herb Robert
Himalayan Balsam st
Holly
Hollyhock lf
Ivy
Japanese Knotweed
Juniper lf
Lady's Mantle
Lavender lf
Lemon Balm
Lilac fl
Lime lf
Magnolia fl
Mallow
Meadowsweet lf
Mint
Moss
Mugwort
Nasturtium
Olive lf
Parsley
Passionflower

Pine
Plantain
Poplar lf
Pot Marigold
Ribwort
Rose fl
Rosemary
Rue
Sage
Self-Heal
Shepherd's Purse
Stinging Nettle
Sweet Cicely lf/fl
Thyme
Violet
Wild Garlic fl/sd
Wild Rocket
Willow
Winter Purslane
Wood Avens
Wormwood
Yarrow
Yellow Dead Nettle

Midsummer — Summer Solstice

Agrimony lf/fl
Bay
Bramble lf
Burdock lf
Catnip
Chameleon Plant
Chamomile
Chickweed
Cleavers
Clover
Comfrey
Daisy
Dandelion

Daylily fl
Dead Nettle
Dock
Enchanter's
   Nightshade
Fennel
Feverfew
Gallant Soldiers
Garlic Mustard lf/sd
Geranium
Grapevine lf
Ground Elder lf
Ground Ivy

Hairy Bittercress
Hazel lf
Herb Robert
Himalayan Balsam st/fl
Holly
Hollyhock lf/fl
Horehound
Hyssop
Ivy
Japanese Knotweed
Juniper lf
Lady's Mantle
Lavender lf/fl

Lemon Balm	Plantain	Stinging Nettle
Lime lf/fl	Pot Marigold	Sweet Cicely fl/sd
Mallow	Ribwort	Thyme
Meadowsweet fl	Rose fl	Violet
Mint	Rosemary	Wild Garlic sd
Motherwort	Rue	Wild Rocket
Mugwort	Sage	Willow
Olive lf	Self-Heal	Wood Avens
Parsley	Shepherd's Purse	Wormwood
Passionflower	Snapdragons	Yarrow
Pine	St John's Wort	Yellow Dead Nettle

Late Summer/Early Autumn — Lughnasadh

Borage	Ground Elder sd	Parsley
Bramble fr	Ground Ivy	Passionflower
Burdock lf	Hairy Bittercress	Plantain
Carob sd	Hawthorn fr	Pine
Catnip	Hazel lf/nt	Pot Marigold
Chameleon Plant	Herb Robert	Ribwort
Chamomile	Himalayan Balsam st/fl	Rose fl/fr
Chickweed	Holly	Rosemary
Comfrey	Hollyhock lf/fl	Rue
Daisy	Hyssop fl	Sage
Dandelion lf/rt	Ivy	Self-Heal
Daylily fl	Japanese Knotweed	Shepherd's Purse
Dead Nettle	Juniper lf	Snapdragons
Dock	Lady's Mantle	Stinging Nettle
Elder fr	Lavender lf/fl	St John's Wort
Enchanter's Nightshade fl/sd	Lemon Balm	Sumac fl/fr
	Lime lf/bd	Thyme
Fennel	Mahonia fr	Violet
Feverfew	Mallow	Wild Rocket
fig lf/fr	Meadowsweet lf/fl/sd	Willow
Gallant Soldiers	Mint	Wood Avens
Garlic Mustard	Mugwort	Wormwood
Geranium	Mullein fl	Yarrow
Grapevine lf/fr	Nasturtium	Yellow Dead Nettle

Autumn Equinox—Mabon

- Apple
- Beech nt
- Bramble fr
- Burdock lf
- Carob sd
- Catnip
- Chameleon Plant
- Chamomile
- Chickweed
- Comfrey
- Dandelion lf/rt
- Dead Nettle
- Dock sd
- Elder fr
- Enchanter's Nightshade fl/sd
- Feverfew
- Gallant Soldiers
- Geranium
- Ginkgo fr/lf
- Grapevine lf/fr
- Ground Elder sd/rt
- Ground Ivy
- Hairy Bittercress
- Hawthorn fr
- Hazelnuts
- Herb Robert
- Himalayan Balsam
- Holly
- Hollyhock sd
- Hops
- Hyssop fl
- Ivy
- Japanese Knotweed st
- Japanese Quince fr
- Lady's Mantle
- Lemon Balm
- Lime bd/sd
- Mallow
- Moss
- Mugwort sd
- Nasturtium
- Oak sd
- Parsley
- Passionflower lf
- Pears
- Plantain sd
- Pot Marigold
- Quinces
- Ribwort sd
- Rocket
- Rose fr
- Rosemary
- Rue
- Sage
- Self-Heal
- Shepherd's Purse
- Snapdragons
- Sorrel
- Stinging Nettle
- Sumac fr
- Sweet Chestnut
- Thyme
- Turkish Hazelnuts
- Violet
- Walnuts
- Wild Rocket
- Willow
- Winter Purslane
- Wood Avens
- Yarrow
- Yellow Dead Nettle

NATURE LORE

Plant lore directory

This section covers over 100 magical and medicinal plants that thrive in European cities. The directory includes street trees, urban weeds, houseplants, and kitchen herbs, highlighting their identifying features, virtues in crafts, herbalism, and magic, and offering notes on foraging or care. Whether you seek insights into plants lining city streets or growing quietly on your windowsill, this guide will help you to embrace urban flora.

Agrimony (*Agrimonia eupatoria* L.)

French: *Aigremoine*; Dutch: *Agrimonie*
Family: Rosaceae

Perennial herb with pinnate leaves with toothed edges, arranged in opposite pairs along a central leaf stem. Small yellow flowers, usually with five petals, which develop progressively up tall, slender flower spikes. May reach 1 m height. Agrimony seed pods are hooked, bristly fruits that cling to passing animals or clothing. Lightly aromatic when bruised and all parts taste mildly bitter.

Virtues

Agrimony has astringent, anti-inflammatory, and diuretic properties. It is used in teas, tinctures, and syrups to help treat digestive issues, such as diarrhoea and indigestion. Topically, it soothes wounds and skin irritations, promoting healing. Additionally, it is effective in treating sore throats, coughs, and urinary tract infections. An Agrimony cold compress (cloth soaked in the cooked tea) may be applied to the forehead, to help relieve migraine. The seeds, leaves, and flowers can be eaten sparingly in salads.

Magical significance

Associated with protection and purification. It is believed to ward off negative energies and encourage clarity of thought. Dried seeds, leaves, or flowers are often used in charms and sachets to bring good fortune and shield against misfortune. Agrimony tea, or incense, can be used to cleanse spaces and objects, promoting peace and harmony. It can enhance dreams and divination, and its seeds are sometimes used in rituals to ensure successful outcomes in projects.

Foraging notes

Find: In hedges, woodland edges, along roadsides and in tall grassland. The yellow flower spikes are quite easy to spot but often confused with other tall yellow flowering plants, like Mullein (*Verbascum* spp.).

When not in flower, Agrimony foliage is easily confused with that of Meadowsweet (*Filipendula ulmaria*).

Harvest: Leaves and flowers, midsummer; seeds, Lughnasadh to autumn equinox.

Alder (*Alnus glutinosa* (L.) Gaertn.)

French: *Aulne*; Dutch: *Als*
Family: Betulaceae

Large conical tree (up to 28 m) with dangling catkins and small, upright cones. Dark bark with light brown twigs, tinged red at growing points and sometimes sticky. Flat-ended leaves are shiny, almost oval, with serrated edges. Alder is said to absorb high levels of soil minerals, perhaps even gold, and it helps other plants to colonise wetlands. Alder leaves are a favourite food of caterpillars, so often are peppered with holes. The catkins are valued by birds and other wildlife.

Virtues

Alder leaves are rich in tannins and taste bitter. They have astringent and anti-inflammatory properties. Alder leaves are used in teas and decoctions to treat diarrhoea, sore throats, tonsillitis, and as a mouthwash. A warm leaf poultice can soothe sore muscles and joints. Alder wood, leaves, and fruit are used to produce dyes. Different parts and seasons yield red, black, brown, yellow, and green stains. Alder wood is water-resistant. It is used to craft clogs and hardwearing tools; trees growing in waterlogged land are best for this.

Magical significance

Associated with water, accumulation, wealth, teamwork, stabilisation, and strength through hardship. The orange–red sap that oozes from cut Alder can be used in blood magic. Chewing the twigs will give a black tongue—perhaps useful in rituals. Use Alder to seek support from water spirits. Alder whistles, made by pushing the pith out from young stems, can be used to call nature spirits to magical work.

Foraging notes

Find: Near waterways and in lowlands. Alder leaves are sometimes confused with Hazel, but Hazel leaves are softer. Look for trees with clear signs of both catkins and cones at the same time.

Aloe Vera (*Aloe vera* (L.) Burm.f)

French: *Aloe vera*; Dutch: *Aloë vera*
Family: Asphodelaceae

Aloe Vera is a succulent with thick, pointed leaves that grow in rosettes. Yellow flowers may develop on spikes, in summer. Clones grow from rootstock when pot-bound. The clear gel and bitter yellow sap are valued for health remedies.

Virtues

The clear gel has anti-inflammatory, vulnerary, antioxidant, and slight analgesic properties. It can soothe sore skin and tired eyes. Internally it calms gut complaints, like heartburn. Try it in smoothies or add to ice cubes. For bug bite relief, blend with a drop of Lavender oil or tincture. Avoid using on fresh burns, as the gel traps heat when it dries. The yellow sap (in green parts) is bitter, antioxidant, antimicrobial, emmenagogue, and purgative. For constipation Aloe bitters can be used occasionally; blend a 2–4 cm length of clean organic leaf (including the skin) into a smoothie. It is used as a laxative and digestive stimulant. Ancient Egyptians used Aloe for parasites. Avoid during pregnancy.

Magical significance

Associated with purification, rejuvenation, protection, love, and fertility. Known as the Plant of Immortality, it features in many ancient texts and funeral rites.

Care and harvesting notes

Care: Prefers well-drained soil, bright sunshine, and indoor protection from frost. Manages well in a pot and enjoys outdoor summer Sun.

Harvest: Occasional whole leaves, extracting the gel by slicing away the green skin. Cut Aloe Vera leaves refrigerate well.

Aloes are protected internationally under CITES; avoid non-sustainable sources. *Aloe vera* (L.) is not threatened.

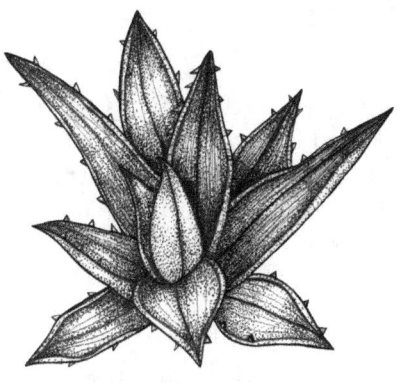

Apple (*Malus* spp.)

French: *Pommier*; Dutch: *Appel*
Family: Rosaceae

Apple trees range from low orchard types to tall Crab Apples (up to 17 m), with oval, toothed leaves and fragrant blossoms. They produce pink–white, Rose-like flowers in the spring. Apple leaves are oval with toothed edges, and the area beneath these trees is ideal for growing herbs. These trees are very valuable to wildlife.

Virtues

The taste and texture of Apple fruit vary widely, from sweet and juicy to tart and dry, while the leaves have a bitter taste. Apples have prebiotic, anti-inflammatory, astringent, and antioxidant properties. Apple leaves and fruit contain valuable compounds, such as quercetin, a phenolic antioxidant also found in Oak and Onion. Apple peel tea may soothe digestive and rheumatic issues. In traditional medicine, apples aid digestion, dentition, and provide a gentle laxative effect. Roasted apples soothe throat and skin inflammations. Apple leaves are sometimes applied as a poultice for their healing properties.

Magical significance

Associated with health, beauty, eternity, joy, companionship, and Druids. In myths, Avalon, the Isle of Apples, represents rebirth. Slicing an apple horizontally reveals a hidden pentagram, a symbol often linked with witchcraft. When harvesting many apples, always leave a few on the tree for the spirits. Wassailing ceremonies honour Apple spirits for fruitful harvests. Apple wood makes an excellent wand, and apples may be buried at Samhain as offerings to guide the spirits of the recently deceased towards Summerland.

Foraging notes

Find: Community orchards, gardens, parks.

Harvest: Autumn Crab Apples for jam, tender spring leaves for tea.

Ash (*Fraxinus excelsior* L.)

French: *Frêne élevé*; Dutch: *Es*
Family: Oleaceae

Medium to large deciduous trees, 30 m+, tall. Compound leaves, spreading branches and black leaf buds. Ash trees have small male or female flowers. Female trees produce large bunches of winged seeds (*keys*). Young Ash bark is smooth and grey–brown. It becomes rougher with age. Compound leaves contain 5 to 13 pinnate leaflets with serrated edges.

Virtues

Ash leaves have a mild laxative effect. They are used for gout, rheumatism, and jaundice. Ash tea or decoction (leaves or bark) helps skin infections, scalp irritation, and dermatitis. The root bark is sometimes used to reduce fevers and to expel worms. As firewood, Ash dries quickly and burns hot. Its fine-grained wood carves easily. Ash seeds are a valuable food source for wildlife.

Magical significance

Ash keys symbolise fertility, solutions, strength, sacred water, protection. In Greek mythology, Zeus created humans from Ash. Yggdrasil, the world tree of Norse Mythology, is Ash, with roots in the underworld and leaves reaching the heavens. Druids carve symbols and charms in Ash. Often grown beside sacred wells. For wand making, choose a straight male or female Ash branch. Carry Ash keys as amulets. Draw protective circles with Ash sticks. Collect sacred water from hollows in Ash trees for rituals and charms. An old Scottish ritual involves feeding sap, which bubbles from burning green Ash wood, to babies, for strength; this may suit initiation rituals for coven members.

Foraging notes

Find: Parks and gardens. Branches grow at odd angles when pruned. Leaves are often confused with Elder and Rowan. Look for the keys.

Harvest: Leaves; young and tender for teas (before midsummer). Older leaves are best for external use. Bark; from pruned branches. Cut cleanly to reduce risk of infection by Ash dieback fungus.

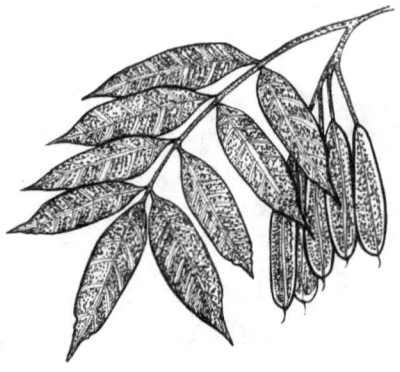

Avocado (*Persea americana* Mill.)

French: *Avocatier*; Dutch: *Avocado*
Family: Lauraceae

Medium tree, 15–20 m tall in warm climates, with long elliptical leaves. Also thrives as a houseplant. In spring, it produces yellow flowers that develop into pear-shaped fruit with large stony pits. These are a relic of its ancient dispersal by now-extinct animals. Avocados have been cultivated for over 10,000 years.

Virtues

Avocado fruit is a valued food. In Middle and South America a poultice from the leaves or grated stone is used to soothe rheumatism, joint pain, headaches, and skin disorders. Avocado oil soothes skin. The fruit pulp may treat intestinal worms, softens skin, draws out impurities, and supports wound healing. It is also very nutritious. An infusion of older leaves is traditionally used to treat colds, flu, cough, high blood pressure, and stomach issues like diarrhoea. It may also inhibit *Herpes simplex* virus. Do not consume young Avocado leaves, as cthey can cause heart palpitations. Use older leaves sparingly as tea.

Magical significance

Associated with love, beauty, fertility, vitality, and prosperity. Ancient Mayan and Aztec cultures considered Avocado to be a sacred tree. The Aztecs called the fruit *āhuacatl*, meaning testicle, and ate it to bring on lust. To attract love and passion, try growing an avocado plant, preferably from seed, and eat the fruit regularly.

Foraging notes

Find: Sunny gardens or houseplants. Prefers temperatures above 2°C.

Harvest: Older, large dark leaves, and fruit from mature trees (use an apple catcher). Beware look-alike houseplant Umbrella Plant (*Schefflera*), which is mildly poisonous to humans but seriously toxic to Cats and Dogs. Choose organic, Fair Trade Avocados, or grow your own to reduce social and environmental harm.

Bay (*Laurus nobilis* L.)

French: *Laurier*; Dutch: *Laurier*
Family: Lauraceae

Evergreen tree with smooth, dark green to brown branches. It produces small white flowers spaced beneath the branches, which later develop into seeds. Tough ovate leaves release a spicy fragrance when rubbed or crushed.

Virtues

Bay has antimicrobial, digestive, and emmenagogue properties. The leaves, buds, flowers, and fruits are spicy and aromatic. Bay can help arthritic pain and digestive disorders. Try making a friction rub or pain-relieving oil using infused Bay oil, or bathe in water infused with Bay. Add a Bay leaf to autumn or winter tea blends, and include in natural incense. Crush a fresh Bay leaf in your hand and inhale the scent to lift your spirits and clear your mind. Fresh Bay leaves will crackle and spark when burned. Bay branches can be woven into crowns and wreaths, and Bay is a popular kitchen herb. Avoid during pregnancy.

Magical significance

Associated with protection, healing, chastity, and creative achievement. Romans celebrated Saturnalia with Bay crowns, while Greeks linked it to the healing gods Asclepius and Apollo. The myth of Daphne and Apollo tells how the water nymph Daphne was transformed into a Bay tree to protect her from the unwanted advances of Apollo. Bay crowns, in the "baccalaureate" ceremony, honour success. Use Bay leaves in spells, charms, and as a protective wash. Write intentions on Bay leaves and burn them in spells. Place Bay leaves under a pillow to inspire creativity, or dip in rosewater first to help predict future love. Carried for safe travels.

Foraging notes

Find: In hedges and gardens, often planted in pots beside doors.

Harvest: Leaves, sparingly any time; branches at winter pruning.
Avoid toxic look-alikes like Portuguese Laurel (*Prunus lusitanica*) and Cherry Laurel (*Prunus laurocerasus*).

Beech (*Fagus sylvatica* L.)

French: *Hêtre*; Dutch: *Beuk*
Family: Fagaceae

Large, stately tree with spreading branches. Leaves are copper or green, smooth and shiny. Trunk is smooth. Some trees retain leaves through winter. Sharp, pointed leaf buds in winter—these push any dead leaves off the branches in spring. Wind-pollinated and attractive to wildlife. Prickly Beechnut cases hold three-sided nuts inside. When the nuts ripen, the cases open their wings and fall to the ground as "Beech mast". Heavy falls happen only every few years.

Virtues

Beech bark has antiseptic properties. It is used to treat wounds, coughs, and colds. Beech twigs (from the Beech timber industry) may have anti-cancer benefits when taken as a herb tea. Beech wood is used in traditional glassmaking. Young leaves taste mild, mature leaves are bitter. In Italy, young Beech leaves are sometimes sautéed with Garlic and Olive oil. Beechnuts are edible and nutritious.

Magical significance

Associated with balance, protection, nourishment, community, grace, and wisdom. Beech does not settle for second best. Linked with spirit travel. Write a wish on Beech wood and bury it, to help it manifest. Known as the "Mother of the Woods" or "Beech Queen", Beech often grows near the "Oak King". Carrying Beech wood is believed to bring good luck.

Foraging notes

Find: Growing in city hedges or as stately trees in parks. They grow well in shaded areas and are often found among other tree species. Beech leaves resemble Hornbeam (*Carpinus betulus* L.), although are less silky when young. Hornbeam leaves can be used similarly.

Harvest: Tender, silky young leaves in spring. In mast years, pick the small nuts from their mast cases, eat raw or roast. Avoid exposing Beech trunks and branches to direct sunlight, as it can damage or even kill the tree.

Birch (*Betula* spp.)

French: *Bouleau*; Dutch: *Berk*
Family: Betulaceae

Graceful tree (to 30 m) with pale bark and pendulous branches. Its ovate leaves flutter in the wind. Young bark is smooth and golden brown. With age it turns white and papery, eventually splitting to reveal the dark craggy bark. Mature Birches often have bark-covered "toes" at their base. White Paper Birch bark is shed as the tree trunk expands, and may litter the ground. Birch is wind-pollinated, with catkins. In spring, clear sap (Birch blood) rises through the tree. Birch trees release a wintergreen-scented chemical when harmed, which can trigger nearby Birch trees to increase their chemical defences.

Virtues

Has purifying and nutritive properties. Birch sap is a spring tonic. Tea made from leaves or twigs is mildly laxative and detoxifying. It can help cystitis and joint pain. Birch leaf-infused oil, soaks, or compresses help joint pain and skin infections. The bark is waterproof and wound healing, and the wood is used in saunas. Birch twigs were previously used in corporal punishment ('birching') and Birch bark was used for crafting sacred manuscripts.

Magical significance

Associated with the Moon, silver, purification, new beginnings, and hope. Traditionally used in marriage ceremonies (jumping the broom), and Birch twigs make good broomsticks. Write spells, incantations, or intentions on collected Birch bark. Birch wood is used to make Scandinavian runes. In Britain, bundles of Birch twigs were used to mark district boundaries at Yuletide. The bright white bark glows in moonlight, symbolically helping us focus on the path ahead.

Foraging notes

Find: In gardens, parks, and woodlands. Note: People with Apple allergies may also be allergic to Birch.

Harvest: Sap in early spring (cut the end of a small branch, collect the drips). Avoid tapping the trunks of urban trees—it stresses them. Leaves, later spring when fresh and young.

Bramble (*Rubus fruticosus* L.)

French: *Ronce Commune*; Dutch: *Braam*
Family: Rosaceae

Strong, thicket-forming, prickly shrub. Up to 2 m in height and spreads vigorously. Leaves are palmately compound with 3–7 oval, serrated-edged leaflets. Pale pink flowers appear in clusters at the ends of stems, with five petals and showy stamens. Blackberries ripen in late summer. Buds form along stems throughout the year.

Virtues

Boiled roots, shoots and leaves are astringent and vitamin C-rich. They can help settle diarrhoea, heavy periods, skin conditions, coughs, and loose teeth (as a gargle/mouthwash). Young leaves and tips taste mildly fruity. Use Blackberries in jams, pies, mead, and wine. Young prickle-free shoot tips can be cooked or eaten raw. Ferment leaves and shoots, or use as tea. Bramble can also be used for fibre dyeing. Weave long stems into baskets, after stripping off the prickles with very strong gloves. Provides shelter and food for wildlife.

Magical significance

Symbolises strong, active protection. Walking or passing under a Bramble arch while reciting charms has been considered good luck. Use the prickles in rituals, to pierce and protect. Keep in a small jar on your altar, or place cut Bramble stems around boundaries. Sweet ripe Blackberries are useful in attraction magic. A simple magical ink can be made by dipping a sharp stick or nib into the purple juice. The leaves, perhaps as a tea, can also be used in health and protection magic. Knobbly old Bramble roots can be cleaned and used for display or in sympathetic magic.

Foraging notes

Find: In neglected areas and hedges. Go prepared for Blackberry foraging with thorn-proof clothing and gloves, and collection tubs. Avoid mouldy fruit and damp locations.

Harvest: Young leaves and buds, year round; berries, when ripe and sweet (Lughnasadh to Mabon). Freeze any surplus.

Broom (*Cytisus scoparius* (L.) Link)

French: *Genêt à balais*; Dutch: *Brem*
Family: Fabaceae

Shrub with long, straight, narrow stems. Produces a mass of sweet-scented yellow flowers in early to high summer, resembling small yellow butterflies with their side wings, hood, and lip petal arrangement. The flowers grow in pairs or alone on long, straight, flexible, slender green stems, which remain vibrant through winter. The leaves are alternate on the stems, usually three-lobed with a short leaf stalk. Seeds form and spread by exploding pods on warm summer days.

Virtues

Broom is not edible and no part of this shrub should be ingested. <u>It contains strong alkaloids and can be highly poisonous</u>. Broom stems can be used for broom making and basket weaving. A yellow dye is made from the flowers and green dye from the bark. Historically, Broom was used as a diuretic and until recently, in the Canary Islands, Broom honey was used for diarrhoea. A salve can be made from the flowers, for painful joints. Broom flowers are very attractive to Bees, and Slugs eat the leaves.

Magical significance

Associated with protection, endurance, strength, and purification. To energetically cleanse spaces, sprinkle Broom-infused water or collected dew. It is said to enhance psychic powers. Use in charms to brush away unwanted energies. A Suffolk saying advises against sweeping with Broom in May. Sometimes used in Pagan marriage rituals for "jumping the broom". Broom flowers were amulets for bodyguards in France and England. Used in rituals to protect magical tools and circles.

Foraging notes

Find: In gardens and parks.

Harvest: Young pale green growth and flowers in spring for dyeing or spellcraft. Avoid older growth, as its higher toxicity can be absorbed through skin contact.

Caution: Do not ingest Broom; it is toxic.

Burdock (*Arctium lappa* L.)

French: *Grande bardane*; Dutch: *Grote klit*
Family: Asteraceae

Biennial plant with taproots over 50 cm long. In its first year, large heart-shaped leaves grow from basal rosette. Leaves are downy with wavy edges. By the second summer, it becomes bushy, up to 2 m tall. Thistle-like flowers mature into burrs for seed dispersal. The plant dies after setting seed. Attractive to Bees and Butterflies.

Virtues

Burdock supports detoxification, promoting healthy blood, skin, liver, and immunity. As tea or food, it stimulates digestion. Poultices and creams treat eczema, psoriasis, and bruises. Roots can be decocted fresh or dried and infused in tonic wines. Pound seeds before use to break their tough coats. Often paired with Dandelion for enhanced detoxification. Mature Burdock leaves are very bitter, but roots and seeds are milder. Peeled stalks are tasty when sautéed, and large leaves are useful food wraps. Burdock root is popular in Asian cuisine, often used in soups, casseroles, and stir-fries. Avoid during pregnancy, with blood-thinning issues, or a sensitive stomach. Diabetics should use cautiously, as Burdock may lower blood sugar.

Magical significance

Associated with deep cleansing and purification, both physically and spiritually. Necklaces, made from dried Burdock root, guard against enchantment. Carry seeds in a locket or pouch to protect you from aches and pains. Say health and success charms as you harvest seeds from the prickly burrs. Always be sure to spread some of the seeds, after collecting burrs.

Foraging notes

Find: Parks, waste ground, and hedges. Look-alike Rhubarb has very large toxic leaves. When mature, Burdock is a huge plant.

Harvest: Small leaves (spring/summer); stems before hollowing (late spring); seeds when burrs brown (late summer–autumn); roots (autumn of the first year to early spring of the second year). Ideally, harvest roots during a Waning Moon.

Cacti (various species)

French: *Cactus*; Dutch: *Cactussen*
Family: Cactaceae

Highly specialised plants adapted to arid environments, with swollen stems, spines instead of leaves, and colourful flowers. Cacti vary greatly in shape, from barrel-shaped to tall, slender, flat, or fuzzy forms. Often confused with Euphorbia, which has corrosive sap. Popular varieties include *Schlumbergera* (Christmas Cactus).

Virtues

Some species provide nutritious flowers or fruit, e.g. Prickly Pears, rich in antioxidants and other beneficial phytochemicals. Also used as forage for animals, a water source in desert emergencies, and as natural fencing for property and livestock. Hallucinogenic species like Peyote and San Pedro are valued for vision work. Barrel Cacti (*Echinocactus* species) have been used medicinally for their antiseptic qualities, and their spines have been used as fish hooks.[10] Cactus skeletons are sometimes repurposed into furniture.

Magical significance

Associated with boundary protection, resilience, strength, and banishing negative energy. In some Native American traditions, certain cacti also represent warmth, hospitality, and protection. Cacti are absorbers of negative energy, so gently rinse in rainwater, to cleanse them. Cacti help us tolerate the prickly traits of others. Placing cacti in the bedroom may repel love energy, so beware if that works against your intentions. For Peyote or San Pedro cacti, care for them and welcome them into sacred spaces. Their living presence encourages intuition and dreamwork.

---

[10] A. Shetty et al. Cactus: A medicinal food. *J Food Sci Technol*. (2012) 49(5): 530–6. doi: 10.1007/s13197-011-0462-5.

Care and harvesting notes

Find: In bright, sunny, dry conditions.

Care: Occasional watering and annual repotting in gritty soil. Avoid watering when flowering.

Harvest: Collect fallen spines for sympathetic magic. Avoid harming hallucinogenic cacti.

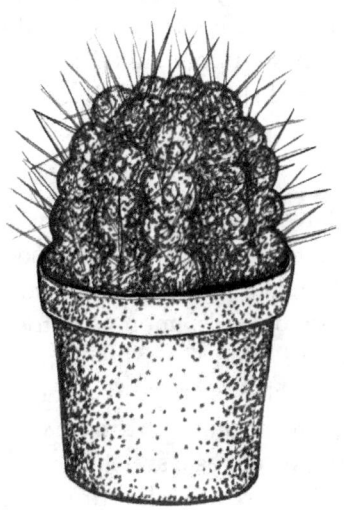

Carob (*Ceratonia siliqua* L.)

French: *Caroubier*; Dutch: *Johannesbroodboom*
Family: Fabaceae

Description

Medium tree with evergreen leaves, small fragrant flowers, and edible seed pods. These resemble large, flattened Broad Bean pods. It thrives in Mediterranean regions. Spain is a leading producer of organic Carob. Carob trees grow well in conditions suited to Citrus trees, so if you can cultivate Citrus, you can likely grow Carob too.

Virtues

Carob seeds and pods have a sweet, earthy flavour with a hint of chocolate. In the Mediterranean, Carob is used to treat diarrhoea, and is often brewed with Cinnamon and Lemon. Carob has also been shown to help reduce blood sugar and cholesterol levels, improve nutrient absorption, and aid heartburn and digestive health. Carob was eaten during famines and used as pig feed. Carob molasses or syrup is often sold in Mediterranean grocery stores. Portuguese, Italian, and Turkish cuisine uses Carob extensively. Try using Carob powder as a sweetener or chocolate substitute in desserts, smoothies, and cakes by grinding dry, ripe pods to a fine powder.

Magical significance

Associated with resilience, ancient wisdom, wealth, grounding, humility, health, and protection. Carob oil, extracted from the pods, was used in Egyptian mummification, and Carob seeds, with their consistent weight of 0.18 g, inspired the carat standard in gemstone measurement. So consider also incorporating Carob in magic related to consistency. Place Carob seeds on your altar, in charm bags, or use them symbolically as currency in ritual practices and money charms.

Foraging notes

Find: In sunny streets and gardens.

Harvest: Ripening pods turn from green to red–brown. Gather fallen ripe pods from the ground, pick or gently shake from the trees. Discard and compost any insect- or mould-damaged material.

Catnip (*Nepeta cataria* L.)

French: *Cataire*; Dutch: *Kattenkruid*
Family: Lamiaceae

Aromatic perennial. With square flower stems, grows to 30 cm height. Small blue hood and lip flowers. Leaves are grey–green, downy, with toothed edges. They are arranged in opposite pairs along the stems. The foliage has an earthy-minty scent. Catnip is valuable to pollinators and small mammals.

Virtues

Has digestive, antiviral, anxiolytic, and antibacterial properties. Catnip is used for respiratory infections, nervous headaches, and to ease trapped gas. Useful for children's health issues, such as colic, ear infections, and restless sleep. Enjoy as tea, infused honey, or syrup. In medieval times, Catnip poultices soothed boils and painful swellings. About 50% of Cats are receptive to Catnip (others react to Valerian root or certain Honeysuckle vines). Sensitive Cats enjoy rolling in it or chewing the stems and leaves. These contain essential oils that mimic feline sex pheromones. A useful plant to grow for feline companions. It can also attract them to gardens. Catnip is used in some Cat toys.

Magical significance

Associated with attracting good fortune, kind spirits, and Cats. Place dried Catnip around the home in sachets, or use as a light spray, to entertain and bond with neighbourhood Cats. Historically, large Catnip leaves were pressed and used as bookmarks in magical texts. Chewing the root is said to agitate even the calmest mind, so a pinch can be added to magical concoctions and spells to shake things up, when needed. A good deterrent of pests, Catnip can be used in protection and deterrent spells. Consider adding to love sachets or tea, with Rose petals.

Foraging notes

Find: Parks and streetside edges. Most roadside Catnip is unsuitable for consumption. So try growing from cuttings, for cleaner plants.

Harvest: When strong—spring equinox to autumn equinox.

Chameleon plant (*Houttuynia cordata* Thunb.)

Chinese: *Yu xing cao*; Korean: *Wonchuri*;
French: *Poivre de Chine*; Dutch: *Moerasanenoom/Viskruid*

Herbaceous perennial with a strong scent and heart-shaped leaves. Eye-catching flowers with four white petals surrounding a central cone of stamens and stigma. The leaves are attached by stalks to red stems, at swollen joints. This plant often becomes invasive. It spreads via white shallow roots.

Virtues

Has antiseptic properties. Rich in healing phytochemicals, Houttuynia-infused oil is useful for skin care and is used in TCM as a "heat-clearing" herb, for congested phlegm conditions and infections. It is also effective externally, as an antiseptic poultice or skin wash. All parts are edible and popular in Asian cuisine and traditional medicine. The leaves are uniquely aromatic, somewhat fishy when raw but fresh-tasting when cooked or dried. The leaves, flowers and roots are easily stir-fried; tougher stems are best used for teas, decoctions, and ferments.

Magical significance

Associated with healing, clearing, clairvoyance, exorcism, and protection. This plant helps repel unwanted influences and purge negative energies. Keep a fresh Chameleon Plant in a small vase at home, where it will grow roots and help keep the space cleansed. It can be a focal point for healing and cleansing rituals. This is one of my favourite herbs to sprinkle, powdered or as a tea, along boundaries, to ritually cleanse and protect.

Foraging notes

Find: Gardens, parks, and escapes. It thrives in damp, semi-shaded areas. Try growing in pots, for a steady supply of roots.

Harvest: Leaves and stems, summer while in flower; roots, in autumn after the foliage begins to fade.

Chamomile (*Matricaria chamomilla* L.; *Chamaemelum nobile* (L.) All.).

French: *Camomille sauvage*; Dutch: *Echte kamille*
Family: Asteraceae

Low-growing plant with feathery, finely divided leaves and small Daisy-like flowers that bloom repeatedly throughout summer. *Matricaria* is an annual plant that self-seeds, while *Chamaemelum* is biennial or perennial, returning reliably each year from strong roots. Both species are sweetly aromatic. *Chamaemelum* is often used to scent lawns and barefoot paths, owing to its tolerance for being trampled. It also tolerates drought so often thrives in roof gardens and tree pits.

Virtues

The flowers and leaves of both types of chamomile taste slightly bitter. Chamomile helps us to relax, sleep, and digest food. It also helps us fight infections. When making Chamomile tea, cover the brew to capture the volatile oils. Well-strained and cooled tea can be used to gently rinse wounds and inflamed eyes. Angry eczema and insect bites often respond well to Chamomile creams and compresses too. A vinegar infusion of Chamomile can act as a mild blonding hair rinse, or skin lotion. Chamomile adds aromatic bitterness to beverages like mead and ale.

Magical significance

Associated with protection, purification, and attracting positive energies such as love and prosperity. Use in rituals to ward off negativity and harm. Historically it was placed inside homes at midsummer, to protect against thunderstorms. Fresh Chamomile flowers can help us to calmly enter a liminal state. Unless sensitive, try chewing a single fresh flower when your state of mind needs to be quickly shifted. Chamomile features in many old charms and incantations.

Foraging notes

Find: Gardens and neglected spaces. Often around lamp posts near gardens. Look-alike Pineapple weed (*Matricaria discoidea*) is also edible, medicinal, and worth learning about.

Harvest: Flowers, pick individually (mid to late summer).

Chickweed (*Stellaria media* (L.) Vill.)

French: *Mouron blanc*; Dutch: *Vogelmuur*
Family: Caryophyllaceae

Low-growing annual, 10 cm tall, spreading up to 45 cm wide. Forms a loose mound of bright green foliage. Flowers are tiny, white and star-shaped. Each with five deeply split petals, which resemble ten. Leaves in opposite pairs. A single line of tiny hairs runs along the length of each stem, shifting slightly at each leaf joint.

Virtues

Chickweed has a mild flavour that appeals to many people and birds, hence the English name. It is used as a rinse, infused vinegar, or in baths for itchy skin, minor wounds, warts, and eye irritations, or as a poultice to draw infection out of the skin. Chickweed can ease rheumatic and muscle pains, used both externally and internally. This plant makes a tasty addition to salads, smoothies, tea, pesto, and soups. Contains saponins, which are toxic although rarely irritate when consumed. Saponins are broken down by cooking. Avoid during pregnancy.

Magical significance

Associated with prosperity, and community. Chickweed helps restore or maintain our ability to live well with others, while promoting healthy boundaries. It is used in love spells and rituals to promote fidelity. If seeking connection with local birds, carry dried Chickweed as an amulet or use fresh in spells and charms. Weave into enchanted meals for loved ones or when trying to bring harmony with healthy boundaries to groups.

Foraging notes

Find: In neglected plant pots, tree pits and street gardens. Chickweed's line of tiny stem hairs is a key differentiating feature. Avoid look-alike toxic Petty Spurge (*Euphorbia peplus*), which has white latex sap.

Harvest: When bright and succulent, year round before seeding. Chickweed becomes stringy and withers in hot, dry weather.

Citrus (*Citrus* species)

French: *Agrumes*; Dutch: *Citrus*
Family: Rutaceae

Shrub-like trees with glossy oval leaves, sturdy stems, and often thorns. Grows 60 cm to 6 m in height. Fragrant, five-petalled white flowers turn into ripe fruit in autumn. Citrus plants thrive with care and attention. Varieties like Lime, Grapefruit, Orange, Yuzu, Kumquat, and Meyer Lemon can all be grown from seed.

Virtues

Vitamin C-rich Citrus fruits have antiseptic, antioxidant, and anticancer properties. Used to ease colds, bronchitis, digestion, and blood pressure. Bitter pith and peel contain bioflavonoids and oils that strengthen capillaries and reduce stress. Citrus leaves are aromatic when crushed. Petitgrain (*Citrus aurantium* ssp. *amara*) is valued as an antidepressant and perfume. Use Citrus for cooking, infuse in honey or spirits, dry for incense, or preserve in alcohol. Diluted Citrus juice brightens hair.

Magical significance

Associated with protection, health, vitality, and balancing bitterness with sweet. Citrus clears the mind and heightens spiritual awareness. Its sourness reinforces boundaries. Use diluted juice for spiritual cleaning, and the peel in charms, spells, or incense. Carry powdered peel in protective vials.

Care and harvesting notes

Find: Sunny climates. Seeds, leaves, and fruit at organic grocers.

Care: Grow in pots as each has a preferred climate. Add fertiliser biweekly in summer and protect from frost. Lemon trees prefer above 10°C and tolerate brief dips to −4°C. Hardy Grapefruit can survive occasional colder weather. Let soil dry slightly in winter to prevent root rot, and place in the sunniest spot available; they thrive outdoors in full Sun during summer.

Harvest: Fruit, whenever ripe. Leaves and stems during annual pruning.

Grow from seeds: Start with plump pips from the tastiest fruits. Mahaut Vidal advises soaking seeds in warm water for a few days, nicking the seed coat, and planting on a pot of free-draining soil with grit or sand. Cover lightly with 0.5 to 1 cm of soil, mist with water, then place the pot in a small plastic bag (with small air holes) to maintain moisture. Keep warm. With patience, seedlings should sprout. Remove the plastic bag once seeds germinate and repot as needed.

Cleavers (*Galium aparine*)

French: *Gaillet gratteron*; Dutch: *Kleefkruid*
Family: Rubiaceae

Annual plant of the Coffee family. Up to 2 m tall. Clings and rambles over other plants and structures. Seeds germinate in autumn and spring, spurting in spring. Bright green leaves grow in distinctive whorls of 4–8 around the stem. This plant is covered in tiny hooked hairs, which enable it to cleave onto clothes, animals, and other plants. Its tiny greenish-white flowers become small, sticky seed balls.

Virtues

Cleavers promotes lymphatic flow, is mildly laxative, and supports detoxification. The plant has a distinctive fresh, somewhat bitter flavour. It can be helpful when treating cystitis, swollen glands, psoriasis, eczema, premenstrual syndrome, lymphedema, and prostatitis. Infuse a small handful of chopped stems and leaves in boiled water and leave until cool. Or add finely chopped Cleavers to smoothies, in place of Spinach. The longer fibrous stems are best juiced or steamed, to soften their texture. The tiny seed balls can be collected when ripe, gently roasted at about 160°C for around 40 minutes, then when cool, ground to a powder. This creates a mild, pleasant coffee substitute, containing traces of caffeine.

Magical significance

Associated with seizing, binding, rapid growth, and movement from darkness towards light. Breaking barriers and energetic flow. Use for ritual cleansing and revitalisation, for spells where vibrancy and positivity are required. Make Cleavers baskets, shaped from a handful of long sticky stems, to hold magical tools, harvested herbs or other precious items. Hold symbolic items together with Cleavers stems, during binding spells.

Foraging notes

Find: In neglected soil, hedges, with nettles, against fences. Look-alikes include Sweet Woodruff (*Galium odoratum*) and toxic Madder (*Rubia tinctorum*).

Harvest: Foliage when young and vibrant, about 30 cm tall (early spring to midsummer). Seed balls, when reddish-brown (after Lughnasadh).

Coffee (*Coffea arabica* L.)

French: *Caféier*; Dutch: *Koffie plant*
Family: Rubiaceae

Tree with glossy, dark green leaves with fragrant white flowers. Up to 9 m tall. Seed pods contain two coffee beans (seeds). Seeds and leaves are aromatic and bitter. Leaves taste milder, earthy, and closer to green tea than coffee. Popular houseplants.

Virtues

Caffeine, in the leaves and beans, can boost mental alertness, physical performance, and is a powerful diuretic. Regular coffee consumption may reduce risk of colon cancer and protect against Alzheimer's and Parkinson's diseases. However, percolated or boiled coffee may harm the heart and raise cholesterol levels. Excessive consumption of any kind can cause nervous system fatigue and aggravate PMS and period pain.

Drinking Kuti (Coffee leaf tea) can support Coffee-growing communities in countries such as Ethiopia and Kenya; Coffee beans are harvested annually, leaving communities with employment issues between harvests. Coffee leaves can be sustainably harvested year round, boosting farmers' employment opportunities. Kuti is said to have a lower caffeine content, is rich in antioxidants, and may help relieve cold symptoms.

Magical significance

Owing to its colonial history Coffee is often associated with money and abundance. However, it is more appropriate to celebrate the way Coffee stimulates the mind and body, and can support spiritual awakening. Sufi mystics use it to enable longer and more ecstatic prayer sessions. Try weaving Coffee into spiritual rituals, where you want to be wide awake and sharp. Of course, beware of overuse.

Harvesting notes

Find: In warm climates, or as houseplants.

Harvest: Annually, one third of its foliage can be pruned for harvest (if organically grown). Ripe or unripe beans can be separated from the pulp, soaked, dried, and roasted. Avoid using non-organic houseplants. Grow seedlings organically for two years before considering a home harvest.

Coleus/Indian Nettle (*Coleus barbatus* (Andrews) Benth. ex G. Don.)

French: *Coléus de l'Inde*; Dutch: *Coleus*
Family: Lamiaceae

Aromatic semi-succulent plant. Mature stems are four-sided with vertical markings. Leaves are downy, ovate, and pointed at the tip. They grow in opposite pairs. Plant leaf is 14 cm long and 8–10 cm wide when mature. Leaf hairs release scent when touched. Blue hood and lip flowers annually.

Virtues

Coleus is used to soothe inflammation, allergies, asthma, wheezing, and eczema, and to support wound healing. However, it contains forskolin, a potent compound that may lower blood pressure, affect insulin and thyroid function, and interact with certain medications. This plant is closely related to Makandi, an Ayurvedic herb, as well as Queen of Herbs or Mexican mint. With a pleasant sage-mint flavour, it can be enjoyed as a tea or used sparingly in cooking as a substitute for Mint.

In regions where *Coleus* grows outdoors, it is sometimes used as a "toilet paper plant". The palm-sized, soft, aromatic leaves easily snap off and make an ideal biodegradable and gently medicated toilet paper. So in times of shortage, consider Coleus.

Magical significance

Associated with eternity, immortality, health, friendship, wealth, and success. The large leaves can symbolise bank notes in money spells, and the scent of the leaves can be used in place of incense, to direct intentions to the spirit realm.

Harvest and care notes

Find: Dry, warm, semi-shade conditions, and houseplants.

Care: Can adapt to cool spaces but is killed by frost and bleached by strong sunlight. Water when soil dries or leaves droop. Repot annually in fresh soil, or fertilise in summer. Prevent legginess by trimming branch tips. To clone, plant a mature stem in slightly moist soil; roots form quickly if not overwatered.

Harvest: Leaves sparingly year round. Dry leaves stacked in a paper bag.

Comfrey (*Symphytum* spp.)

French: *Consoude officinale*; Dutch: *Smeerwortel*
Family: Boraginaceae

Herbaceous perennial. Large, hairy, heart-shaped leaves. Bell-shaped white–blue flowers. Several species grow in towns and cities, some tall, others forming dense ground cover. Leaves and stems are mucilage-rich. Beneficial to wildlife, attracting Bees and providing shelter for animals.

Virtues

Comfrey leaves have a pleasant taste and cucumber-ish scent. Historically it was eaten cooked, similar to Chicory, however, owing to pyrrolizidine alkaloids (PA) toxicity concerns, internal use is no longer permitted in some countries. Comfrey species contain allantoin, mucilage, and other constituents that can support wound healing. Root and leaf used to promote skin, bone, tendon, and ligament healing. Apply on unbroken skin as a poultice or ointment. As the leaves fall and decay, they provide a nutrient-rich mulch to topsoil. Used in home fertiliser blends.

Magical significance

Associated with deep healing, repair, smoothing things over, and growth. Comfrey is particularly suitable when working magic to resolve deep-seated issues like broken trust or wounded relationships.

Foraging notes

Find: In hedges, neglected land, and urban plantings. Creeping Comfrey is used for ground cover, while Russian and Common Comfrey are more common in community gardens for wildlife and mulch.

Beware confusion with poisonous look-alike Foxglove (*Digitalis*).

Harvest: Foliage in spring to autumn—snap off cleanly. Roots in autumn. Leave developing flowers for pollinators. Hang-dry for best results.

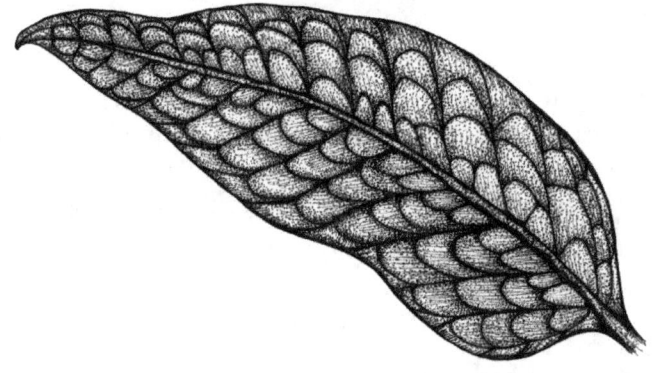

Daisy (Bellis perennis L.)

French: *Pâquerette*; Dutch: *Madeliefje*
Family: Asteraceae

Small, evergreen perennial with rosettes of small dark green, spoon-shaped leaves. Its typical Asteraceae flowers feature a central yellow disc composed of numerous minute individual flowers, surrounded by pink-tipped white petals. Each flower stem supports a single flower or flower bud that opens on sunny days.

Virtues

Daisy is a wound herb, with anti-inflammatory, vulnerary, and mild analgesic properties. It can be applied as a juice, poultice, compress, or cool tea rinse for bruises and minor wounds. Daisies have also been used to ease aches, pains, sprains, and mouth ulcers. The flowers and young leaves can be cooked in soups and casseroles or added to tea blends. Flower buds can be pickled, as a substitute for capers. The leaves and flowers of Daisy have a slightly bitter and aromatic taste.

Magical significance

Associated with hope, love, and innocence. Use in love charms, spells, and divination rituals. Plucking Daisy petals, muttering "She loves me, she loves me not," is a folk divination practice. Wear as protective amulets—try Daisy chain bracelets, or tucked into clothes, lockets or pouches. The flower has also been linked with death. It is said to bring comfort for bereaved mothers. Daisies often grow well in cemeteries, giving rise to the phrase "Pushing up the daisies". An old name for Daisy was "Day's eye".

Foraging notes

Find: In parks, lawns, and along path edges. Usually in full Sun and compacted soil. Look-alike Mexican Fleabane (*Erigeron karvinskianus*) often grows in pavement cracks.

Harvest: On sunny days (spring to autumn). Wash thoroughly before use. Daisies are usually cooked before consumption, particularly in polluted urban environments.

Dandelion (*Taraxacum officinale* F.H. Wigg.)

French: *Pissenlit*; Dutch: *Paardenbloem*
Family: Asteraceae

Herbaceous perennial, with yellow mop-head flowers, deeply toothed leaves. The hollow stems hold milky sap, and pom-pom seedheads aid dispersal. Dandelion leaves form a rosette above the long tapering taproot. They are smooth and hairless. The flowers open on sunny days and close at night.

Virtues

Dandelions support liver health, stimulate bile, and act as diuretics. Roots contain inulin, which supports gut health. They are laxative if eaten in excess and can lower blood sugar levels. Eaten raw, steamed or preserved, Dandelion leaves, flowers and stalks are nutritious and somewhat bitter. The flowers emit ethylene, ripening nearby fruits.

Magical significance

Associated with opportunism, strength, and resilience. Blowing Dandelion clocks, to tell the time, is playful divination. In mythology, Hecate gave dandelions to Theseus, to prepare for his challenge with the Minotaur. Dandelion flowers gathered before dawn are most potent.

Foraging notes

Find: In pavements, lawns, and parks. Often treated with toxic herbicides. They can thrive in tall plant pots. Look-alike Mouse-ear Hawkweed (*Pilosella officinarum*) is hairy, medicinal but not toxic.

Harvest: Leaves and flowers, mid spring to early winter. Leaves are best before flowering time; roots, early winter.

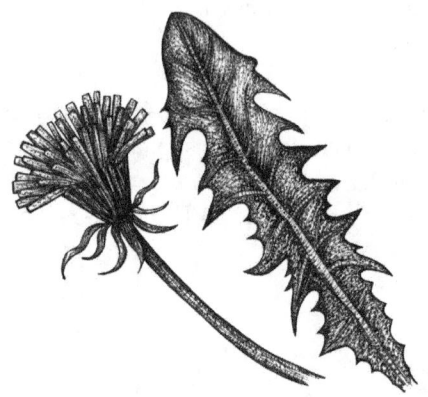

Daylily (*Hemerocallis fulva* (L.) L.)

Chinese: *Huánghuācài*; Dutch: *Daglelie*; French: *Lys d'un jour*
Family: Asphodelaceae

Herbaceous perennial, growing in clumps from rhizomes. Green shoots emerge in spring, becoming lanceolate leaves that snap easily. Flower spikes grow up to 1 m with clusters of buds and large flowers (peach, orange, or yellow). Each flower lasts one day. They resemble Lilies but are unrelated.

Virtues

The flowers and rhizomes are used in China to clear heat and dampness, detoxify, and relieve depression. Citrusy petals can be added to salads, or used in tea or insect repellent. Traditional recipes favour the flower buds: blanching before being either steamed, dried, pickled, fried in batter or added to soup. A Chinese friend recommends that if consuming closed flower buds, the ovaries should be snapped off and discarded, before blanching and steaming—this works well. Avoid gastric distress by cooking Daylily rhizomes and shoots in several changes of water, and eat all parts sparingly. Daylily buds are integrated into marriage rituals, in some regions. Daylily vinegar is both beautiful and delicious.

Magical significance

Tightly closed Daylily flower buds symbolise purity, beauty, and expectation whereas the open flowers symbolise happiness, flirtation, and opportunity, and can be used in rituals to help us move on from hardship and sadness. By incorporating Daylily flowers at different stages of maturity, we can work with life cycles and rebirth. Daylily is well suited to spells aimed at increasing resilience, or recovery.

Foraging notes

Find: Street planting, parks.
 Poisonous look-alike Lilies have leafy flower stems whereas daylily flower stems are smooth.

Harvest: Flower buds, during night or early morning; Open flowers, at dusk when insects have pollinated them; Rhizomes, early winter, when foliage dies back; green shoots, in spring: cut as you would asparagus, and ensure fully cooked before eating sparingly.

Dead Nettles (*Lamium* spp.)

French: *Lamier*; Dutch: *Dovenetel*
Family: Lamiaceae

Dead Nettles, such as (White Dead Nettle, Yellow Dead Nettle, Purple or Red Dead Nettle) are perennial herbs characterised by square creeping stems and opposite heart-shaped leaves that do not sting, unlike their namesake. As they approach flowering, stems grow upward and develop whorls of showy hooded and lipped flowers in colours ranging from white to purple, depending on the species. When leaves are crushed or rubbed, they emit an aromatic scent, which fades when dried.

Virtues

Dead Nettles are useful wound herbs, with astringent and aromatic properties. They can help stop bleeding and speed healing. White Dead Nettle may ease leucorrhoea and other female reproductive complaints. Purple Dead Nettle is best for wounds, while Yellow Dead Nettle is used to lift spirits and combat melancholy. As a cooled tea, all can be used as a healing mouthwash. The flowers contain sweet nectar at their base. They are visited by many pollinators so are best left on the plants.

Magical significance

Yellow Dead Nettle is associated with money, abundance, and prosperity. Use especially when your mood needs to be lifted. Yellow Dead Nettle has potent energy, so be careful what you wish for!

Foraging notes

Find: White and Purple Dead Nettles in edges and hedges as occasional weeds. Purple Dead Nettle is often cultivated and found in flower beds. Yellow Dead Nettle (*Lamium galeobdolon*) grows vigorously, often taking over gardens. This is the best species to harvest.

Harvest: Flowers, sparingly (spring—Samhain); foliage, Yellow Dead Nettle possible year round, more tender and cleaner in spring.

Devil's Ivy/Ivy Arum (*Epipremnum aureum* (Linden & André) G.S. Bunting)

French: *Pothos*; Dutch: *Drakenklimop*
Family: Araceae

A climbing, creeping tropical plant originally from the Society Islands. Devil's Ivy has glossy, heart-shaped leaves, which may be variegated or pure green. This plant is very easy to grow and is an excellent green companion spirit. When well tended and given support, it will grow to over 2 m. Grow as a trailing plant or trained along railings, wires, bookshelves, and ceilings. It seeks to create the forest habitat that it comes from. Devil's Ivy is rather like a green Labrador: if suited to your home it will become a wonderful companion.

Virtues

This plant is poisonous, so don't try to eat it or use it in external remedies. Devil's Ivy has excellent air cleansing properties and can create a wonderful indoor forest aesthetic. Tending the plant is very rewarding too. This is a classic way to bring biophilia into your home.

Magical significance

Associated with success, harmony, cleansing, clothing, shielding, invisibility, protection, and poison. Avoid damaging the plant for rituals, instead bring it along to your magical workspace, or better still, grow it there. Develop a relationship with the plant spirit.

Care notes

Grow this plant in a bright or partially shaded spot, but keep it out of direct sunlight. Provide well-drained soil and opportunities to clamber around. Spray occasionally and water when the soil begins to dry out. Repot in fresh soil or provide diluted organic fertiliser in the spring–summer growing season. Cuttings can be placed directly in water, then potted when a good root system develops.

NB: The sap within Devil's Ivy can irritate eyes and skin. Its foliage and sap are toxic to people and companion animals, such as Cats and Dogs, so should never be ingested.

Dock (*Rumex* spp.)

French: *Oseille*; Dutch: *Zuring*
Family: Polygonaceae

Tough, herbaceous perennials with wide oval-shaped leaves that taper to a point. Some species may have wavy leaf edges and develop rust-coloured spots as they mature, owing to oxalic acid content. Leaves develop from a deep taproot. A tall central flower stem forms as the growth season progresses. Inconspicuous, densely clustered flowers eventually form seeds. These turn rust-coloured by autumn. The foliage withers in winter, leaving seed spikes.

Virtues

Medicinally, Dock is valued as a blood purifier, laxative, and liver stimulant. It is used for skin issues like eczema and psoriasis. Dock can be eaten and tastes sour, though caution is advised given the often high oxalic acid content. Decoctions of Dock seeds have been used for respiratory complaints, and they make a welcome find in winter. The mucilage in many Dock seeds can be useful for thickening soups, stews, or sauces. Dock leaves may be sautéed, steamed, added to casseroles or used to wrap butter and food packages, serving as a natural food holder or plate. Avoid during pregnancy for the laxative effect.

Magical significance

Associated with purification, cleansing, and flow. Dock transforms negativity, making it useful in recovery magic. Their sour nature historically repels (being opposite of sweet, which attracts) and in Irish folklore, Dock seeds are carried for fertility. Dock leaves are often said to help relieve Nettle stings, especially when practised with the incantation: "Nettle in, Dock out." Dock seeds are easily gathered and stored for spellwork and amulets.

Foraging notes

Find: In neglected urban areas, near hedges, in long grass, near trees.

Harvest: Seeds, autumn through winter; young leaves, in spring are best for taste; roots, in autumn under a Waning Moon.

Elder (*Sambucus nigra* L.)

French: *Sureau noir*; Dutch: *Vlier*
Family: Adoxaceae

Shrub-like tree with crooked, brittle branches and rough bark. Large, rather unpleasantly scented compound leaves, with 7 to 9 leaflets. Fragrant cream-coloured flowerheads. These develop into black Elderberries. Hosts the Jelly Ear fungus (*Auricularia auricula-judae*) on dying branches. Green parts (leaves, seeds, bark, and twigs) contain amygdalin, a cyanogenic glycoside. This toxic compound is deactivated by heat, so cook Elderberries before use and apply other green parts of the Elder tree externally.

Virtues

Elderflowers soothe colds and respiratory infections, and encourage sweating. As a compress they relieve sore, puffy eyes and skin blemishes. Elderberries boost infection resistance. Elder leaf infused oil soothes bruises, sprains, and chilblains. The flowers and berries can be used in wines and mead, and add a unique flavour to sweet foods, syrups, and pancake batter. The pith inside Elder branches can be used as a soft cork material, and was formerly employed to mount biological specimens.

Magical significance

Associated with protection, health, and wisdom, featuring prominently in European folklore. The Elder Mother (Hyldemoer), believed to dwell within the Elder bush, is still revered and respected in Northern Europe. Foragers should seek her permission before harvesting from the tree. And, never burn or cut Elder without her consent. Use Elder pith to cork spell bottles and include the leaf oil in flying ointments.

Foraging notes

Find: In hedges, parks, and gardens.

Ground Elder (*Aegopodium podagraria*) resembles Elder foliage but is edible, while Elder leaves are not. Elderflowers and berries are sometimes confused with Meadowsweet and Viburnum species.

Harvest: Elderflowers (Beltane—midsummer); berries (midsummer—Samhain); leaves (spring to late summer).

Elm (*Ulmus* L.)

French: *Orme*; Dutch: *Iep*
Family: Ulmaceae

Tall street trees, with greyish bark becoming fissured with age. Almost heart-shaped leaves with serrated margins. Small wind-pollinated flowers are followed by papery seed cases. These rustle in the breeze then carpet the streets. "Spring Snow" is a tourist attraction in Amsterdam, where 39,000 Elms grow. Each seed case contains a green seed.

Elms were common across Europe until Dutch Elm Disease (DED). It has caused around 30 million Elm deaths since the 1960s. Those that survived in cities like Amsterdam and Brighton are well-managed and monitored. The responsible fungus, *Ophiostoma novo-ulmi*, is carried by Bark Beetles that tunnel beneath the inner bark of Elms. The disease causes yellow, wilting leaves in summer, dying twigs, and eventual death. Healthy Elms also have a tendency to drop their dead branches quite suddenly.

Virtues

Elm seeds are a valuable food source for wildlife and foragers. They can be eaten raw, steamed, or made into a paste, and taste good in spring pesto or salt-fermented. *Ulmus macrocarpa* seeds are used in China to treat intestinal parasites. Elm wood was traditionally used for coffins, and the inner bark of Slippery Elm (*Ulmus rubra*) is valued for its soothing mucilage. Owing to sustainability concerns, Marshmallow root (*Althaea officinalis*) is commonly used as a substitute.

Magical significance

Associated with melancholy, death, determination, whispers, and wealth. Incorporate spring snow in spells and rituals focused on cutting ties and silencing idle chatter. The coin-sized seeds are also an excellent choice for money spells.

Foraging notes

Find: Lining city streets.

Harvest: Seeds (mid April–mid May). Gather the greenest seeds as they fall. Elm seeds taste best when pale green but store best when brown. To help protect the Elm population, avoid harvesting living material and report any signs of DED to your local council.

Enchanter's Nightshade (*Circaea lutetiana* L.; *C. alpina* subsp. *alpina*)

French: *Herbe aux sorcières*; Dutch: *Heksenkruid*
Family: Onagraceae

Herbaceous perennial. Creates dense yet delicate ground cover, in shady areas. It has opposite oval leaves and spikes of delicate pinkish-white flowers, each with two strongly notched petals and protruding stamens. Small seed burrs cling to clothes and animal fur. Brilliant white roots creep a few centimetres underground. Enchanter's Nightshade belongs to the Willowherb family, rather than the Solanaceae (Nightshade family).

Virtues

A mild astringent, Enchanter's Nightshade is considered a wound herb. It can be used as a poultice or compress to speed healing of bruises, sprains, and minor cuts. Enchanter's Nightshade is very attractive to small pollinating hoverflies.

Magical significance

Associated with persistence, just reward, return, fairness, karma. The scientific name comes from both Circe, a sorceress of Ancient Greece expert in spells and herbs, and Lutetia, an old name for Paris, which was then known as Witch City. I consider Enchanter's Nightshade essential for many magical workings, so add drops of tincture, or a few dried seed burrs to most spells and rituals. The plant symbolises the cycle of giving and receiving, the consequences of actions—"What goes around comes around." In magical practices, the ripe seedheads are used in rituals, gatherings, and potions after harvest and drying.

Foraging notes

Find: Shady edges, hedges, woodland, parkland shrubberies.

Harvest times: Leaves until midsummer; flowers until Lughnasadh; burrs until Mabon. Ripe burrs are coated with citric acid so, when licked, taste rather like sherbet and are a treat to find during walks. The edibility of the herb isn't widely known, so consume only small amounts of the leaves and flowers, preferably cooked. Best as a ritual herb.

Fennel (*Foeniculum vulgare* Mill.)

French: *Fenouil*; Dutch: *Venkel*
Family: Apiaceae

Hardy perennial. Fennel has compound umbels of tiny yellow flowers, hollow ribbed stems, and feathery, highly aromatic leaves that release a sweet, anise-like, and slightly spicy scent, when bruised. Grows into a statuesque plant, with flower stems radiating from the same point on the main stem. In some areas it may reach 2 m tall.

Virtues

Fennel calms the digestive system, relieves trapped gas, and can help to calm an agitated mind. Chewing Fennel seeds, which taste far stronger than the bulb and stem, freshens breath and helps heavy meals to settle. In some regions, Fennel seed infusion is used as eye drops for treating conjunctivitis and styes. All above ground parts of the herb can be eaten raw or cooked. The stem and bulb taste delicious in Fennel–Quince Electuary and Mullein–Fennel Infused Wine; these two recipes are mentioned in the medieval manuscripts of Hildegard von Bingen. Records of the use date from the earliest herbal texts.

Magical significance

Associated with strength and pride, and historically has featured in charms to protect homes from fire and enchantments. The ancient Greeks associated it with health, efficiency, and clear thinking. We could follow the example of Prometheus, and use Fennel sticks to light fires. The sweet spiciness of Fennel makes it suited to use in abundance magic.

Foraging notes

Find: In open sunny positions. Grows well in pots, and is popular in community gardens.

Harvest: Leaves, sparingly throughout the growing season. Avoid disturbing developing flower spikes; seeds, when brown and ripened in late summer.

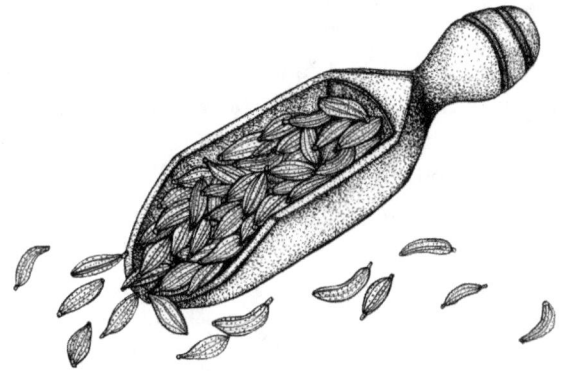

Feverfew (*Tanacetum parthenium* (L.) Sch. Bip.)

French: *Grande Camomille*; Dutch: *Moederkruid*
Family: Asteraceae

Herbaceous perennial with flat indented leaves, similar to Parsley or Chrysanthemum, and small Daisy-like flowers with white petals around a flat yellow central disc. Feverfew leaves may be downy or smooth. The plants can reach 60 cm tall before tending to collapse and regrow. Bruising Feverfew leaves or flowers releases a strong Chrysanthemum-like, pungent, Citrus scent.

Virtues

Above ground parts taste bitter and aromatic. This plant has a long history of use to treat headaches, migraine, menstrual and menopausal issues, to promote digestion, calm nerves, and to relieve coughs and colds. Add the juice to insect bites to calm inflammation. When eating a small amount of raw foliage, combine with foods, to prevent it causing mouth ulcers. Use small amounts of flowers or leaves to season meals, in tea blends, or infuse in wine or honey. Since the Middle Ages, Feverfew has helped to clear melancholy, and is thought to attract Toads to gardens, which in turn helps to keep Slug populations down. Containing pyrethrin, this plant is repellent to insects, including Bees and is apparently self-pollinating.

Magical significance

Associated with purification and protection. Used to purify magical tools, and placed near crystals and divination materials to encourage clarity. Include in rituals and charms to invoke the energies of Toads (good fortune, transformation, fertility, and protection of witches). Grow where you wish to keep invasive, chaotic energies out. In pots, they can be placed around areas of magical working. Create a spray from infused Feverfew to help dispel intrusive energy.

Foraging notes

Find: Gardens, nearby pavement cracks.

Look-alike Chamomile has finer leaves, a sweeter aroma and flowers with a conical central disc.

Harvest: Leaves and flowers when in peak condition (Beltane to Mabon).

Fig (*Ficus carica* L.)

French: *Figuier*; Dutch: *Vijgenboom*
Family: Moraceae

Tree up to 4 m tall with large leaves and smooth bark. Leaves and branches release a milky latex. The cup-shaped inflorescence contains hundreds of tiny flowers, pollinated by Fig Wasps that become trapped inside. Fertilised flowers mature into sweet purple–green fruit, with the remains of flowers visible inside.

Virtues

Figs can be eaten fresh, dried, or as syrup, all mildly laxative. The fruit pulp softens skin and reduces inflammation. In the Canary Islands, cobwebs and Fig wood ash are used to soothe Spider bites. The latex is analgesic, used externally for warts and corns (but can irritate skin). Fig leaves make a refreshing drink when infused in syrup, and Fig bark is used in traditional medicine for wounds and bruises.

Magical significance

Fruit is associated with sweetness, attraction, nourishment, nakedness, and seduction. However, *Ficus carica*, is part of an enormous plant genus that includes the mystical Bodhi tree (*Ficus religiosa*), and Banyan trees. The Hindu god Krishna is said to live within the Banyan leaf. Weeping Fig (*Ficus benjamina*), a popular houseplant, is closer to those sacred species and better used in magic related to success, prosperity, creating ritual space, and deity worship. Rubber Plants (*Ficus elastica*) are well suited to binding and boundary magic. Try growing close to your altar and, of course, include figs in rituals whenever you can; They are very useful in post-ritual feasts.

Foraging and care notes

Find: Sunny gardens, streets, or as houseplants.

Care: Repot annually and protect from cold when young. *Ficus* prefers sunlight, well-drained soil, and occasional misting. Best grown in large terracotta pots, with occasional tepid showers to clear dust.

Harvest: Leaves in late summer (before they drop); fruit when plump and tender. They ripen over winter and spring.

Gallant Soldiers (*Galinsoga parviflora* Cav.)

French: *Galinsoge à petites fleurs*; Dutch: *Kaal knopkruid*; Columbian: *Guascas*
Family: Asteraceae

Delicate annual plant with bright green, sprawling foliage, reaching 75 cm tall, when undisturbed. Its aromatic leaves grow opposite each other, with short stalks and toothed margins, giving them a slight hairy texture. The plant produces small flowers with 3–8 short white ray-petals (florets) surrounding a central yellow disc, with small gaps between each white floret.

Virtues

Gallant Soldiers are traditionally used in Middle America to help close wounds and calm Nettle stings. The plant arrived in Europe in the late 1700s. It dries easily for longer-term use and adds a pleasant mild flavour to dishes when raw or cooked. It is an essential ingredient in Colombian ajiaco soup (*guascas*) and empanadas, and can be added, if clean, in salads, pastas, potato dishes, casseroles, soups, and teas. Found street seedlings can be potted to mature and set seed at home.

Magical significance

Associated with opportunity, fertility, invisibility in plain sight, spiciness, community, success, and prosperity. It can help us thrive, almost invisibly, in urban environments. Use to embody resilience and success, despite adversity.

Foraging notes

Find: In neglected, polluted urban locations such as tree pits, and at the base of road fences and poles.

Harvest: From the cleanest locations. Nip off sections of foliage using fingernails, (midsummer to Samhain).

Garlic Mustard (*Alliaria petiolata* (M. Bieb.) Cavara & Grande)

French: *Alliaire officinale*; Dutch: *Look-zonder-look*
Family: Brassicaceae

Biennial plant, which is often invasive and can grow up to 120 cm tall in its second year. It starts life as a rosette of kidney-shaped leaves, gradually developing into a tall plant with heart-shaped leaves. Clusters of white flowers form progressively at the top of central flower stems, from mid-spring. Each flower has four petals, in the cross pattern characteristic of the Cabbage family. Long slender seedpods, each containing about 20 edible seeds, develop throughout the flowering season. The leaves emit a robust pungent scent when bruised and the flowers attract Cabbage White butterflies (*Pieris rapae*).

Virtues

Has warming antiseptic properties. Used for sore throats, gums, and mouth ulcers. A poultice can be made by pounding the leaves. Garlic Mustard is said to strengthen digestive powers when eaten cooked. Leaves taste of Garlic and Mustard—and are increasingly fiery and bitter after the flower spike appears. Leaves and flowers can be used in pesto, sauces and soups, and are traditionally eaten with fish. Dried seeds can be ground with vinegar, to make an alternative to Mustard. Add leaves to a warming footbath for headaches and colds.

Magical significance

Associated with growth and warmth. Use to spice things up, when needed. The tiny seeds are very portable. Try weaving them into love spells, herb pouches, and rituals that need warmth.

Foraging notes

Find: In shade, near fences, buildings, and trees.

Ground Ivy (*Glechoma hederacea*) has leaves similar to first-year Garlic Mustard, but grows from creeping stems rather than a central rosette.

Harvest: Leaves, best in spring of the second year. Winter leaves are edible but less appetising. Harvest sparingly in winter to allow plants to mature and flower in spring. Seeds and flowers (Beltane to Mabon).

Geranium, Cranesbill (*Geranium sylvaticum* L.)

French: *Géranium des bois*; Dutch: *Bosooievaarsbek*
Family: Geraniaceae

Perennial, usually evergreen in mild winters. Rosette- and then clump-forming, growing up to a 30 cm tall, with scented leaves on stalks, emerging from a central rosette. Leaves and stems are covered in fine hairs. Geranium leaves are round but deeply divided, cleft, and toothed. The flowers bloom mainly from mid spring to summer. They have purple–pink petals with purple veins. Flowers develop into long, beak-shaped seed capsules. There are many species of Geranium, which can be used interchangeably, including *Geranium pusillum* (Small-flowered Cranesbill), which often grows unnoticed in lawns.

Virtues

Geranium is traditionally used to help treat haemorrhoids, internal bleeding, heavy periods, and diarrhoea. It is also useful as a gargle to tone gums. Can be infused in wine, oil, or honey, and makes a delicious tea or syrup. With a reputation as a mild aphrodisiac, aromatic Geranium flowers and leaves can be used in sweet treats or used for body massage. The flowers are very attractive to pollinating insects, and the clumps of foliage provide welcome urban shelter for wildlife.

Magical significance

Associated with love, heartache, and happiness. The seed capsules symbolise long-beaked birds and are useful in charms seeking connection with city Herons and Storks.

Foraging notes

Find: In urban shrubberies and streetside planting, and small species in parkland lawns.

Harvest: Leaves, year round, but best in spring to midsummer, before the main flowering phase begins. Winter leaves catch air pollution in their hairs. Flowers, harvested whenever present, usually Beltane to Mabon.

Ginkgo (*Ginkgo biloba* L.)

French: *Arbre aux quarante écus*; Dutch: *Japanse notenboom*
Family: Ginkgoaceae

Tall, elegant, deciduous tree with Duck feet-shaped leaves that flutter and turn apricot-yellow in autumn. The leaf form resembles flattened bunches of conifer needles. Female Ginkgos produce pairs of round, fruit-like sarcotesta. These fall, rot, and smell very unpleasant. They possibly attracted dinosaurs. One of the oldest tree species in the world. Examples have survived catastrophes such as nuclear war.

Virtues

Seeds are used in Traditional Chinese Medicine to treat senility, phlegmy coughs, colds and discharge, and strengthen the lungs. TCM makes little use of the leaves, but in the West, they are used as a nootropic to boost memory by improving brain circulation. Green Ginkgo leaves are toxic and should be left on the tree; yellow leaves are safer. The seeds can be cooked, after removing the toxic sarcotesta. Soaking overnight loosens the flesh, which can then be rubbed off with rubber gloves. Alternatively, bury in the ground until the flesh decomposes. When clean, the seeds are roasted until golden, with translucent pistachio-green centres. They are eaten in moderation during Chinese and Japanese autumn festivals. Avoid Ginkgo if taking medications, breastfeeding, or pregnant.

Magical significance

Associated with survival, resilience, hope, health, wealth, old age, wisdom, elders, ancestors, and clear thinking. Feature Ginkgo leaves in autumn displays, press them in magical texts, wrap them around magical tools where their qualities are called for and spend time near Ginkgos when studying, or seeking creative inspiration.

Foraging notes

Find: Parks and gardens.

Harvest: Leaves, when they fall in autumn. Yellow Ginkgo leaves are less toxic and better tolerated; seeds fall as fruit in autumn–winter. Wear protective gloves when harvesting the fruit, and be aware that those allergic to Mango are likely to be allergic to Ginkgo.

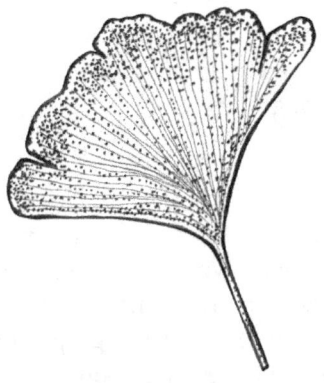

Grapevine (*Vitis vinifera* L.)

French: *Vigne cultivée*; Dutch: *Wijnstok*
Family: Vitaceae

Deciduous, woody climbing vine. Up to 30 m. Forked tendrils attach to fences and branches. Large palmate leaves. Clusters of yellow flowers develop into bunches of grapes.

Virtues

Enjoy grapes fresh, juiced, dried as raisins or fermented into wine. Tender leaves can be eaten raw; mature leaves improve with blanching in hot water, or preserved in brine. They are popular in Mediterranean dishes, such as Dolmades. Eating fresh grapes may ease urinary tract infections, and support convalescence. Sour grapes relieve sore throats, while raisins ease constipation. Vine leaves can be added to Mustard foot baths to help relieve headaches and hangovers. Grape seed extract, a potent antioxidant, can be added to homemade potions to prolong their shelf life. Vine sap has been used to treat minor wounds, and is found in some skincare products. Vine leaf poultice reduces inflammation, pain, and bleeding. Grow against buildings for heat insulation.

Magical significance

Associated with balance, perseverance, strength, joy, productivity, wealth, growth, mental clarity, and community. Vines and ripe grapes amplify magical work. Use sweet grapes, juice or raisins for spells related to attraction; sour grapes and leaves to help repel unwanted influences. Tender Vine growth can be woven into green crowns for ritual and ceremony. Include Vine leaves in meals aimed at growth, success, and abundance.

Foraging notes

Find: South-facing walls, fences, and occasional public spaces. Help neighbours with summer pruning. Look-alike Virginia Creeper (*Parthenocissus quinquefolia*) is toxic, with five-pointed leaves, tiny berries, and high levels of oxalic acid.

Harvest: Young delicate leaves late spring, mature leaves until autumn chill; sour grapes from midsummer, sweet grapes in autumn.

Ground Elder (*Aegopodium podagraria* L.)

French: *Égopode podagraire*; Dutch: *Zevenblad*
Family: Apiaceae

Herbaceous perennial. Tall leaf stems and compound leaves divided into 3 to 9 oval, toothed leaflets. This was once a popular garden vegetable in the Middle Ages. It is now invasive. Flower stalks (up to 60 cm) with white, umbrella-shaped flowerheads. Visited by hoverflies.

Virtues

Traditionally used as a diuretic to treat gout. Nowadays, it is commonly eaten as a foraged vegetable, rich in antioxidants, but it unfortunately causes photosensitivity in some people. The leaves have a fresh Parsley–Carrot flavour, the seeds are similar to the spice Ajwain, and the roots taste somewhat pungent. Ground Elder leaves can be used in countless late spring recipes. Try steaming and seasoning, wrapping around balls of rice, with Nettle in pesto, or adding to soups. The dried seeds can be used as a seasoning. Cosmetic makers have begun using Ground Elder extracts in anti-aging skin preparations.

Magical significance

Associated with power, defence, strength with flexibility, determination, dominance, vigour, and youthfulness. This is a potent herb and should not be used lightly. It is most potent when the seedheads are green and can be used when success and takeovers are involved. Try infusing, to use as a sprinkling water, make wine, and add Ground Elder seeds to spell pouches. Any part of this plant can be used.

Foraging notes

Find: Gardens and parks in both sunny and shady areas. Look-alikes Dog's Mercury (*Mercurialis perennis*) and Elder tree foliage are toxic.

Harvest: Tender leaves from spring to midsummer; seeds midsummer to autumn; roots, autumn.

The plant's chemical profile becomes more intense when harvested for a long time, or when the flowers are developing. Externally or internal exposure can then cause tingling, photosensitivity, and a laxative effect. Light harvesting and consumption is advised.

Ground Ivy (*Glechoma hederacea* L.)

French: *Lierre terrestre*; Dutch: *Hondsdraf*
Family: Lamiaceae

Aromatic perennial, often evergreen. Long, trailing square stems that root at intervals. Kidney-shaped leaves. Slightly hairy with aromatic glands underneath. Small purple–blue hood and lip flowers grow in whorls around the stems during spring and summer.

Virtues

To clear congestion in the head, lungs, ears, throat, and gut. Ground Ivy compress or poultice can speed the healing of abscesses, bruises, and black eyes. This herb was used by the Physicians of Myddfai in Wales for fever, Snake bite, and eye inflammation, while Renaissance painters are said to have drunk the tea and used Ground Ivy poultice to help clear their bodies of lead, from contaminated paints. The leaves, flowers, and stems are edible. They taste minty and bitter. Useful in salads, tea, or infused in honey. Before Hops became popular, Ground Ivy was used in ale brewing, hence an old name for the plant, Alehoof. Adds flavour to broths, beer, sauces, and soups. The flowers are a spring favourite of Bees. Avoid during pregnancy.

Magical significance

Associated with protection, removal of negative or stagnant energy, clearing, clairvoyance, and clairaudience. Use Ground Ivy infusion or fresh leaves to cleanse magical tools and spaces. Hildegard von Bingen recommended Ground Ivy to prevent ill humours entering the head. A protective spray for the body and environment can be made from Ground Ivy tea or tincture.

Foraging notes

Find: Under trees, shrubs, and hedges. In parks, gardens, and neglected locations. Look-alikes include first-year foliage of Garlic Mustard (which grows as a rosette rather than on trailing stems).

Harvest: Year round, although best during peak growth season, when flowering spikes are visible (mid spring–summer).

Hairy Bittercress (*Cardamine hirsuta* L.)

French: *Cardamine hirsute*; Dutch: *Kleine veldkers*
Family: Brassicaceae

Small annual. Smooth leaves, resembling watercress, from a central rosette. Has a strong spicy aroma when bruised. White flowers, with four petals, form in clusters at the top of the flower stem. Ripe seedpods explode upon touch. Hairy Bittercress has a very short life cycle: seed-to-seed in just 12 weeks.

Virtues

Hairy Bittercress is a tasty, abundant, locally growing spice, which warms and stimulates, in a similar way to Mustard. Add a handful of leaves to a warming foot bath at the first signs of headache or a cold. Hildegard von Bingen suggested using Bittercress as a warm poultice, for fever treatment. The leaves and flowers can be eaten raw or lightly cooked, similar to Watercress, and add wild spice to salads, soups or sandwiches.

Magical significance

Associated with warmth, stirring up of stagnation, seizing opportunities, wealth, speed, and relocation. Hairy Bittercress has a vibrant playful energy. It grows quietly, yet quickly. It is barely visible and then explodes to take over an area. Plant its seeds in rituals where rapid growth is needed. It is very helpful for those who feel unnoticed. Include Bittercress foliage as a pungent reminder of the cumulative power of small habits.

Foraging notes

Find: Between paving stones, bricks, and in bare ground. Where one plant sets seed, dozens will quickly grow.

Harvest: Year round except droughts. Tastes more spicy in hot, dry weather. Wash well, as the leaf hairs tend to collect dust.

Hawthorn (*Crataegus monogyna* Jacq. and *C. laevigata* (Poir.) DC.)

French: *Aubépine monogyne*; Dutch: *Meidoorn*
Family: Rosaceae

Small thorny tree, 5–15 m tall. Cream-white flowers (some hybrids pink) and rough bark. Clusters of red fruit. Flowers, leaves, and fruit may emit decay-like scents. Roots host nitrogen-fixing bacteria, helping Hawthorn thrive in poor soils.[11] Pollinated mainly by flies.

Virtues

Hawthorn is a popular hedging tree. A heart tonic, it protects the heart and blood vessels, reduces stress, and lowers inflammation. Ripe haws taste like starchy apples and can be used in fruit leather, infused in honey, or brandy, or added to casseroles. Flowers and leaves taste nutty and green, best in the first flush. Seeds are inedible. Though safe, consult a professional before medicinal use.

Magical significance

Associated with protection, boundaries, love, fertility, Beltane, Samhain, twilight, Fairies, tolerance, resilience, adaptability, and witches. Hawthorn energy adapts to obstacles, rather than fighting them. Using Hawthorn increases our strength, tolerance, and courage, and makes us more adaptable and loving. Hawthorn wreaths, made from pruned branches, can be hung outside to deter unwanted energies (bringing them indoors is considered bad luck). Use the flowers in fertility rites and late spring headdresses. Smear dew from Hawthorn on the skin at Beltane to protect our inner and outer beauty. Invite Hawthorn to spells and rituals related to heartbreak, bereavement, and other matters of the heart. Lone Hawthorns near water often become clootie trees (where strips of fabric are tied to symbolise wishes), or are visited at twilight to speed connection with the spirit realm.

---

[11] N. Diagne et al. Use of *Frankia* and actinorhizal plants for degraded lands reclamation. *BioMed Res Int.* (2013): 948258.

Foraging notes

Find: Hedgerows, edges, and street plantings.

Harvest: Leaves (spring equinox to midsummer); buds, blooms, and leaves (around Beltane, as "Bread and Cheese"); haws (Lughnasah to Samhain, when red and tasty). Spit out the seeds.

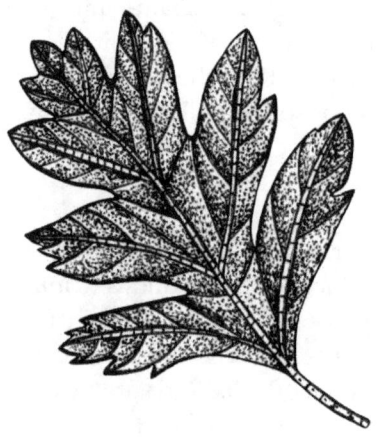

Hazel & Filbert (*Corylus* L.)

Family: Betulaceae

Wind-pollinated trees. Long catkins and flowers, which form on the same tree. Eventually flowers become nutritious nuts.

Turkish Hazel (*Corylus colurna* L.; *Noisetier de Byzance*; *Boomhazelaar*)
Tall street tree (up to 25 m). Stress-tolerant. Produces many nuts in large elaborate nut cases, which hail down on parked cars in early autumn.

Hazel (*Corylus avellana* L.; *Noisetier*; *Hazelaar*)

Filbert (*Corylus maxima* 'Purpurea' Mill.; *Noisetier de Lambert*; *Lambertsnoot*).
Hazel and Filbert are bushy and grow in woodland. They have crooked branches and multiple stems growing from their base. Filberts have longer tubular casings (involucres) than Hazelnuts.

Virtues

Leaves have astringent, anti-inflammatory, and vulnerary properties. As a poultice, or infusion, they ease bruises and diarrhoea, or help cold symptoms. Leaves taste slightly bitter, but can be eaten cooked, fermented, dried, or fresh. Hazelnut oil is used for threadworms in children. The nuts can also be made into a delicious syrup. Catkin tea is useful for coughs and colds. Coppiced branches are woven into strong fence panels (hurdles) and baskets.

Magical significance

Associated with water, whipping, shaking things up, protection, listening, responsiveness, and clear flowing energy. Coppiced Hazels (hard pruned to the ground) yield some of the best wands and staffs available; they are straight, easy to craft, and have a clear energy. Forked Hazel rods are used for water divination.

Foraging notes

Find: Streets, parks, gardens, hedges.

Harvest: Turkish Hazels are the easiest. Street cleaning teams often remove them to compost or burn so scoop up the cleanest when you can.

NB: Avoid using Hazel or Filbert leaves, nuts, or wood if you have nut allergies.

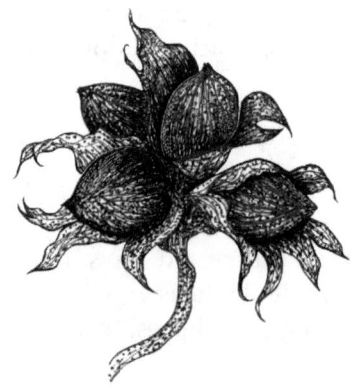

Herb Robert (*Geranium robertianum* L.)

French: *Géranium Herbe à Robert*; Dutch: *Robertskruid*
Family: Geraniaceae

An annual or biannual herb starting as a spring rosette. Grows to 80 cm wide and 40 cm tall. Its feathery, palmate leaves (6 cm mature) develop a rusty hue by Lughnasadh before seeding and dying back. Has red stems, green–red veins, and small pink–purple flowers. The plant emits a strong scent, earning the name "Stinking Bob".

Virtues

All parts are edible and dry well. Its scent improves upon drying. Use in tea, salads, omelettes, syrups, and ferments. Traditionally used for wound healing, bleeding, stomach issues, and ear, nose, and throat ailments. Herb Robert may also enhance chemotherapy and aid radiation recovery. It repels insects and can support nearby plants. Avoid if taking blood-thinning medication.

Magical significance

Associated with protection and good fortune through quiet persistence. It can be used to repel unwanted attention and is useful in spells and charms to heal heartbreak or attract love. This plant is said to encourage connection with Fairies and the bird Robin, known for its fieriness, bravery, and defence of boundaries.

Foraging notes

Find: In shady, untended locations; near hedges, quiet edges, and garden fences. If growing in strong sunlight, the stems become crimson red, without green.

Harvest: Foliage, Beltane to midsummer; flowers, Beltane to Mabon. The shallow roots pull easily from the soil, so take care not to destroy the whole plant when foraging and allow it to set seeds for next year.

Himalayan Balsam (*Impatiens glandulifera* Royle)

French: *Balsamine de l'Himalaya*; Dutch: *Reuzenbalsemien*
Family: Balsaminaceae

Tall annual (up to 2 m). Translucent, grooved stems, red-tinged at leaf and flower joints. Ovate, serrated leaves. Cave-like pink and white flowers, where Bumblebees shelter. Ripe, club-shaped green seedpods explode to release seeds. Highly invasive.

Virtues

The leaves and flowers have a neutral taste. As the seeds ripen, their taste progresses from buttery, through nutty, to rancid. Try making tea, syrup, or colourful infusions from the flowers. The hollow stems make fun drinking straws, and Balsam seeds can also be used to thicken jams and spreads. The plant is used in homoeopathy for anxiety, and as a Bach flower remedy for impatience, frustration, and irritability. Traditionally, it has been used to treat skin inflammation, warts, bug bites, sore skin, and Poison Ivy rash. The flowers can be ground into a paste for skin care, and the plant sap is anti-inflammatory. Himalayan Balsam's high antioxidant content makes it popular with nutrition supplement producers.

Magical significance

Associated with explosive force, rapid growth, monopoly, impatience, and irritability. Himalayan Balsam is also useful where sensitivity is needed. Stem straws can be blown through, to rekindle smouldering embers, or to blow out candles, spread powders or infusions, to add magical intention to those actions.

Foraging notes

Find: Near water, disused land.

Harvest: All parts (midsummer to autumn equinox); seedlings (Imbolc and spring equinox). Avoid spreading the seeds. It is illegal in some countries like the UK. Eat leaves sparingly owing to potential calcium oxalate.

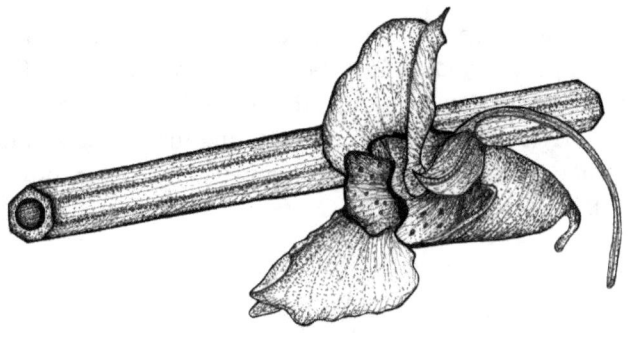

Holly (*Ilex aquifolium* L.)

French: *Houx*; Dutch: *Hulst*
Family: Aquifoliaceae

A slow-growing evergreen tree that can live up to 300 years. It may grow tall in dense woodlands or be clipped into a hedge. The glossy leaves often have sharp points, though some are smooth-edged. Bright red berries appear in autumn, creating the classic winter image. The tree's bark is smooth with brown warts. Branches often trail to the ground.

Virtues

Holly leaves and bark were once used to encourage sweating and treat rheumatism, coughs, colds, urinary issues, and fever. The leaves contain saponins and alkaloids, including traces of caffeine and theobromine. Leaves can be pounded into a poultice or used as tea. Holly leaves are mildly stimulant, but far less than South American relative *Ilex paraguariensis*, from which Yerba Mate is made. However, this should be done cautiously, as ingesting too much can cause intestinal distress. Holly berries are toxic and can lead to violent vomiting and diarrhoea. Holly is also used for hedging and winter decorations.

Magical significance

Associated with protection, good luck, strength, blood, defence, winter, alertness, and luminescence. Grow at entrances and along property boundaries to deter intruders and lightning. The leaves were sometimes called Bat's wings in medieval times. Use in spells where a watchful, alert barrier is needed. The Holly King is said to rule winter alongside the Ivy Queen, after dethroning the Oak King at Herfest. Variegated Holly is said to be feminine. The evergreen branches of Holly are useful in Yuletide decorations. They featured in Saturnalia, the midwinter festival of Ancient Rome. Holly leaves may also be used as natural gift labels at Yuletide.

Foraging notes

Find: Hedges, woodlands, parks, gardens.

Harvest: Leaves, year round. Leave the berries for wildlife. Avoid eating the berries.

If Holly berries are taken home, perhaps on branches for winter decorations, return them to hedgerows, to potentially grow into new plants.

Hollyhock (*Alcea rosea* L.)

French: *Rose trémière*; Dutch: *Stokroos*; Chinese: *Shu kui*
Family: Malvaceae

A biennial or perennial plant with stunning flower spikes. Often grown near walls. First-year growth forms a rosette, reaching up to 2 m in its second summer. Leaves are broad, rough, and round with indented edges. Funnel-shaped flowers range from white to deep purple, with silky petals and showy fused stamens, blooming mid to late summer. Seeds cluster like small Dutch cheeses. Hollyhock flowers attract Bees.

Virtues

Hollyhock leaves and flowers are soothing and aromatic. The tea is used to treat sore throats, coughs, and damaged skin. Valued since ancient times in cosmetics and medicine. Believed to have been used in Neanderthal funeral rituals. Try infusing the colourful flowers in honey or syrup. Apply a poultice to sore skin. And make textile dye from darker flowers. The leaves and flowers can also be simmered in wine, or added to cooked dishes.

Magical significance

Associated with enchantment, protection, abundance, and healing. Hollyhocks are gateways to other planes. Grow as part of a protective forcefield, to keep prying eyes outside of private spaces such as your home or garden. Soft-gazing at the flowers can help us to enter liminal states. The unusual seedheads, known as "fairy cheese", can be collected on city walks for later use in spells and rituals. Many historical recipes include Hollyhock, to help us connect with benevolent spirits. Try combining with Calendula flowers, Hazel leafbuds and Thyme, to make an anointing infusion.

Foraging notes

Find: In pavement cracks, near buildings, lamp posts, or railings. Boost local stocks by scattering seeds and pressing them gently into the soil.

Harvest: Leaves, before flower spikes bloom; flowers, when fully open. Leave plenty for seeds to form.

Hyssop (*Hyssopus officinalis* L.)

French: *Hysope*; Dutch: *Hyssop*
Family: Lamiaceae

Aromatic, semi-evergreen subshrub. Bushy plants, 60–80 cm high. Square stems and aromatic leaves. The flowers, which bloom from summer to early autumn, come in shades of blue, deep purple, red, pink, and white. They form dense whorls around the stems where the leaves join.

Virtues

This aromatic and bitter plant is a stimulating expectorant that helps loosen phlegm. It aids digestion by relieving trapped gas and bloating. Often made into infusions, elixirs, and syrups for respiratory complaints, such as coughs and asthma. As a compress, poultice, or soak, Hyssop eases bruises and rheumatism. It is sometimes seen as a cure-all. This plant is very popular with wildlife, and is often grown alongside waterways, where it helps to strengthen the edges.

Magical significance

Associated with strength, purification, forgiveness, and regaining innocence. It is used in rituals for cleansing and clearing away worries, such as in ritual baths or after-shower rinses. It is also used for anointing the forehead in rituals to help us move forward and release worries.

Foraging notes

Find: In warm, sunny locations. It is often grown as a low hedge or border by municipalities, and is easy to spot when in bloom. Strong Hyssop plants can tolerate being cut back by about a third, twice per year. Better to freeze any leftover Hyssop, after harvesting and using, as dried Hyssop lacks many of its aromatic oils and magical potency.

Harvest: For medicinal use, around midsummer, when in flower; leaves and shoot tips, possible to harvest year round.

Ivy (*Hedera helix* L.)

French: *Lierre grimpant*; Dutch: *Klimop*
Family: Araliaceae

A climbing evergreen with dark green or variegated, three-pointed leaves. Ivy can trail or climb up to 30 m using small stem suckers, often on trees or buildings. The yellow–green flowers provide Bees with their last nectar of the year, and develop into berry clusters, essential winter food for wildlife like Pigeons. While misunderstood as harmful to trees, Ivy benefits ecosystems by offering habitat, insulation, and greenery.

Virtues

Ivy berries are toxic to humans, however its leaves are used medicinally. Ivy leaf infused Olive oil can gently stimulate skin circulation. It is used in many anti-cellulite treatments. Leaves can also be used in teas and syrups, to relieve catarrhal complaints. The poultice is also used to treat corns, warts, eczema, boils, and abscesses. Ivy stems can be woven into garlands, crowns, or seasonal decorations. Ivy berries provide important winter sustenance for birds and other wildlife. Ivy irritates some people's skin. It may be narcotic in high doses.

Magical significance

Associated with protection, cleansing, purification, and community. It is also associated with fertility, fidelity, and attachment, and can provide a shielding or concealing effect, much like an invisibility cloak. Ivy is a Moon herb, with a silver energy about it. This quiet, graceful plant is particularly lovely to be around at night. Ivy is traditionally used in Yuletide decorations, and was associated with Bacchus, the Roman God of Wine. Ivy crowns were worn by partygoers, apparently to protect them from intoxication and poisoning. This old use can be worked into protection and hex-breaking rituals.

Foraging notes

Find: Year round on walls, trees, or as houseplants.

Harvest: Prune gently to avoid damage, focus on unattached growth. This plant is not related to Poison Ivy (*Toxicodendron radicans*).

Japanese Knotweed (*Reynoutria japonica* Houtt.)

French: *Renouée du Japon*; Dutch: *Japanse duizendknoop*; Chinese: *Hu Zhang*; Japanese: *Kojiyo*
Family: Polygonaceae

Vigorous herbaceous perennial growing from rhizomes, reaching up to 4 m tall. Its tall, green stems have magenta/pink joints, with heart-shaped, alternate leaves. These mature to deep green and 8 cm across. Small cream–white flowers bloom on upright spikes from summer to autumn. In spring, shoots emerge resembling Asparagus spears. The plant dies back in winter, leaving brittle stems.

Virtues

Tastes sour when cooked, similar to Rhubarb, and can be used in sweet and savoury dishes. Growing parts contain mucilage, which is noticeable when snapped or crushed. This can be utilised in preparations such as leaf and stem syrups, ferments, and vinegars. In Traditional Chinese Medicine the root, seen as bitter and cold, is used to support the cardiovascular, respiratory, and nervous systems. Knotweed is also used to treat minor skin infections, and constipation. Knotweed contains high levels of resveratrol, a potent antioxidant, now sold in many food supplements and cosmetics. This herb is not suitable during pregnancy.

Magical significance

Associated with binding, fidelity, multiplication, fortune, and money. Knotweed can be used in magic where potent, fertile, and dominant qualities are needed. Use the seeds or syrup in money spells, and where there is a need to take over space, or push something out.

Foraging notes

Find: Near waterways, parks, gardens, and derelict sites.

Harvest: Young shoots in spring; mature stems in spring/summer. Repeated cutting weakens the plant, aiding control.

Highly invasive and difficult to eradicate, follow local regulations carefully. Do not compost, disturb roots, or spread material. Clean tools thoroughly after harvesting.

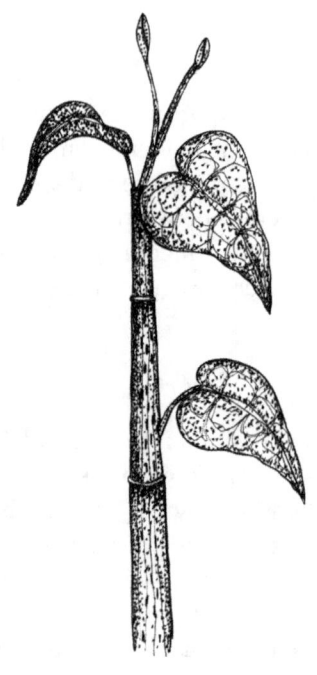

Japanese Plum/Loquat (*Eriobotrya japonica* (Thunb.) Lindl.)

French: *Néflier du Japon*; Dutch: *Loquat*; Chinese: *Pí pá*; Japanese: *Biwa*
Family: Rosaceae

An evergreen shrub reaching up to 10 m. It has long, serrated leaves up to 25 cm. Young leaves are fuzzy and toxic; they form at branch ends. Mature leaves are dark and glossy above, hairy below. Sweet-tart, nutritious fruit with shiny seeds, popular in Asian and Mediterranean cuisine. In climates with year round temperatures of 15–30°C, Loquats fruit in spring/summer after flowering in autumn/winter.

Virtues

Biwa tea, made from mature Loquat leaves, has several purported health benefits, including skin health, anti-inflammatory effects, and support for respiratory issues. It is used in Traditional Chinese Medicine (as *Pi Pa Ye*) to relieve coughing and wheezing. Steep 1 teaspoon of dried, crumbled mature leaves in hot water for 3 minutes. Loquat fruit is rich in vitamins A, C, and E, antioxidants, and fibre. It can support digestion, immunity, and blood sugar control. Use in jams, jellies, and desserts.

Caution: Young leaves contain toxic cyanogenic glycosides and must never be consumed.

Magical significance

Associated with creativity, fertility, success, resilience, protection, youthfulness, and prosperity. It also represents sweetness and opportunism, and can help us grow metaphysical roots in the ground of our new hometowns. The seeds can be saved from store-bought Loquat fruit. They are smooth, shiny, and sit nicely in the palm. Useful for altars, amulets, and charm bags. Mindfully eat the fruit then push the seed into the ground, to encourage intentions to manifest. A large mature Loquat leaf can be used as a portable, biodegradable altar.

Foraging notes

Find: Gardens and parks.

Harvest: Only mature leaves, sparingly. Avoid toxic young leaves. Consider growing your own Loquat trees.

Japanese Quince (*Chaenomeles japonica* (Thunb.) Lindl. ex Spach)

French: *Cognassier du Japon*; Dutch: *Japanse sierkwee*
Family: Rosaceae

Spiky, deciduous shrub often pruned as a hedge. With dark branches, sharp spikes, and small glossy green leaves that fall in autumn. Deep pink–red, Rose-like flowers bloom in late winter to early spring, developing into small Quince-like fruit, which are hard and yellow–green.

Virtues

The fruit have astringent, anti-inflammatory, antiviral, and antibacterial properties. It is used to treat ailments such as coughs, sore throats, and digestive issues. Often used as a tea to boost the immune system. Japanese Quince tastes very sour when uncooked. When slow cooked and sweetened, it becomes highly aromatic and soft. Try in jam, fruit leather, porridge, smoothies, pancakes, or other dishes. This plant features in Japanese art and culture, especially in festivals like Hinamatsuri (Doll's Festival) for the health and happiness of little girls.

Magical significance

Associated with protection (particularly of children), winter, rebirth, and transient beauty. Japanese Quince is also believed to fight demons and bring good luck. Use any part of this plant in boundary protection work. It is especially useful where a quiet watchful eye is needed throughout the year. Try cleaning, slicing and drying the golden quinces, or leaves. Then powder and add a pinch to spell jars and charm bags. Include in feasts and sprinkle finely along boundaries.

Foraging notes

Find: In hedges and urban landscaping.

Harvest: Fruit, when yellow or yellow–green; flowers in late winter/early spring. Leave plenty of flowers for wildlife and to develop into fruit.

Juniper (*Juniperus communis* L.)

French: *Genévrier commun*; Dutch: *Jeneverbes*
Family: Cupressaceae

Slow-growing evergreen conifer. Up to 15 m tall. Whorls of grey-tinged, needle-like leaves surround its stems. Branches grow upward, forming a compact cone shape. Some varieties spread or grow into wind-sculpted shapes. Male plants bear yellow flowers, females produce small flowers that develop into blue–black, berry-like cones. New foliage is soft, but mature growth becomes spiky.

Virtues

Juniper berries and needles have warming, stimulating, diuretic, and antiseptic properties. Used sparingly in tea, salves, and soaks, to ease urinary tract infections, arthritis, gout, and rheumatism. Avoid during pregnancy, breastfeeding, or kidney disease. It is often found in hair products that stimulate the scalp. Hildegard of Bingen recommended it for pain relief and respiratory issues. Juniper berries are used to flavour gin, hearty casseroles, soups, and jams.

Magical significance

Associated with warmth, spice, magical protection, cleansing, and intuition. Often used in anti-theft, exorcism, and detoxifying spells. The foliage and cones can be used in powerful incense blends. It was traditionally used in Europe to protect from plague and to break hexes. Mundane folk also believed that Juniper bushes could slow down witches, owing to their need to count every leaf on the plant. I certainly find them mesmerising, so it may well work! Make Juniper water to cleanse magical spaces and tools. Add a few dried berries to charm bags and press small lengths of foliage in books.

Foraging notes

Find: In parks, gardens, and exposed locations. Juniper is endangered in many areas.

Harvest: Berries (cones) sparingly when blue and ripe. Dry in a paper bag and crush as needed. Collect young needle tips in spring or summer for a milder resinous flavour.

Purchase organic plants or berries. Do not be tempted to harvest from the wild.

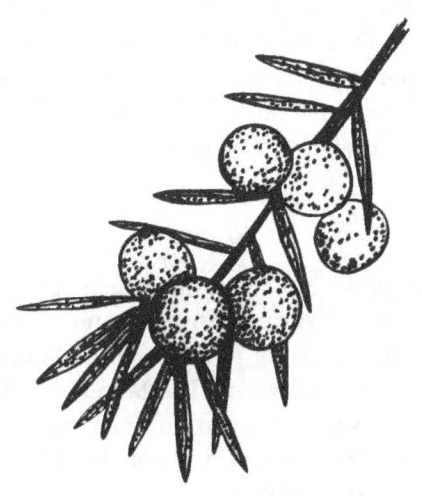

Lady's Mantle (*Alchemilla* spp.)

French: *Alchémille*; Dutch: *Vrouwenmantel*
Family: Rosaceae

Low-growing perennial. About 30 cm in height. Leaves are palm-shaped, and downy. Each has 7 or 9 folds and crinkly edges. Produces frothy sprays of delicate yellow–green flowers, which are petal-less. The leaves collect dew, and sap which is pumped out by special cells when the plant is saturated with water.

Virtues

Lady's Mantle has mild bitter and astringent properties. It is traditionally used for its sleep-inducing, wound-closing, healing, and tightening effects. It is used for many women's ailments, particularly menstrual and menopausal issues. The tannin-rich tea can help calm inflammation, when used as a skin or mouth rinse. It also has a reputation for helping to tighten skin and restore beauty. Lady's Mantle oil, salve, and poultices are traditional preparations for this. The leaves and flowers can be eaten in salad and risotto, or infused into dairy products.

Magical significance

Associated with protection and transformation. The crystal dew collected on Lady's Mantle leaves has long been thought to possess magical properties. Historically, it was used to cure bewitchment and played a role in alchemy, hence its scientific name. Alchemists believed it was an essential ingredient in their quest for the Philosopher's Stone. Dew collected at Beltane, under the Full Moon is particularly potent for use in beauty essences. Use Lady's Mantle in rituals and spells related to restoring boundaries, and preventing invasion or harm.

Foraging notes

Find: In parks, gardens, and pavement cracks. Often in municipal planting. Wild examples are rare.

Harvest: Leaves, when looking healthy and vibrant, spring through summer; flowers, sparingly when fresh and yellow–green (Beltane). Scatter seeds, when found, to proliferate local stocks. Dew: use directly or collect clean drops with a small pipette and preserve with brandy.

Lavender (*Lavandula angustifolia* Mill.)

French: *Lavande*; Dutch: *Lavendel*
Family: Lamiaceae

Highly aromatic evergreen. A perennial shrub (up to 1.5 m) with soft, grey, needle-like leaves. Mature stems are gnarled, with loose bark. Tall, square-angled flower stems with blue–purple flowers. They mature into fragrant blue–grey seedheads by late summer. Lavender has a slightly sprawling growth habit.

Virtues

Helps ease anxiety, depression, and inflamed skin conditions like eczema. An old English saying, "As Rosemary is to the spirit, so Lavender is to the soul," highlights how it can clear gloomy thoughts. It has a strong minty, aromatic flavour. Use sparingly to flavour cakes, biscuits, sugar, and honey. Infuse in vinegar, oil, or tea for headaches and tension relief. Lavender jelly is more delicious than it may sound. Try cooled Lavender tea, as a gargle for throat infections. The volatile oil is useful for minor kitchen burns, relaxation, pain relief, digestion, asthma, and as an insect repellent. A popular ingredient in potpourri and deodorants. Lavender's name derives from "lava," meaning to wash—it has a long history of use in washing and perfumes. Lavender water is a calming room spray. This herb is highly attractive to Bees and Butterflies.

Magical significance

Associated with cleansing, purification, and expelling unwanted spirits. Easy to use in purification rituals, as a hydrosol or essential oil spray. Weave flower stems with ribbons into a saining bundle. Bunches of dried Lavender seed stems make a useful ritual broom, for use in small spaces. Hanging this in an apartment, perhaps on a wall, will also help to purify the space and protect.

Foraging notes

Find: In sunny pavement gardens, parks, or street plantings.

Harvest: Blue–grey seed stems from Lughnasadh; leaves sparingly from spring to autumn, taking only new growth. Avoid winter harvests to protect the plant.

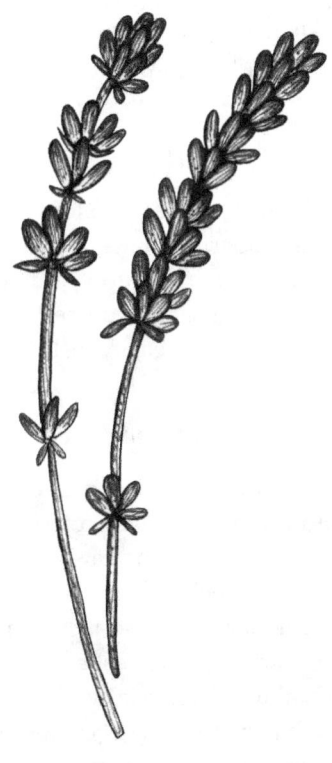

Lemon Balm (*Melissa officinalis* L.)

French: *Mélisse officinale*; Dutch: *Citroenmelisse*
Family: Lamiaceae

Lemon-scented perennial. Square stems, small opposite leaves with a wrinkled surface and slightly toothed edges. To 20 cm high when in flower. Flowers are small, white, two-lipped and tube-shaped, arranged in whorls around the stem at leaf joints.

Virtues

This plant is used to calm nervous tension and anxiety, and help lower blood pressure. Antiviral properties make it useful in cold sore-relieving lip balms. It can be used as a skin rinse, foot, or hand soak. Lemon Balm tea is mentally uplifting. Try in salads, desserts, and to flavour mead. The plant dries well, but its scent is easily lost.

Magical significance

Associated with health, happiness, abundance, community harmony, and youthfulness. Lemon Balm has a deep connection to spirit, and communication with Bees. This herb is associated with Melissae, the Greek Goddess of Bees, protector of beekeepers, their hives, and honey. Use in spells and rituals that seek harmony and respect in relationships, especially between humans and the other aspects of nature. Fresh foliage can be rubbed on magical tools, especially wooden ones, to remind us of the constant need for balance and respect, as we use them. Use when seeking to communicate between the spiritual and physical planes. Try growing the plant, or regularly sprinkling dried leaves around your working area, to enhance your connection with spirit, and the effectiveness of your magical work.

Foraging notes

Find: Semi-shaded areas in gardens, woodlands, and municipal plantings. Easily identified by its Lemon scent and square stems.

Harvest: Beltane to autumn equinox. Take occasional stems from larger plants, leaving flowers to set seed.

Lilac (*Syringa vulgaris* L.)

French: *Lilas commun*; Dutch: *Sering*
Family: Oleaceae

Large shrub, 4–5 m tall. Smooth oval or heart-shaped leaves. Produces large pyramid-shaped "panicles" of small tubular flowers. White to purple, with a strong sweet scent. Short blooming period.

Virtues

Traditionally, Lilac has been used for irritated skin, as a fever tonic, and against intestinal parasites. It is also mildly anxiolytic. Lilac flowers are edible and can be used to make mead, cordial, or added to milky dishes such as ice cream, infused cream, and rice pudding. They are used in decorations and bouquets for their intoxicating scent. Lilac wood is good for carving.

Magical significance

Associated with protection and communication with the spirit realm. Lilac should be grown near homes. Purple Lilacs, in particular, are believed to keep malevolent spirits away. White Lilac flowers have been linked with bad luck, death, and disease. So, you may want to keep it away from sick people. The scent of Lilac can help drive out unwanted energies and spirits; it can also enable us to enter a liminal state. I find that having Lilac with me on the physical plane can act as an anchor, guiding me back home, at the end of spiritual journeys. Lilac's brief flowering period is also symbolic of the shortness of life in full bloom. Giving Lilac to another signals that you wish to end the relationship.

Foraging notes

Find: In parks and gardens. Seek out neglected Lilacs in public spaces.

Harvest: Flowers (early summer), sparingly from strong shrubs with many blooms. Use sharp tools to snip whole flower panicles, minimising damage. Light pruning during harvesting can promote healthy growth and more flowers the next year.

Lime/Linden (*Tilia* spp.)

French: *Tilleul*; Dutch: *Linde*
Family: Malvaceae

Large deciduous trees. Heart-shaped leaves and pale grey–brown ridged bark. Tufts of hair grow at leaf vein joints. Suckers grow from the trunk's base; these retain leaves until hard frosts. Lime blossom, at midsummer, is rich in nectar. Lime is an important food source for city Bees. Its round seeds turn brown when ripe. Leaf Aphids produce sticky honeydew, often leading to sooty mould on leaves. Limes can thrive in polluted air. They are often pruned to provide terrace shade.

Virtues

Lime can tame tempers, ease anxiety, and help with easier breathing. The leaves are mild and tender compared to other trees. They can be eaten directly from the tree when clean and release a soothing mucilage when chewed. The flowers taste very sweet on sunny days. These can be dried or infused directly in water or honey. Green Lime seeds can be roasted and blended into a tasty paste. Sitting beneath midsummer flowering Limes can bring a gentle sense of intoxication, as if drunk from the blossom scent. Tender leaves can be eaten as a salad or sandwich filling. Sprinkle the flowers on desserts. Pour Lime blossom syrup over midsummer cakes.

Magical significance

Associated with shelter, rest, calm, happiness, community, Bees, and clean air. They are often planted as memorial trees. The heart-shaped leaves lend themselves to love spells, and the flowers attract good fortune. Picnic under Lime blossom for a heady experience.

Foraging notes

Find: Streets and parks; Amsterdam alone has almost 30,000 Limes.

Harvest: Tender leaves, spring equinox to Samhain; buds from trunk burrs year round; flowers around midsummer; unripe seeds, midsummer to Lughnasadh.

London Plane (*Platanus* x *hispanica*)

French: *Platane*; Dutch: *Plataan*
Family: Platanaceae

Fast-growing tree with large palmate leaves (similar to Sycamore), wind-pollinated flowers, and seed balls that hang through winter and fall in spring. Its bark scales off, revealing pink and grey mosaic patterns, aiding survival in polluted areas. Seed hairs and pollen, often released together, can trigger allergies. Commonly boulevard trees. They absorb harmful gases and heavy metals, making them valuable urban air cleaners.

Virtues

London Plane timber, called Lacewood, is used for indoor furniture. The tree supports urban wildlife and provides much-needed shade. Its sap resembles that of Sycamore, but its leaves, while potentially antimicrobial and anti-inflammatory, are not suitable for use owing to pollution. Autumn leaves are ideal for ephemeral art, and bark shedding may inspire creative projects.

Magical significance

Associated with adaptation, tolerance, abundance, and resilience. Spend time with Plane trees, examining the mosaic bark patterns and branch shapes. Shed bark can be used as a writing or drawing surface. If reachable, and if you are not sensitive to allergens, collect a few pom-pom seed balls in winter, dry them whole in bags, and use in rituals to attract abundance. The seeds and pollen represent irritation. Try immersing a seed ball in a small jar of honey or syrup, not to eat but to use in spells calling for tolerance. Write symbols and intentions with this syrup on London Plane leaves.

Foraging notes

Find: Street tree, parks, and gardens.
   Avoid visiting during pollen release.

Harvest: Seed balls for rituals, early winter; leaves for colour in autumn, and fresh for poultices in late spring. Shed bark, for rituals can be collected from beneath trees throughout the year; it often resembles litter, and feels dirty.

Magnolia (*Magnolia* L.)

French: *Magnolia*; Dutch: *Beverboom*
Family: Magnoliaceae

Elegant, angular tree with large, glossy, oval leaves, smooth bark. Impressive goblet or star-shaped flowers, pollinated by small crawling insects. Petals range from white to cerise pink.

Virtues

Magnolia leaves, flowers, and bark are used to help relieve stress, anxiety, pain, and depression. Dried, steamed Magnolia bark, is bitter, warm, and drying. It is traditionally used in China and Japan to clear phlegm, relieve bloating, dampness and wheezing. Try using the leaves as a compress or poultice. Magnolia flowers help clear sinus congestion, and headaches. The central flower parts are covered in irritating hairs, so strain infusions with two muslin cloths. Petals taste fragrant and spicy, and can be eaten straight from the tree; each species has a slightly different taste. Petals and young leaves can be dried, powdered, or infused fresh in honey, syrup, or water. Used in tea, they can bring restful sleep. Avoid taking Magnolia during pregnancy.

Magical significance

Associated with clarity, dignity, elegance, stability, perseverance, and personal growth. The flowers are also symbolic of spicy, irresistible attraction. Use Magnolia to guide your magical work in the direction you want. Spend meditative time with the tree at any time in the year; sketch its form, study its bark and buds. If plentiful in your area, consider using a bowl-shaped Magnolia bloom to symbolise a cauldron in Beltane rituals. Sprinkle a pinch of Magnolia petal or leaf powder into candle flames and write intentions on the leaves.

Foraging notes

Find: Parks and gardens.

Harvest: Take 1–2 petals per flower to preserve beauty; use soon after harvest. Collect leaves sparingly during the growing season. Bark can be removed from pruned branches.

Mahonia (*Berberis aquifolium* Pursh (Mahonia)) Barberry (*Berberis vulgaris* L.)

French: *Épine-vinette*; Dutch: *Mahonie, Zuurbes*
Family: Berberidaceae

Evergreen shrubs with tough, glossy leaves. Mahonia (Oregon Grape) grows 1–4 m tall, with Holly-like, prickly leaves. It has large, bright yellow flower racemes in midwinter to spring, maturing into sour, dark purple berries. Barberry has oval or spoon-shaped leaves with sharp spikes, and clusters of yellow flowers and red berries. Both shrubs have inner bark yielding bright yellow sap.

Virtues

Both Mahonia and Barberry contain berberine, an antimicrobial, anti-inflammatory, and liver-supportive phytochemical. They are used to treat skin disorders, and support wound healing, gastrointestinal issues, fungal infections, and fevers. They are also used to treat respiratory issues and sinusitis. The dried berries, rich in vitamin C, are used in syrups, honey, and jams. The berries and flowers can add a sour and bitter taste to syrups and jams. The flowers can be eaten (sparingly) directly from the plant. They taste rather like marmalade. The root and stem bark can be used as a sustainable substitute for Goldenseal (*Hydrastis canadensis*), which is an overharvested herb. Goldenseal is also berberine-rich. Avoid during pregnancy, breastfeeding or if taking medications.

Magical significance

Associated with protection and positive energy. Carry as amulets. Use where strength in community is required. Barberry helps particularly with staying alert and vigilant.

Foraging notes

Find: Parks and gardens. Mahonia's showy winter flowers are easy to spot.

Harvest: Flowers, winter; berries, summer; bark sparingly from pruned branches or roots. Remove bark with a vegetable peeler or pocket knife.

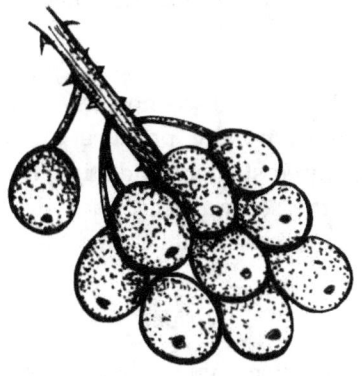

Mallow (*Malva sylvestris* L.)

French: *Grande Mauve*; Dutch: *Groot kaasjeskruid*
Family: Malvaceae

Biennial plant, up to 90 cm in its second year. A basal rosette of glossy, kidney-shaped leaves eventually produce tall flower stems. Five-petalled flowers with fused stamens and stigmas bloom progressively, from midsummer in the second year. Each develops into a round, cheese-like seed pod (as with Hollyhock and Marshmallow).

Virtues

Contains mucilage with a soothing, slightly laxative effect. Medieval Abbess Hildegard of Bingen advised a cooked Mallow with Plantain poultice to heal broken bones and soothe skin complaints. Mallow leaf-dew was smeared on eyelids to improve eyesight. The leaves combine well with Thyme, in elixirs for coughs and colds. Infuse in water, honey, glycerol, or syrup. Used as a skin wash to soothe rashes and sensitive skin. Take it as tea for gut irritation. The seeds taste nutty, similar to peanuts. Mallow leaves and flowers work well in salads or can be cooked like spinach. Unrelated Jute Mallow (*Corchorus olitorius*) contains far more mucilage. It is used in bakoula, a Turkish dish, and molokhia from Egypt.

Magical significance

Associated with clear vision, clairvoyance, and removing obstacles. In France, Mallow has been used to keep evil spirits away from homes and gardens. It has also been used as an antidote to aphrodisiacs and love potions. Use this plant in magical work to smooth the way, in situations where obstacles need to be softened, making them easier to remove. Mallow is one of the seven herbs in Irish folklore that no evil could harm. In England, it was used for strewing and weaving into Beltane garlands.

Foraging notes

Find: Along waterways, in neglected spaces. Sow the seeds in sunny areas to increase numbers.

Harvest: Spring equinox—midsummer, tender leaves and stems; Beltane—Mabon flowers and seedpods sparingly.

Meadowsweet (*Filipendula ulmaria* I (L.) Maxim.)

French: *Reine-des-prés*; Dutch: *Moerasspirea*
Family: Rosaceae

Herbaceous water-loving perennial. With creamy, frothy, Almond-scented flowerheads. These form on tall, reddish, and hairless stems at midsummer. Emerges from shallow water or damp ground in spring, with strong stems that eventually reach about 1.5 m. Leaves are pinnate with multiple pairs of lanceolate to ovate, serrated leaflets, and a larger terminal leaflet at the end. Each leaf underside is usually paler than the top, and slightly hairy.

Virtues

Has anti-inflammatory and analgesic properties. Used for gut health, rheumatism, joint pain, fever reduction, respiratory issues, and skin conditions like shingles. Meadowsweet is the plant from which Bayer developed aspirin in 1897 owing to its high salicylic acid content. It can reduce hyperacidity, calm gut cramps, and improve mood. Popular in bridal bouquets, mead flavouring, and as a strewing herb. Useful in jams and soups.

Magical significance

Associated with love, fidelity, fertility, and protection, water spirits, flowing energy, and happiness. Known as Queen of the Meadow, it is a sacred Druid herb with uplifting and mobilising energy. Traditionally used in divination charms, and for protection against malevolent energy.

Foraging notes

Find: In fertile damp soil, along the edges of ponds, ditches, and waterways.

Harvest: Sparingly, flowering tops, usually top third of a plant including leaves, at midsummer, ideally as the flowers begin to open. Avoid disturbing the root systems, which support waterway edges. Avoid plants affected by mildew. At home, allow time for secretive insects to leave the complex flowerheads, before processing.

Mint (*Mentha* spp.)

French: *Menthe*; Dutch: *Munt*
Family: Lamiaceae

Hardy perennials with tender square stems and opposite pairs of leaves. Each variety has a slight difference in appearance and scent. Usually grows 60 cm tall when in flower. Spreads easily, sending out roots when trailing stems touch the ground. When approaching blooming, Mint produces handsome spikes with small pink, white, or Lilac-coloured flowers arranged in whorls. Flowers are visited by many pollinating city insects while the leaves are the preferred food of others, including the eye-catching Green Mint Beetle (*Chrysolina herbacea*).

Virtues

Has antispasmodic, antimicrobial, and anti-inflammatory properties. Mint soothes coughs, colds, indigestion, IBS, and Nettle stings, eases breathing, freshens breath, and relieves joint pain in rubs. It also deters Mosquitoes. Use cautiously with ulcers or reflux. Mint leaves and flowers are edible, cool, and spicy. They enhance salads, teas, desserts, and sauces, and are popular in Mint jelly, syrup, and puddings. Mint tea helps regulate body temperature and pairs well with Yarrow and Elderflower.

Magical significance

Associated with protection, love, prosperity, and health in various cultural traditions. Historically, it was used in charms and rituals to secure lasting love, ward off evil, and attract good fortune. Sacred to the Druids, Mint was also a common strewing herb to repel pests like Fleas, Moths, and Mice, symbolising purity and protection.

Foraging notes

Find: In pots, gardens, parks. Often available as a potted grocery/market herb.

Harvest: Young growth, pinch out top leaves to encourage side growth. Shaded plants have stronger flavour. Avoid disturbing the roots, especially near waterways, as Mint plants help stabilise banks. Harvest Water Mint (*Mentha aquatica*) above the waterline to minimise risk of taking waterborne pathogens home with you. Avoid mildew-covered leaves.

Moss (Bryophytes)

French: *Mousses*; Dutch: *Mos*

Small, non-vascular plants that absorb water and nutrients through their tissues. They thrive in damp, shaded areas, forming dense green mats or clumps. They adapt well to urban environments, colonising many spaces. Species like Bryum Moss tolerate full sun, growing in cracks, roofs, and gutters.

Virtues

Sphagnum Moss was used in WWI for its antiseptic and absorbent properties.[12] It remains valuable for outdoor survival situations. The high absorbency of Moss makes it a substitute for sanitary products and toilet paper. Moss improves air quality, stabilises soil, and prevents erosion. It also acts as a rain reservoir. It is essential in creative projects such as terrariums, Kokedama, and fairy gardens. Moss provides soft bedding for nesting birds and supports many bugs and microbes. Moss-watching is a popular hobby in some cultures. Being around Moss is very calming and grounding.

Magical significance

Associated with stability, fertility, growth, healing, protection, resilience, adaptability, and calm. It has magical and symbolic significance across many cultures. Use in rituals aimed at environmental connection, or finding your niche in life. Nurture Moss in environments where negative energy, or excess, needs to be absorbed. Moss heals emotional or spiritual wounds and is seen as a bridge between the physical and spiritual realms; being near Moss can enhance intuition and connection to the spirit realm. Included in potions, charm bags, or amulets focused on fertility, protection, or simply to deepen connection with nature.

---

[12] P. Ayres, Wound dressing in World War I—The kindly Sphagnum Moss. *FieldBryology* (2020) 110: 27–34.

Harvesting and care

Find: In damp, shaded areas (tree trunks, paving cracks, walls, and roofs).

Harvest: Spring, gathering loose Moss dropped by birds. Moss grows slowly, so harvest sparingly.

Care: Replicate woodland conditions; mist with rainwater indoors.

Mugwort (Artemisia vulgaris L.)

French: *Armoise commune*; Dutch: *Bijvoet*
Family: Asteraceae

Shrubby, perennial herb up to 2 m tall. Fresh green foliage emerges by Beltane. Downy, grey–green leaves with silvery undersides and smooth, dark green tops. Reddish, grooved stems develop into spikes of tiny clustered flowers by midsummer. Over winter, Mugwort stems shelter insects.

Virtues

A bitter, aromatic emmenagogue. Mugwort is a versatile herb with edible foliage, flowers, and seeds. It supports digestion, stimulates the stomach and gallbladder, improves circulation and respiration, and helps female reproductive issues. Mugwort helps calm anxious minds, clears gut parasites, and revives tired feet. It can be used in place of Sage (*Salvia officinalis*) in cooking and combines well with Rose, Chamomile, and Calendula. A traditional flavouring for ales. Mugwort tea develops a dramatic purple colour. In Japan, where it is called Yomogi, Mugwort is commonly used in soups, stews, teas, mochi and onigiri. Avoid during pregnancy.

Magical significance

Associated with divination, protection, and prophetic dreaming. It was used for washing magical tools, saining (especially at midsummer), and creating garlands for protection. In German tradition, a chaplet of Mugwort was worn and then burned in a bonfire to dispel ill-luck. Mugwort sticks, cut when fresh, are used for divination. This is a dream herb, mildly narcotic, and closely linked with midsummer. Hang over doors for protection against evil spirits. Named after Artemisia, the Moon goddess, Mugwort was historically valued for its protective qualities and connection to childbirth.

Foraging notes

Find: Waste ground, hedges, sunny spots.

Harvest: Tender growing tips and flower buds (most potent at midsummer). Dry and crumble leaves to use.

Nasturtium (*Tropaeolum majus*)

French: *Capucine*; Dutch: *Oost-Indische kers*
Family: Tropaeolaceae

Annual climbing plant, grown easily from seed. Large, round, green or variegated leaves with radiating veins. Peppery scent when bruised. Flowers are yellow, orange, red, or variegated, with nectar-filled spurs. Seeds are large, green before ripening to sand-brown.

Virtues

A versatile edible plant with a hot, spicy flavour, suited to salads and steamed dishes. Excellent capers can be made by pickling the green seeds, in vinegar or brine. Traditionally, Nasturtium has been used as a mild laxative, and for treating scurvy, respiratory issues, haemorrhoids, and infections. It has antiseptic properties and is rich in vitamin C and iron. Sometimes used in hip baths to help regulate periods. As a lotion, it stimulates the scalp, and soothes psoriasis.

Magical significance

Associated with passion, purification, protection, abundance, and joy. Nasturtium is considered an aphrodisiac as it stimulates playful sensuality. Use in rituals where things need spicing up, motivating, and helping along.

Foraging notes

Find: Thrives in full sun in parks and gardens, self-seeding in nearby areas.

Harvest: Leaves and flowers, summer–late autumn. Leave plenty to ensure self-seeding and a good supply for capers. Beware pesticide use.

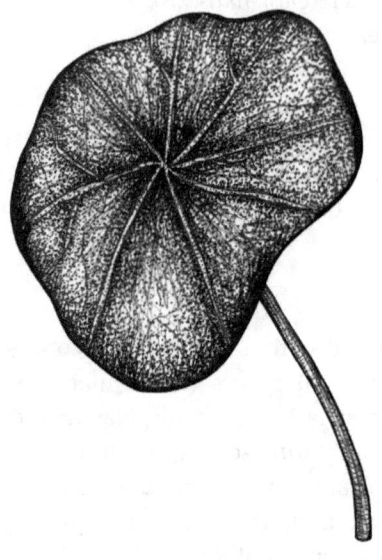

Nettle (*Urtica dioica* L.)

French: *Ortie*; Dutch: *Brandnetel*
Family: Urticaceae

Robust perennials with heart-shaped, serrated green leaves, growing up to 2 m tall. Stems are square in cross-section and covered with stinging hairs. Nettle flowers appear from midsummer to autumn, with both male and female plants. Nettle thickets provide food and shelter for wildlife, including butterflies and small mammals.

Virtues

Nettles are incredibly versatile, with edible leaves, stems, seeds, and roots, each offering distinct flavours, from the nutty seeds to the rich, green leaves. Nutrient-rich Nettles are high in iron, vitamins A, C, E, and fibre, making them ideal for treating anaemia, hay fever, and allergies. They also promote healthy skin and scalp, and are used for benign prostate disorders, rheumatism, and fluid retention. Culinary uses include Nettle tea, soups, stews, pasta sauces, smoothies, and even nettle wine. Nettles can also be powdered, salted, or pickled, and Nettle purée is a versatile base for many dishes. Anointing the head with Nettle infused oil is a medieval treatment for forgetfulness. Nettle stems contain long strong fibres. They are valued by traditional fabric weavers and paper makers.

Magical significance

Associated with protection, nourishment, and resilience. Nettles may be used in rituals related to developing clarity and purging negative emotions. In spells Nettle seeds were historically used in aphrodisiac potions. Linked with Beltane and May customs in Britain and Ireland, Nettle also symbolises humility and simplicity, helping align things in the right place. Use Nettle infused oil, or juice, in spells to help find lost possessions. This is a very grounding herb, also useful as a strong tea or in food after rituals.

Foraging Notes

Find: Waste ground, quiet corners, and waterways.

Harvest: Wear gloves. Young tops, Imbolc to Beltane. Seeds, around Lughnasadh; roots, autumn equinox to Yule. Leave plenty for wildlife.

Oak (*Quercus* L.)

French: *Chêne*; Dutch: *Eik*
Family: Fagaceae

Majestic, round-topped tree with wavy-edged, tannin-rich leaves. Oaks are wind-pollinated, with male and female flowers on the same tree. Acorns are spread by mammals, such as Squirrels, which bury them to leach tannins into the soil. There are various Oak species, including the Cork Oak, English Oak, and Holm Oak. Oaks are common in cities, growing quickly and thriving in urban areas. Mature Oaks may recover from lightning strikes after appearing dead for years. However, the fight against the Oak Processionary Moth (*Thaumetopoea processionea*) is leading to the felling of many Oaks near populated areas.

Virtues

Oak's tannin-rich parts are used for waterproofing and disease protection. Oak remedies include a snuff for nasal polyps, and an infusion (with Sage) to tighten gums. Oak bark tea helps prevent stomach ulcers. Acorn flour, after leaching tannins, is delicious. Oak barrels are used to keep wines safe, while deepening flavour. Oak leaf wine is very tasty. Acorn flour is delicious: leech out the tannins by securing shelled acorns in a laundry mesh bag. Place it inside of a toilet cistern and use the toilet as usual. Each soak and flush will help purify the acorns. When the water runs clear (usually a couple of weeks) the acorns should be tannin-free and ready to dry, grind, and use.

Magical significance

Associated with strength, pride, bitterness, reliability, fertility, protection, and regeneration. The Green Man (or Oak King) is portrayed with an Oak leaf crown. He rules nature between spring equinox and autumn equinox. Use pruned Oak stems in crowns and carry an Oak leaf or acorn as a fertility or protection amulet.

Foraging notes

Find: Streets, parks.

Harvest: Fallen acorns in autumn, young leaves in spring.

Olive (*Olea europaea* L.)

French: *Olivier*; Dutch: *Olijf*
Family: Oleaceae

Small evergreen tree with slim, oval leaves. White flowers bloom in spring, followed by oil-rich olives. Olive trees thrive in warm, dry Mediterranean climates but can adapt to colder, wetter conditions. They need protection from harsh winters, especially when young.

Virtues

The leaves and fruit are used to soothe our body, soul, and taste buds. Olive oil, pressed from the seeds, is mono-unsaturated. The leaves can be decocted, made into tea, dried and powdered, or cooked in a little water. They have a smooth, savoury taste. Olive leaves are used to support the skin, digestive, nervous, and immune systems. A Canary Islands remedy for hangovers is to decoct Horehound (*Marrubium vulgare*) with young Olive leaves. Olive oil is a key ingredient in healthy Mediterranean diets. Use directly, or infused with Garlic, to soothe earache and many skin disorders. It stays fresh and potent for longer than most other plant oils. Twisted Olive wood is full of character and can be crafted into spoons, wands, boards, and bowls.

Magical significance

Associated with peace, love, calm, good fortune, youthfulness, and fertility. Use any part of the Olive tree in harmony spells, rituals, and feasts. Olive brings people together and smoothes differences. Carry Olive wood as a calming amulet. Scatter the leaves inside ritual spaces, and lay them under doormats to welcome harmony into your home. Place them in charm bags to harmonise the other ingredients. Anoint spell candles with a dab of Olive oil and use this as a herb in its own right, rather than simply a carrier to be infused with other plants. Use Olive wood tools where wisdom and peace are called for. Weave branches into crowns.

Foraging notes

Find: Gardens, Mediterranean restaurants, terrace pots.

Harvest: Pruned branches. Harvest ripe olives when tender.

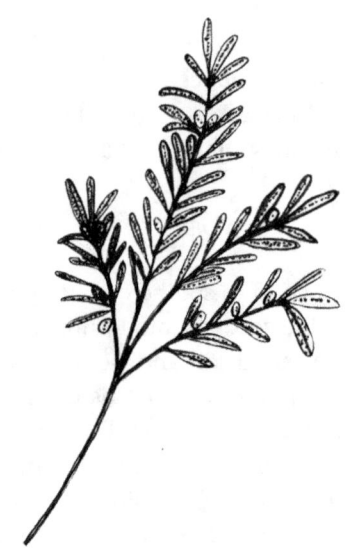

Parsley (*Petroselinum crispum* (Mill.) Fuss)

French: *Persil*; Dutch: *Peterselie*
Family: Apiaceae

Biennial plant with bright green, feathery, finely divided leaves. Grows from a rosette and can reach 15–60 cm tall. May remain green year round. Flowers are tiny and white, on tall umbrella-like structures. The stems become tough when the plant sets seed.

Virtues

Parsley has anti-inflammatory and antimicrobial properties. It is used to ease digestion, stimulate menstrual flow, as a diuretic, and to treat gout. Parsley has edible leaves, stems, roots, and seeds. It is rich in vitamins A, C, E, and iron. It has a fresh, lightly spicy, and peppery flavour. In the kitchen, it is commonly used in salads, sauces, risottos, mixed vegetables, and smoothies, and its roots can be used for cooking or powdered for vibrant colours in syrups, vinegar, or spirits.

Magical significance

In ancient Greece and Rome, Parsley was associated with death and funeral rites, believed to bring bad luck if transplanted and often used to decorate tombs. It was thought to be the only food needed by the dead, and was traditionally planted or moved on Good Friday to avoid misfortune. Parsley is also considered protective, especially when grown alongside Rue, and linked with many superstitions, such as allowing it to be "stolen" rather than given away to avoid magical issues. Folklore suggests that birds avoid Parsley, possibly owing to its reputed harmful effects on them.

Foraging notes

Find: In gardens and kitchen pots. Unlikely in the wild. Avoid confusing with local poisonous members of this plant family, such as Fool's Parsley (*Aethusa cynapium*).

Harvest: Collect individual leaves and stems, year round. Seeds when ripe (turning brown).

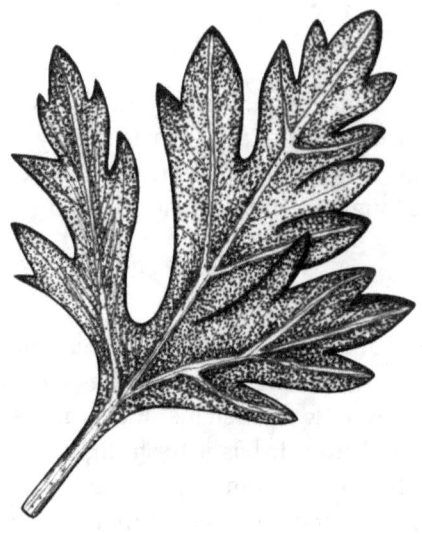

Passionflower (*Passiflora caerulea* L.)

French: *Fleur de la passion*; Dutch: *Blauwe passiebloem*
Family: Passifloraceae

Hardy perennial or semi-evergreen climber (up to 10 m). With vine-like stems and tendrils for climbing. It produces fragrant flowers from early summer until autumn, with 10 white sepals, blue and white filaments, and a cross-shaped arrangement of stamens. Orange-peach fruit ripen in late summer, containing sweet gel-covered seeds. The plant dies back in winter but retains some greenery year round.

Virtues

Passionflower is known for its sedative and calming properties. It can reduce anxiety, promote sleep, and calm nervous tension. It is a potent sedative, and overuse can cause a hangover-like state. The ripe fruit is sweet and edible, and can be used to make jelly or syrup. The leaves can be used in teas, syrups, and tinctures. Avoid during pregnancy and breastfeeding.

Magical significance

Associated with peace, calm, hypnotism, and protection. Passionflower has a very beguiling shadowy energy. It likes to be tended and repays its carers by whispering warning messages and keeping them safe. Grow at home entrances and boundaries, to mesmerise nosy visitors, and keep them away. It also makes a beautiful backdrop to outdoor altars. Use in rituals to encourage growth through rest, and to calm anger. A weak leaf or flower tea can be used to help enter a liminal state.

Foraging notes

Find: Planted against fences and walks in residential streets.

Harvest: Surreptitious pruning, focusing on neglected, very overgrown plants. Cut 30–50 cm from trailing stems of strong plants, in the growing season. Work neatly, with scissors or secateurs. Harvest sparingly to maintain the plant's health and vigour.

Pine Family (Pine, Fir, and Spruce)

Pine (*Pinus*): French: *Pin*; Dutch: *Dennenboom*
Fir (*Abies*): French: *Sapin*; Dutch: *Zilverspar*
Spruce (*Picea*): French: *Epicéa*; Dutch: *Fijnspar*

Family: Pinaceae

Evergreen conifers with needles and cones, all releasing a citrus and resin scent when bruised.

Pine: Long needles that grow in groups rather than being evenly spaced along branches. Pine cones, usually large and cylindrical.

Fir: Needles, evenly spaced, attached to branches by tiny suction cups. Needles cannot be rolled between fingers. Cones grow upright like candles.

Spruce: Short, sharp, four-sided needles attach singly to peg-like structures on branches. Strongly scented. Cones ripen slowly and hang down after pollination.

Virtues

Needles, cones, inner bark (bast), and resin are used for survival food. Pine inner bark is rich in carbohydrates, fibre, vitamin C, and minerals; a useful antimicrobial for sinus relief. Spruce resin is used medicinally and for turpentine, and beer. The wood is used to make violins and guitars. Fir needles have a resinous medicinal scent; useful in syrups and honey. Recently the Pine family have become popular in mixology and gastronomy; young shoots and needles can add flavour to carriers like gin, butter, and chocolate. Or dry, grind, and use as a spice. Canary Islanders traditionally use Pine charcoal to treat food poisoning.

Magical significance

Associated with strength, longevity, and health. Pine has spiritual significance in Scandinavia and North America, where traditional harvesting practices honour tree spirits and help to protect the trees.

The scented evergreen foliage is popular in Yuletide decorations. Pine family resin can be used in incense or to attach stones onto magical tools.

Foraging notes

Find: Parks, gardens. Organic Christmas trees.

Harvest: Young scented growing tips of foliage, in spring. Fallen cones after storms or on low branches; resin from naturally damaged trees.

NB: Avoid confusing young Pine/Fir/Spruce foliage with poisonous Yew (*Taxus*). Only eat needles from Christmas trees if organically grown (many are treated with toxic chemicals).

Plantain and Ribwort (*Plantago*)

Plantain (*P. major*); French: *Grand Plantain*; Dutch: *Grote weegbree*
Ribwort (*P. lanceolata*); French: *Plantain lancéolé*; Dutch: *Smalle weegbree*

Family: Plantaginaceae

Perennial herbs with leaves growing from basal rosettes. Ribwort has lanceolate, ribbed leaves, while Plantain has broader, fleshy leaves. Both grow upright if undisturbed, but lie flat when mowed or suppressed. Tall flower stems form spikes of green seeds. Plantain has a shallow root system, and thrives in compacted soil.

Virtues

Plantain is used to heal skin wounds, irritations, stings, burns, and to soothe the respiratory system. It draws foreign bodies and pus from the skin, so is often used in salves or poultices. As tea or syrup it can treat coughs and colds during winter. Is also useful for allergies. Plantain leaf sap is anti-inflammatory and vulnerary, often used directly on foot blisters and gout. Ribwort can be used as a substitute for Plantain, and has similar properties. Some carnivorous Elf Cup fungi are known to live within its leaves. Try a *Plantago* poultice on the forehead, to relieve headaches. Plantain is more practical for culinary use, as the leaves have more flesh and less stringy ribs.

Magical significance

Associated with grounding, resilience, and rootedness. Both can help us feel at home in new environments. Many old divination practices featured *Plantago*, such as counting leaf veins to determine the number of lies told in a day. Hildegard von Bingen recommended drinking Plantain juice to relieve a love enchantment. Ribwort was part of a ritual to assess the quality of hay in Welsh farming communities. It was also part of the Nine Herbs Charm of the Anglo-Saxons.

Foraging notes

Find: In compacted soils near paths and walkways, well-trodden urban areas.

Harvest: Leaves or seed stalks, not entire plants. Year round, when looking verdant.

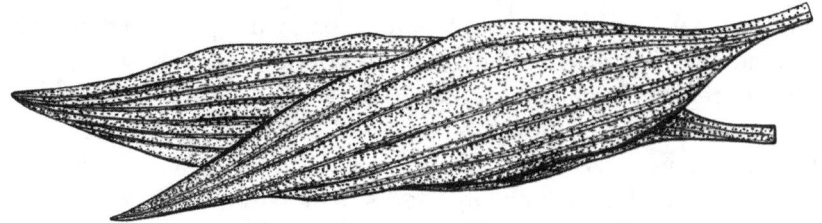

Poplar (*Populus* L.)

French: *Peuplier*; Dutch: *Populier*
Family: Salicaceae

Majestic trees (up to 30 m) with an upright form. Roughly triangular leaves with long leaf stalks that tremble in the wind. Sharp leaf buds, often aromatic and sticky (sticky buds). Long wind-pollinated catkins. Tolerate high winds, so often grown as windbreaks. However, heavy Poplar branches are brittle and can easily snap in storms. Most species have deep red–purple flower buds and red catkins (on separate trees), which are hard to see owing to the height of most Poplars. Some species have smooth bark with large "eyes" on the trunks where branches were shed. The white outer bark of some species splits as the trunk expands, revealing rough mature bark. Closely related to Birch and Willow. Often has a scent of balsam.

Virtues

Poplar leaves and buds are strongly anti-inflammatory and antiseptic, often used in compresses or skin balms to soothe bruises, swelling, painful joints, support wound healing, and ease coughs. Various species are favoured by different cultures but all have similar properties. Infuse leaf buds in Olive oil, then thicken with beeswax to make a soothing balm.

Magical significance

Associated with air, wisdom, power, growth, sacrifice, communication, resilience, and oversight. The rustling leaves of species like Aspen (*Populus tremula*) are said to carry messages from spirits. The long red catkins may represent fingers. These trees often reach the heavens, symbolising a connection between the spirit and earthly realms. Listen to air whispering through Poplars whenever possible; watch the leaves dance in the wind and enjoy their bright colour. The many leaves of Poplar are often linked to wealth and success.

Foraging notes

Find: Streets, near tall buildings, as windbreaks beside wide waterways and farmland.

Harvest: Sticky buds, spring; leaves during the spring–summer growing season. They resemble Linden leaves but are glossier.

Pot Marigold (*Calendula officinalis* L.)

French: *Souci officinal*; Dutch: *Goudsbloem*
Family: Asteraceae

Annual or biennial plant. 50–70 cm high and 30 cm wide, often sprawling. Can survive mild winters. Has aromatic, slightly sticky leaves owing to its oils and resins. Yellow and orange Daisy-shaped flowers. Easy to grow; prefers full Sun and well-drained soil. Self-seeds readily.

Virtues

Has anti-inflammatory, antiseptic, detoxifying, and vulnerary properties. Used to heal skin wounds, fungal infections, insect stings, and bruises. It can also soothe gastrointestinal inflammation and pain. Commonly used in salves, rinses, baths, and teas. Pot Marigold is also useful for menstrual pain and is often included in baby skin preparations. It tastes bitter and is useful in soups, stews, and herbal stock cubes. Pot Marigold can be grown as a companion plant, to maintain soil moisture and deter some pests. Slugs seem attracted to it.

Magical significance

Associated with sunshine, persistence, and success, it symbolises wealth, warmth, and strength. Its uplifting qualities make it a positive and resilient herb, as reflected in Shakespeare's reference to it as "Merrybuds". Pot Marigold is also considered a protective and healing herb, often used in rituals for its sunny and positive energies.

Foraging notes

Find: In gardens and allotments.

Harvest: Flowers, on sunny days year round. More in summer. Leave some to self-seed. Leaves, best in spring and summer.

Primrose and Cowslip (*Primula vulgaris* Huds. and *P. veris*)

French: *Primevère commune*; Dutch: *Steutelbloem*
Family: Primulaceae

Perennial, often in small groups. Rosettes of long, ovate leaves with prominent midribs. Primrose flowers are usually yellow, though many hybrids exist. Cowslip has a tall stem with a cluster of yellow flowers resembling a bunch of keys, at the top.

Virtues

Cowslip roots are strong expectorants, helpful for flu, colds, sore throats, and clearing phlegm. The leaves share similar properties. Flowers are milder but still useful for their antispasmodic and sedative effects. They make a pleasant bedtime tea. The plant has been used to treat rheumatism, skin conditions, and inflammation both internally and externally. Primrose is more commonly used for its leaves and flowers, in sedative teas and remedies for rheumatism and gout. However, caution is needed as it can act as an anticoagulant. Useful and attractive in jellies, salads, and syrups. Beware of most traditional recipes, which require large, unsustainable quantities of the flowers. Avoid if pregnant, breastfeeding, or taking blood thinners.

Magical significance

Associated with protection, playful fairy energy, and for safeguarding secrets. Both plants are symbols of spring and renewal. Traditionally, Primrose balls were hung in Irish and English homes to deter witches and bring good fortune. Hildegard von Bingen recommended placing Primrose on the skin near the heart to ward off airy spirits. In Yorkshire, Primrose hoops were placed over doorways for protection. Use Primroses or Cowslips in rituals and spells related to locks, keys, and hidden matters.

Foraging notes

Find: Endangered through overharvesting; grow your own from seeds, or buy organic plants.

Harvest: Roots, leaves, and flowers sparingly in spring.

Red Clover (*Trifolium pratense*)

French: *Trèfle*; Dutch: *Klaver*
Family: Fabaceae

Low-growing perennial with trifoliate oval leaves, often marked with a "V." It produces ball-shaped clusters of pink to red tubular flowers from Beltane to Lughnasadh. Flowers contain sweet nectar, attracting Bees.

Virtues

Red Clover is valued in treatments for chronic skin conditions such as eczema and psoriasis. It is also used for mild anxiety and hormone-related disorders, owing to its isoflavones. Clover also has some anti-cancer activity. Traditionally, it has been used to treat coughs and other respiratory disorders. Try the flowers in soothing tea blends, salves, and syrups. Red Clover is beneficial in gardens; it is a leguminous plant that fixes nitrogen, improves soil fertility, and prevents soil erosion. Clover is also an important nectar source for bees and other pollinating insects.

Magical significance

Associated with luck, and protection from evil forces. Clover is sacred to Druids; the trifoliate leaves connect to Celtic triads and the three aspects of the divine. Four-leaf Clovers, a rare variation of the plant, are especially lucky. If found, dry and keep as charms. They attract prosperity and positive change. Use Red Clover in magical work related to protection, fortune, abundance, healing, and luck. Add to charm bags. Try Clover-infused syrup in money spells, and float Clover flowers in ritual baths. Use dried flowers in candle dressing blends.

Foraging notes

Find: Park and garden lawns.

Harvest: Summer but leave flowers for wildlife and be cautious when foraging to avoid confusion with non-edible Trifolium species.

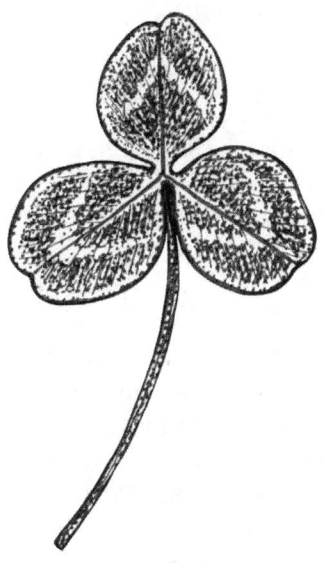

Rocket (*Diplotaxis tenuifolia*)

French: *Roquette*; Dutch: *Grote zandkool*
Family: Brassicaceae

Perennial with long, narrow, deeply toothed leaves with central white veins. Leaves grow in a rosette from a central root. Yellow flowers with four petals in a cross shape, typical of the Brassicaceae family. Flower stems reach about 60 cm.

Virtues

The fresh younger leaves are tasty in salads, sandwiches, smoothies, and as garnishes. They can also be lightly cooked but are best enjoyed fresh. Blend with oil and garlic to make a spicy pesto. When crushed, Rocket seeds release a strong, spicy scent and flavour. They can be used to make a Mustard-like condiment. Rocket has been used in cough syrups. The leaves and seeds can be included in foot soaks for tired feet. They combine well with grated Onion, Ginger, and Black Pepper.

Magical significance

Associated with warmth, tolerance, movement, transformation, and clearing stagnation. Use to increase opportunism and wealth. Spicy Rocket seems to grow where there is nothing; it literally turns sand, rain, and air into gold. Try using it in work where transformation seems almost impossible.

Foraging notes

Find: In neglected, usually sunny exposed locations and often in sandy soil. Often grows between paving stones and at path edges.

Harvest: Year round, preferably younger leaves before flowering (for a milder flavour). The peppery heat intensifies as they age. Rocket tolerates regular light harvesting of leaves but should be left with enough foliage to maintain strength and ability to flower and seed. Harvest seeds when ripe; flowers, individually and sparingly.

Rose (*Rosa* spp.)

French: *Églantier*; Dutch: *Roos*
Family: Rosaceae

Shrubs in various forms, including rambling, climbing, and standard varieties. Common in urban landscapes, providing summer colour and scent. *Rosa rugosa* (Beach Rose or Japanese Rose) is particularly street-tolerant. It has large, fragrant flowers, woolly stems, and fewer thorns than other Roses. *Rosa rugosa* flowers are pink or white, blooming throughout summer. The ripe hips are large, ruby red, with easy-to-separate pulp and seeds. Climbing Roses often feature large scented flowers, but may fail to produce hips. Dog Rose (*R. canina*) forms a large prickly bush. It has smaller flowers and hips, and is best left for wildlife.

Virtues

Tender young leaves and supple stems from all Rose species are astringent and may be used as tea to cleanse wounds, and settle upset digestion. Use Rose flowers similarly, and to soothe the emotional heart. Rose hips contain many nutrients that boost immunity and skin health. Try preserving Rose hip flesh in honey, syrups, or elixirs. The seeds, when hair-free, can be used in skin care. Rose petals can be dried, made into syrup, jam, or infused vinegar, and used to decorate food.

Magical significance

Associated with protection, love, romance, beauty, luxury, and serenity. In languages of flowers, Rose colours have various meanings, and these can be worked into rituals. Rose thorns represent secrecy and protection; Carefully pick them from Rose stems, dry in paper bags and use for protection work. Use in witch bottles and charms. Lay thorn-covered Rose stems around vulnerable boundaries. Grind and powder thorns in hex-breaking rituals.

Foraging notes

Find: In parks, gardens, and city planting. *R. rugosa* is the easiest to forage.

Harvest: Flowers in summer, sparingly. Hips from late summer to autumn. Leaves in spring.

Rosemary (*Salvia rosmarinus* Spenn.)

French: *Romarin*; Dutch: *Rozemarijn*
Family: Lamiaceae

Bushy aromatic evergreen shrub. Up to 2 m tall, with needle-like leaves and woody stems, similar to Lavender and Sage. Small blue flowers bloom throughout the year. It prefers well-drained soil and full Sun, thriving near buildings that reflect warmth. Regular pruning is needed to maintain shape and health.

Virtues

Rosemary is used for a range of purposes including varicose veins, hair growth stimulation, and as a painkiller. It has antimicrobial, anti-inflammatory, and sedative properties. It can also aid in memory, alleviate anxiety and bronchial asthma, and provide relief for rheumatic conditions and muscle pain. Rosemary is also used to improve mood, digestion, and respiratory health. Medieval texts advised applying the juice of Rosemary root to ease toothache. The young, softer growth can be used in cooking for its deep aroma and flavour. Rosemary stems can be used as skewers. The wood from mature shrubs can be carved into tools. Infused Rosemary oil and salves are used for various skin and muscle conditions.

Magical significance

Associated with remembrance, protection, memories, and happiness. It is traditionally used at funerals, placed on or inside coffins, and included in funeral wreaths. Rosemary is known as a "Spirit Stopper", protecting against theft, evil, and malevolent witchcraft. A form of divination involves sprinkling flour beneath a Rosemary bush. Any marks found in the flour the next day are then interpreted. The wood is gnarly and aromatic, well suited to whittling small magical tools such as amulets and stirring sticks.

Foraging notes

Find: Parks and gardens.

Harvest: Year round but very sparingly in winter. Soft growth at the stem ends. Avoid harvesting from plants infested with Rosemary Beetles, which weaken the plant.

Rue (*Ruta graveolens*)

French: *Rue des jardins*; Dutch: *Wijnruit*
Family: Rutaceae

Hardy evergreen shrub. 20 to 90 cm tall with woody lower stems and pale green–grey foliage. Leaves are bi- or tri-pinnate, smooth, deeply divided and rounded. Rue has unusual yellow flowers with 4 or 5 petals. Seedheads are light brown. The plant is strongly aromatic.

Virtues

Rue has antimicrobial properties and is traditionally used for coughs, respiratory issues, and digestive stimulation. It can be a potent emmenagogue and is known to affect the uterus, so it must be used carefully, and avoided during pregnancy or breastfeeding. It can also be used for various ailments such as toothache, low appetite, sprains, skin disease, eye problems, and menstrual disorders. Rue oil is used for calming rage and tension, and can be used to stop nosebleeds. In small amounts, Rue adds a unique flavour to stews and casseroles. Used sparingly owing to its bitterness and potential toxicity. Rue was used in plague remedies, and as an antidote to jail fever.

Magical significance

Associated with protection, increasing psychic powers, and love spells. It is a symbol in Italian witchcraft and used for its protective qualities. Rue is said to improve vision, both physical and inner, and is useful in spells requiring precision. Historically, it was used to ward off witches, and is known for its ability to clear melancholy and aid in spiritual clarity. Rue is also used in cleansing rituals and charms for accuracy and protection, and in protective charms and potions.

Foraging notes

Find: Parks and gardens. Prefers sunny, Mediterranean-like locations.

Harvest: Lightly, year round, preferably in the morning. Gather the young, fresh growth before it flowers.

NB: Be cautious of photosensitivity. Protect skin when harvesting, as exposure to sunlight afterward can cause blisters or rashes.

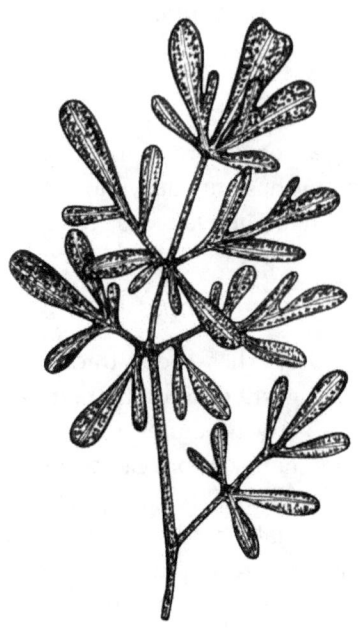

Sage (*Salvia officinalis* L.)

French: *Sauge officinale*; Dutch: *Salie*
Family: Lamiaceae

Hardy evergreen, aromatic shrub. Bushy, up to 80 cm tall. Sage has square stems, grey–green oval leaves, and blue–purple flowers. The variety *Salvia officinalis 'Purpurea'* has purple leaves.

Virtues

Sage is used to relieve headaches, PMS, infections, cold sores, and some symptoms of Alzheimer's. Sage can help cognitive performance. It helps dry up breast milk, and should not be used during pregnancy and breastfeeding. Sage adds savoury flavour, stimulates appetite, and is used in throat gargles, teas. and tooth powders.

Magical significance

Associated with immortality, wisdom, and protection. It is traditionally used in spells and rituals related to memory, understanding, healing, and calm. It has a historical association with Toads. According to folklore, it is bad luck to plant Sage for yourself; the task should be done by someone else. Sage is used in various forms of divination and magical practices. Try writing intentions on Sage leaves then tuck under your pillow, or bury them.

Foraging notes

Find: Gardens and parks.

Harvest: Leaves, sparingly year round. Ancient Romans avoided using iron tools for harvesting Sage. It is said to react with iron salts. Use your fingernails or bronze tools, especially for ritual harvests.

Do not confuse Sage with Russian Sage (*Salvia yangii*), which is toxic and often found in gardens.

Self-heal (*Prunella vulgaris*)

French: *Brunelle commune*; Dutch: *Gewone brunel*
Family: Lamiaceae

Low-growing perennial with square stems and opposite pairs of leaves. Dense clusters of purple flowers arranged neatly in whorls around an upright stem. It grows 15–30 cm tall, with a spread about 30 cm. Often develops runners. The stem is deeply grooved, sturdy, and somewhat rough to the touch. Self-heal blooms all summer and is loved by Bees and other insects.

Virtues

Self-heal has astringent and styptic properties, making it excellent for stopping bleeding and healing wounds, both internally and externally. It has powerful anti-inflammatory actions, soothing the skin and throat, and is used to treat conditions such as IBD and internal bleeding. Historically, it was revered as one of the best wound herbs, often used in simple salves made from pounded leaves and flowers mixed with honey. It is also used in infusions, gargles, washes, soaks, and decoctions for wound rinsing, burns, and bruises. Self-heal has a long history of being prized by ancient herbalists, and is mentioned in many historic herbal texts for its healing powers.

Magical significance

Associated with protection and healing energy. Linked with the "Heart of the Earth", Self-heal is often used in rituals and spells to heal the Earth, also to encourage self-care. In Irish folklore, Self-heal is one of the seven herbs that no evil could harm. It represents the power of healing oneself, and is used for protection, to stop the destruction and bleeding of the Earth's resources.

Foraging notes

Find: In gardens and parks. Mainly lawn edges, in damp, well-drained soil. Prefers shade.

Harvest: Leaves and flowers, spring–autumn. Best when in flower.

Shepherd's Purse (*Capsella bursa-pastoris*)

French: *Capselle bourse-à-pasteur*; Dutch: *Herderstasje*
Family: Brassicaceae

Annual plant, with white flowers and heart-shaped seed pouches. Flower stems are smooth. Tiny flowers (each with four petals) develop up the flower stem. The leaves form a basal rosette close to the ground initially, then grow upward as the plant matures, emitting an acrid, mildly Cabbage-like smell. Shepherd's Purse is a common weed, often found in urban environments, even in poor soil conditions, and can be seen year round.

Virtues

Used in herbal medicine to treat heavy bleeding, both internal and external. It is also used to treat severe diarrhoea and urinary disorders. Shepherd's Purse tea has a Cabbage-like aroma and is not particularly pleasant to taste. This herb is also used to ease nausea, either by boiling in spring water or eating raw in salads.

Magical significance

Associated with protection, resilience, and the ability to tolerate unpleasant circumstances. The heart-shaped seed pouches symbolise love, safeguarding, and invisibility. Its medicinal use for stopping bleeding can be applied symbolically to prevent waste of resources, or conservation.

Foraging notes

Find: Streets, around lamp posts and poles. Often has dust and debris tangled around it, making it less ideal for food or medicinal use. Most suited to magical work.

Harvest: Leaves, seeds, and flowers, during spring, summer, and autumn.

Snake Plant, Mother-in-law's Tongue (*Dracaena trifasciata* (Prain) Mabb.)

French: *Langue de belle-mère*; Dutch: *Vrouwentong*
Family: Asparagaceae

An evergreen plant with upright, strong leaf blades growing from a basal rosette, 60–120 cm tall. The leaves may be green or variegated, with a snakeskin-like pattern. Flowers occasionally, producing delicate, silver–white blooms and berry-like fruit. Formerly known as *Sansevieria trifasciata*.

Virtues

Often used as a spiky green barrier. It can lift the mood and is sometimes found in airports to absorb water from travellers' bottles. Some African communities use its leaf fibres for ropes and textiles. Snake Plants purify the air slightly but are mildly toxic and may cause dermatitis. Some indigenous populations use them for treating external swellings and skin infections.[13]

Magical significance

The tongue-like leaves of the Snake Plant are associated with truth, honesty, and clarity. It is a strong, sharp, and fiercely protective plant, often used to shield against the evil eye. The unique leaf pattern allows it to blend into its surroundings in the wild, making it suitable for protection work involving invisibility. Grow Snake Plants at entrances and boundaries to repel unwanted energies. Include them in rituals related to clear communication, overcoming barriers, and connecting with the spirit realm. Yellow-edged Snake Plants are especially associated with Oya, the mother goddess, protector, and mistress of storms in the Santeria, Afro-Caribbean religion. This powerful plant is used when fierce, maternal protection is called for.

---

[13] H. Kasmawati et al. Unrevealing the potential of *Sansevieria trifasciata* prain fraction for the treatment of androgenetic alopecia by inhibiting androgen receptors based on LC-MS/MS analysis, and in-silico studies. *Molecules* (Basel) (2022) 27(14): 4358.

Care notes

Easy to grow and tolerant of shade, but these plants do require some light. Water lightly when the soil dries out and avoid them standing in water, which can cause root rot. Repot and divide plants at the base when the pot becomes overcrowded with roots. Wipe Snake Plant leaves clean of dust and pollution occasionally. These plants enjoy spending summers outdoors.

Snapdragon (*Antirrhinum majus* L.)

French: *Muflier à grandes fleurs*; Dutch: *Grote leeuwenbek*
Family: Plantaginaceae

Herbaceous perennial, 50 cm–1 m tall (occasionally 2 m). The leaves are spirally arranged, broadly lanceolate, and can be 1–7 cm long and 2–2.5 cm wide. The stems are often glandular, sometimes woody towards the base. Snapdragons produce flowers on tall spikes, each flower being 3.5–4.5 cm long, with a unique 'lip' structure that gives them their characteristic appearance. Wild Snapdragons typically have pink to purple flowers with yellow lips, but cultivated varieties come in a wide range of colours, from pastel to bright shades of blue, orange, pink, purple, red, white, cream, or yellow.

Virtues

Popular in gardens and as cut flowers. They are also found in traditional medicine, where they have been used as a diuretic, and for treating scurvy, liver disorders, tumours, and various inflammatory conditions. Recent studies have shown Snapdragons possess antimicrobial, cytotoxic, antioxidant, and other biological activities.[14] If grown organically, the flowers and leaves can be used in salads, syrups, or as a bitter green. They are also suitable for use as a beautiful cut flower or as a soothing poultice.

Magical significance

Associated with curse breaking, protection, and guardianship. They are also linked to communication, often used in spells to help with truth-telling or to encourage honest conversations. Grow Snapdragons wherever you can, especially near your home and workplace.

---

[14] J. Seo et al. *Antirrhinum majus* L. flower extract inhibits cell growth and metastatic properties in human colon and lung cancer cell lines. *Food Sci & Nut*. (2020) 8(11): 6259–68. https://doi.org/10.1002/fsn3.1924

Foraging notes

Find: Gardens, streets, between cracks, against walls. Often in mucky locations.

Harvest: Summer, sparingly, to allow the plants to continue thriving. Be cautious with store-bought flowers, as they are usually sprayed with chemicals and should not be consumed. Grow your own if at all possible.

Spider Plant (*Chlorophytum comosum* (Thunb.) Jacques)

French: *Plante araignée*; Dutch: *Graslelie*
Family: Asparagaceae

Evergreen perennial native to seasonally dry tropical climates in Africa. It grows from thick, rhizomatous roots that produce numerous long, thin, green or variegated, striped leaves with a satiny, grass-like texture. This fast-growing, compact plant reaches a maximum height of 50 cm. Small white flowers periodically develop on long stems, which also produce "babies" or "spiderettes" that can be planted separately to propagate new plants.

Virtues

The roots and leaves of the Spider Plant are known for their nutritional and medicinal benefits. The mild, salad-like leaves are eaten as a green leafy vegetable in parts of Africa, and the cut leaves make a pleasant tea. The plant is known to support digestive, respiratory, bone, and sexual health for men and women. There is also much focus on its use to prevent and treat hormone-related acne, menstrual disorders like cramping and PMS, and breast cancer.[15] The plant is closely related to the rejuvenating Ayurvedic herb *Musli*. Additionally, it is a valuable air-purifying plant and is generally considered safe to grow around pets.

Magical significance

Associated with love, prosperity, growth, fertility, happiness, playfulness, and purification. Use Spider Plants in rituals to bring these qualities to life. They are well-suited for growing around an altar.

---

[15] I. Rzhepakovsky et al. Phytochemical characterization, antioxidant activity, and cytotoxicity of methanolic leaf extract of *Chlorophytum comosum* (green type) (Thunb.) Jacq. *Molecules* (Basel) (2022) 27(3): 762. https://doi.org/10.3390/molecules27030762

Harvesting and care notes

Find: As a houseplant.

Care: Water the plant when the soil is dry or when it begins to look wilted (ideally, just before this point).

Harvest: Ensure the plant is organically cultivated. Harvest during an annual trim by gathering the leaves together above the plant and cutting cleanly with sharp scissors.

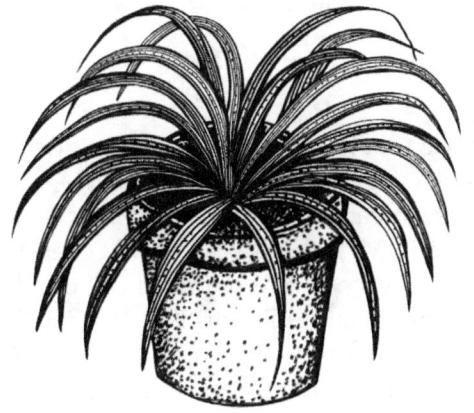

Stag's Horn Sumac (*Rhus typhina* L.)

French: *Sumac vinaigrier*; Dutch: *Fluweelboom*
Family: Anacardiaceae

A large deciduous shrub (3–6 m tall), with velvety branches, especially on new growth. Forms dense thickets by sending up new shoots and has large, lance-shaped leaves that turn bright red in autumn. Sumac produces upright pyramidal clusters of yellow–green flowers that give way to red fruit (drupes) resembling candles. These ripen in early autumn.

Virtues

Stag's Horn Sumac fruit has antimicrobial, antioxidant, and astringent properties. It is rich in tannins and vitamin C. It is used for conditions like diarrhoea, sore throats, and urinary tract infections. The dried fruit is a popular spice in Middle Eastern cuisine, often used as a Citrus substitute. It adds a tangy flavour to dishes and can be used whole or ground. Make a pink lemonade-like drink by soaking the ripe drupes in cold water, then straining and sweetening the liquid. Additionally, the plant has traditional uses in dyeing and as a smoke source for rituals.[16]

Magical significance

Associated with fire, energy, strength, vitality, and passion. Stag's Horn Sumac's upward-moving energy can be used to invigorate a space or ritual. Its bright red fruit clusters can be used in place of candles to maintain a symbolic flame. Stag's Horn Sumac lemonade can bring a little passion and energy to rituals.

Foraging notes

Find: In gardens or nearby hedges.

Look-alikes: Poison Sumac (*Toxicodendron vernix*) and Varnish Tree (*Toxicodendron vernicifluum*). Stag's Horn Sumac has upright red drupes and yellow–green flowers.

---

[16] T. Liu et al. Composition analysis and antioxidant activities of the *Rhus typhina* L. stem. *J Pharm Analy.* (2019) 9(5): 332–8.

Harvest: Late summer, collect vibrant red fruit before heavy rains, which can wash away flavour and cause mould. To check ripeness, wet your fingers, touch the berries, and taste for acidity. After harvesting, leave fruit on a light surface for a few hours to allow insects to escape. Avoid washing the fruit before making lemonade to preserve flavour.

St John's Wort (*Hypericum perforatum*)

French: *Millepertuis*; Dutch: *Sint Jans Kruid*
Family: Hypericaceae

Herbaceous perennial, up to 30 cm tall. A compact plant with small, simple leaves arranged in opposite pairs. In summer, oil glands fill with a red oil, visible when held to the light. Bright yellow flowers with showy stamens, in clusters at the top of the stems. A related species, Tutsan (*Hypericum androsaemum*), is larger with woodier stems. Tutsan can be used interchangeably with St John's Wort for magical purposes and in making skin oils and salves.

Virtues

Has bitter, analgesic, antiviral, and antidepressant properties. Used to ease muscle pain, encourage detoxification, lift mood, and help fight infections. Infused in water, oil, and footbaths. However, it should be used cautiously when taken internally, as it can speed the clearance of certain medications from the body. Tutsan was historically used for similar purposes.

Magical significance

Associated with protection and midsummer magic. St John's Wort brings sunshine, happiness, and health into rituals. The plant is often added to wreaths hung over doors, incorporated into saining bundles, or used in natural incense blends. Its infused water is sprinkled around working circles and used to cleanse magical tools. Tutsan can also be used in these practices, with its larger size making it particularly suitable for creating protective hedges in garden settings.

Foraging notes

Find: In neglected sandy soils, field edges, in full sun. Tutsan is a popular garden plant, often grown as a low hedge.

Harvest: Midsummer, ideally on sunny days. Hold up to light, red oil-filled leaf glands indicate potency. St John's Wort is often mistaken for Ragwort (*Jacobaea vulgaris*), which is toxic and dangerous to livestock, especially when dried and mixed into hay.

Succulents (Various)

French: *Plantes succulentes*; Dutch: *Vetplanten*
Family: mainly Crassulaceae: *Sempervivum, Aeonium, Sedum, Hylotelephium*

Plants with fleshy roots, stems, or leaves that store water in dry conditions. They vary from native species to those imported from arid regions. Unfortunately, some succulent species are threatened by over-harvesting and unsustainable practices.

Virtues

Some species are used to treat wounds, while others can cause irritation. Many have medicinal properties. Money Tree (*Crassula ovata*) can help wound healing, Houseleek (*Sempervivum* spp.) was used to soothe earache, and Rhodiola (*Rhodiola rosea*) can improve physical and mental endurance. Ice Plant (*Hylotelephium telephium* (L.) H. Ohba) is an edible perennial, grown in many cities. Euphorbiaceae family plants look similar to succulents but they contain toxic, corrosive sap.

Magical significance

Generally associated with wealth, abundance, good fortune, and preparation for tough times. Some have a rich history of folklore, such as Houseleeks (known as *Donderblad* or Thunderleaf in Dutch), which are said to protect homes from misfortune, e.g. lightning. Succulents can be grown in pots or on living roofs for protection. Try prominently displaying a Money Plant (*Pilea peperomioides* or *Crassula ovata*), which are long associated with prosperity and success.

Care notes

Tender succulents from warm climates need indoor care, especially in sunny spots. Replicate their native dry habitats by watering occasionally and ensuring well-draining soil. Some succulents grow well in pots or green roofs. If you plan to remove a few succulent leaves for rituals, do so during the growing season (late spring to summer).

Sugarcane (*Saccharum officinarum* L.)

French: *Canne à sucre*; Dutch: *Suikerriet*
Family: Poaceae

Upright, grassy plants, up to 2 m tall, from rhizomes. Sugarcane has been cultivated for 8,000–10,000 years and originates in New Guinea. Unrefined sugar was first produced in India around 2,500 years ago. Crusaders brought cane sugar to Europe in the late 1000s. At that time, it was treated as a luxury spice. Well before that time, Sugarcane's labour-intensive cultivation was linked to slavery. Production surged in the 1500s–1800s, when the colonial powers of Europe established plantations, using slave labour, in tropical regions. Still today, cane sugar production is rife with social and environmental exploitation; the process often involves burning plantations to control vermin, very strenuous physical labour, and heavy factory processing. The history of Sugarcane is inextricably linked to domination, pain, and slavery. Cane sugar should be treated as a precious commodity. Only Fair Trade organic sugar should be purchased.

Virtues

Inner fibrous stem contains a sweet and nutritious juice. Unrefined forms of sugar, such as jaggery, rapadura, and oerzoet have a rich scent and flavour. In China Sugarcane was used as a sweet vegetable, as a medicinal plant from around AD 317. European medieval herbals show its use in various remedies, and sugar remains popular in traditional herbal medicine, such as Indonesian Jamu, to balance flavours.

Magical significance

Associated with sweetness and attraction. Use when trying to activate or attract positive energy. Empower sigils and symbols by tracing them with sugar water; when dry the crystals can be burned, buried, or consumed in rituals. In candle magic, sugar can be pressed into warm wax and engraved symbols. Some practitioners stand spell candles in small bowls of sugar, or extinguish flames with sugar water or herb syrup. Layering magical herbs with sugar in a small jar will increase the power of both ingredients.

Harvesting and care notes

Care: Can be grown in well-drained soil with plenty of water and sunshine in summer, and indoor shelter when temperatures drop below about 5°C. The purple *S. officinarum purpurea* is smaller and can grow well in a large pot.

Harvest: Purple canes when at least one season old, and about 6 cm diameter. Larger canes yield more sweetness but the plant can be cut back at any time. Cut a whole cane then chop into shorter sections, about 15 cm long. Slice the outer skin with a long vertical cut then peel it away to reveal the sweet flesh. The lower portions of cane are the sweetest. Protect yourself from the sharp-edged leaves and regularly apply an organic fertiliser to your plants during the growing season.

Sweet Chestnut (*Castanea sativa* Mill.)

French: *Châtaignier commun*; Dutch: *Tamme kastanje*
Family: Fagaceae

Medium to large tree. Wide-spreading branches and long (to 28 cm), glossy, oval leaves, with pointed tips and serrated edges. Can live 700 years in warmer regions. Wind-pollinated flowers and catkins are present on each tree. Edible nuts fall during autumn, enclosed in cases that are velvety inside and prickly outside. At least two nuts are found within each case, but their size and quality vary. Sweet Chestnut trees have smooth grey–purple bark, similar to the related Beech, with long, vertical fissures.

Virtues

Sweet Chestnut leaves are astringent, expectorant, and antimicrobial. They are also used to help coughs and colds, but additionally for diarrhoea and skin complaints. Try making tea from the young leaves for these purposes. The sweet nuts can be eaten fresh, roasted, puréed, ground into flour, or boiled in water or syrup. Add to porridge, cakes, rice, soups, and spreads. Sweet Chestnuts are nourishing and medicinal, and are used in some regions for respiratory complaints.

Magical significance

Associated with fertility, abundance, nourishment, strength, attraction, sweetness, and success. Place in charm bags. Eat Sweet Chestnuts at autumn feasts. In Greek mythology, this tree is associated with Zeus.

Foraging notes

Find: In parks and large gardens.

Harvest: Nuts from fallen cases in autumn; leaves in spring/summer from mature trees. Look for the serrated leaf edge and avoid confusion with Horse Chestnuts (*Aesculus*), which should not be eaten. Horse Chestnut leaves consist of 5–7 large leaflets in a hand-like shape. Sweet Chestnut leaves grow singly along the branches. Horse Chestnut cases are harder, spiny, and contain one large conker. They form from tall clusters of showy flowers.

Sweet Cicely (*Myrrhis odorata* L.)

French: *Cerfeuil musqué*; Dutch: *Roomse kervel*
Family: Apiaceae

Hardy perennial with Anise-scented, fern-like leaves. Emerges early in spring and may persist through mild winters. Grows up to 90 cm, with umbrella-shaped clusters of white flowers that develop into flask-shaped seedpods.

Virtues

Sweet Cicely has carminative and digestive properties. It helps stimulate digestion, relieve trapped gas, and aid in the smooth passage of food through the gut. Leaves, flowers, and seeds have a sweet, musky, Anise-like flavour. Young leaves can be used fresh in salads, or chopped into sauces and desserts. Green unripe seeds can be chewed to freshen breath and ease digestion. Dip the flowerheads in batter for tempura (although better to leave on the plants to set seed). Use foliage to flavour stewed fruits and jams. Sweet Cicely is often used to make schnapps, syrup, or liqueur.

Magical significance

Associated with bringing sweetness, delight, and upliftment. It is often used to impart clarity and cheerfulness, making it a valuable addition to magical practices aimed at enhancing mood and bringing lightness into one's life. In Welsh tradition, Sweet Cicely is often found in graveyards, where it is used to rub on wooden tools and magical items to give a pleasant scent and positive energy. Sweet Cicely is useful in rituals and spells intended to uplift the spirit and bring clarity of mind.

Foraging notes

Find: Shady gardens and woodland edges.

Harvest: Leaves from Imbolc to midsummer; seedpods from Beltane.
Avoid confusion with Poison Hemlock (*Conium maculatum*).

Swiss Cheese Plant (*Monstera deliciosa* Liebm.)

French: *Faux philodendron*; Dutch: *Gatenplant*
Family: Araceae

Large, climbing tropical vine, from Central America (up to 20 m x 20 m). Heart-shaped leaves with fenestrations (holes) and tough aerial roots. Occasional flowers resemble Lords and Ladies (*Arum maculatum*); both plants are in the Araceae. The slow-maturing fruit, known as Banana-Pineapple, is a tropical delicacy. In young plants, the leaves secrete excess water, as drops from the leaf tips. This guttation is natural; the drops may be collected and used in rituals but not on the skin.

Virtues

Green parts are toxic if ingested, owing to calcium oxalate, which painfully irritates mucous membranes. The scientific name, meaning delicious monster, refers to the fruit. *Monstera* filters air, so it should be kept dust-free. It is possible to train them up walls and beneath ceilings, to create green healing spaces. The plant has traditionally been used as both a poison and an anti-inflammatory remedy, but only the ripe fruit is edible. The green parts and sap must be handled with care.

Magical significance

Associated with strength, luck, prosperity, friendships, collaboration, purity, fertility, creativity, growth, longevity, and ancestry. They are ideal for spells aimed at bringing big plans into the world, especially when a slow, steady approach is needed. Growing this plant creates a large, positive presence. Collect guttation drops from the leaves for use in rituals linked to the plant's magical associations.

Care notes

Provide plenty of space and support, in a semi-shade location. Water when the top two centimetres of soil are dry. To prevent root rot, grow in well-draining soil and avoid it standing in water. Occasionally shower with tepid water, or wipe with a damp cloth to remove dust. These special green monsters are easy to care for but should be kept away from leaf-nibbling humans and companion animals.

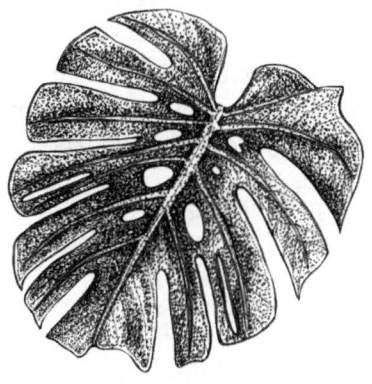

Sycamore (*Acer pseudoplatanus*)

French: *Érable sycomore*; Dutch: *Esdoorn*
Family: Sapindaceae

Large, fast-growing deciduous tree with broad, palmate leaves. Grey–brown bark when young, becoming cracked and scaled with age. Clusters of green–yellow flowers after Beltane, then pairs of winged seeds (helicopters). Seeds germinate quickly, populating gardens and parks. Can regenerate from its roots. Sycamore provides shelter and food for wildlife, including Aphids, which excrete sticky honeydew on the leaves.

Virtues

As with Maple trees, Sycamore has a sweet sap, which rises from the roots to crown and can be tapped from large trunks, in early spring. To create a syrup from this sap, much simmering, time, and fuel are needed. So it is better to drink the sap or dilute the liquid 50:50 with vodka to help preserve it. Sycamore leaves are not very appetising. They can be wrapped around baked goods, such as bread rolls, as they cook, to impart a slight sweetness. Fresh leaves are astringent. They can be decocted and used as a skin wash. Sycamore wood is resistant and durable, and can be crafted into strong tools. Fallen leaves make attractive bookmarks.

Magical significance

Associated with fertility, growth, sweetness, expansion, regeneration, and success. Often grown near exposed buildings for protection. Sycamore is a generous tree, and using it in magic attracts positive energy and nourishment. You may like to create messages and sigils using colourful autumn Sycamore leaves. They can be temporarily glued to surfaces with a dab of honey. Spells and charms can be written directly on the large flat leaves. Sycamore sap can be used as an invisible ink. Ancient Greeks poured wine on the soil by Sycamore tree roots, as an offering.

Foraging notes

Find: In hedges and parks.

Harvest: Seeds in autumn, young leaves in late spring, and sap in spring from a healthy tree.

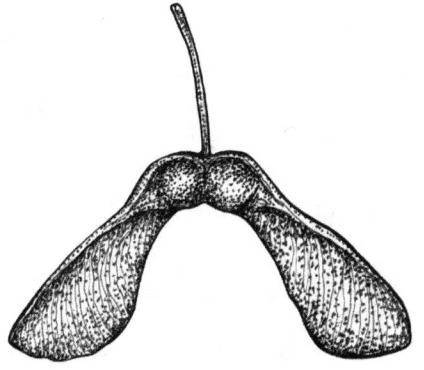

Tea Plant (*Camellia sinensis* var. *sinensis*; *C. sinensis* var. *assamica*)

Chinese: *chá*; Japanese: *cha*; French: *Théier*; Dutch: *Theeplant*
Family: Theaceae

Evergreen shrub or tree, typically kept at 1.5 m but grows taller in the wild. Described by Li Yu (AD 760–780) as having "leaves like Gardenia, flowers like wild white Rose". Dark green, lanceolate leaves grow on strong branches, with pale green tips that are used to make the world's second most popular beverage. Beautiful solitary white flowers with showy stamens bloom in early spring or late winter.

Virtues

Tea contains tannins, caffeine, and antioxidant polyphenols. Matcha, powdered green tea leaves, contains the most concentrated levels of these beneficial phytonutrients. Adding milk reduces how much of it can enter the body. Tea's astringency is useful for calming the gut and treating skin irritations. Cooled, strong tea can be used as a soothing rinse for sore eyelids. Tea has been shown to reduce cancer risk, slow ageing, and support heart health. It is also used for headaches, and as a stimulant (when consumed in the morning) or calming nervine (consumed in the evening). Tea can be used as a hair dye and skin stain. It was popular as a stocking substitute during wartime Europe. Green tea leaves are quickly steamed after plucking. This preserves the green colour and the fresh, grassy flavours of the leaves. The leaves are then rolled and dried. For black tea, harvested leaves are allowed to fully oxidise before drying; this helps develop rich, robust flavours.

Magical significance

Tea has a recent and uncomfortable place in Western magic. It was brought here through colonisation, exploitation, and pain. Some associate it with fortune, but this is inappropriate. Focus instead on Tea's millennia-long tradition of improving health and wellbeing. Notice how it can shift consciousness, and use it as a symbol of courage over adversity. Use in magic that honours origins, respects boundaries, and seeks repair. Tea is a potent reminder of the far-reaching effects of dominance and disregard.

Foraging notes

Find: Rarely in Europe, although popular as Bonsai.

Harvest: Bright green tender young leaves can be harvested twice a year. Harvest some entire leaves, not only leaf tips.

Purchase: Only Fair Trade tea. Slavery and misfortune is still rife in the Tea-trade.

Thuja (Red and White Cedar) (*Thuja occidentalis* L.; *Thuja plicata* L.)

French: *Thuya géant, Arbor vitae*; Dutch: *Levensboom, Reuzenlevensboom*
Family: Cupressaceae

Evergreen conifers with flattened needle-like branchlets. Thuja species vary widely, from towering 70 m trees to small potted varieties. They produce small, aromatic cones with overlapping scales that stand upright in clusters on branchlets. Thuja trees typically have a tidy apex. Their dense foliage and thirst often suppress growth beneath them but they coexist well in forests.

Virtues

Thuja occidentalis is the best-known medicinal species. Owing to its toxic chemicals, internal use is not recommended. Infused or essential oils, used sparingly, may help with respiratory infections, cold sores, skin issues, warts, and joint pain. It should never be used during pregnancy or breastfeeding. Thuja wood and foliage dust can cause irritation or allergies. These trees offer nesting sites for birds and food for some animals. Thuja is significant in Native American culture, being used for totem poles, canoes, and rope.

Magical significance

Associated with protection, cleansing, and purifying. It also offers a form of invisibility, helping us to hide in plain sight. In areas where Thuja grows wild, such as Japan and Korea, these trees are revered as part of the cultural heritage. Thuja branchlets can be tightly bundled and dried for outdoor saining. Avoid inhalation of the smoke as it is toxic. Collect Thuja cones for ritual work; these can also be included in natural incense blends. Thuja tea can be used to cleanse ritual spaces and any magical tools which will not be used for food or drink.

Foraging notes

Find: In parks and gardens. Look for a pyramidal bush, and the characteristic upward-pointing cones. Many hybrids are grown as this is an attractive evergreen for gardens.

Harvest: Cones when found, throughout the year.

Thyme (*Thymus vulgaris* L.)

French: *Thym commun*; Dutch: *Echte tijm*
Family: Lamiaceae

Aromatic, shrubby perennial. Tiny evergreen, oval leaves. Square stems become woody with age. Grows to 10–30 cm tall with small purple flowers that bloom from late spring to summer, attracting Bees.

Virtues

Has antiseptic, antimicrobial, and warming properties. Use in teas to soothe coughs, sore throats, and digestive issues, and in salves and oils for muscle aches and skin conditions. Infuse in bathwater, or foot soaks to help relieve respiratory and rheumatic problems. Thyme is also a useful insect repellent. Its strong, warm, and spicy flavour can enhance soups, stews, sauces, meats, and vegetables.

Magical significance

Associated with healing, purification, protection, and love. Thyme is historically believed to aid in visualising Fairies. It can be used in baths and incense for cleansing purposes, and in love divination, such as placing it in shoes to dream of a future lover. It has also been used to protect against bewitchment, to fumigate orchards, and is sometimes taken when moving house to carry luck. Additionally, Thyme is associated with courage and strength, and in remembrance—it can be thrown on the coffin of a deceased friend as a symbol of wishing them luck on their onward journey. Try sewing sprigs or leaves of dried Thyme into the seams of clothes, to protect the wearer; in Sweden, this was traditionally done for Bridegrooms.

Foraging notes

Find: Parks and gardens, or as a potted kitchen herb.

Harvest: Lightly trim fresh growing tips with scissors or fingers, during the growing season. Winter harvesting often damages plants. Harvest just before full flowering for most potency. Dry the stems, then strip leaves and flowers, or use whole sprigs.

Turmeric and Ginger (*Curcuma longa* L.; *Zingiber officinale* Roscoe)

French: *Curcuma, Gingembre*; Dutch: *Curcuma; Gember*
Family: Zingiberaceae

Closely related rhizomatous perennials with tightly coiled leaves that mature into sturdy, spicy-scented stems. Originally from India, these plants may develop stunning flowers when grown at home.

Virtues

The flowers, foliage, and rhizomes of Ginger and Turmeric can be used in food and remedies. Ginger has anti-inflammatory, antibacterial, and digestive properties. It is useful for colds, flu, colic, nausea, impaired circulation, arthritis, and menstrual discomfort. Turmeric has anti-inflammatory, antiseptic, and cancer-fighting properties. It is used in many skin treatments, though it may stain. Turmeric incense can relieve sinus congestion.

Both feature prominently in Jamu, Indonesian traditional medicine. Add both herbs to diets or make remedies like muscle rubs using fresh Ginger juice and Olive oil. A paste of Ginger, Turmeric, and Aloe Vera soothes aching joints. Ginger soothes sore throats when sucked raw. Both are great in teas and Golden Milk. Regular intake promotes health, but avoid excess Turmeric especially if on blood thinners.

Magical significance

Both herbs are associated with spiciness, energy, growth, and protection from malevolent spirits Use them in rituals intended to heat things up and get things moving. Turmeric is more earthy and grounding than Ginger. Turmeric has been revered since ancient times in Asia, as a symbol of the Sun and light.

Harvesting and care notes

Care: Warm, humid environments like bright bathrooms. Plant organic Ginger rhizomes partly exposed and Turmeric shallowly, but completely buried. Keep soil moist; rhizomes sprout within a month if humidity is maintained (use a plastic bag tent). Remove the tent when stems grow a few centimetres tall.

Harvest: Lift rhizomes in winter after the plant dies back, snapping off portions while leaving the rest to regrow. Trim stems and leaves during the growing season. Enjoy flowers on the plant if they appear.

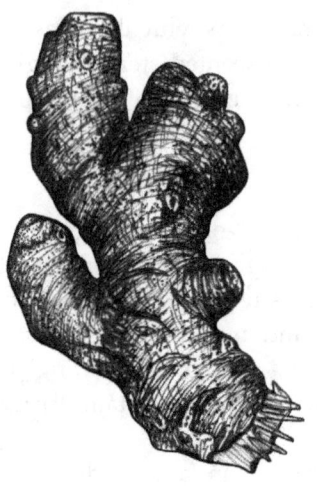

Violet and Pansy (*Viola* spp.)

French: *Violettes et Pensées*; Dutch: *Viooltjes en Hoornviooltjes*
Family: Violaceae

Low-growing, spreading herbs. Violets are evergreen perennials with heart-shaped leaves and small, fragrant, purple flowers. They thrive in shady woodlands. Leaves are pale when young, dark green when mature. Pansies are cultivated hybrids with larger, showy flowers in many colours and patterns. They have rounded leaves. Both plants sprawl and have flowers with two upper petals, two side petals, and a larger lower petal.

Virtues

Violet flowers taste mildly sweet, sometimes a little spicy. Pansies are more grassy than sweet. Both can be added as fresh floating flowers on soups, casseroles, and drinks. Or sugar-coat and use to decorate desserts. Young Violet leaves can be included in salads or brewed into tea. Eaten raw, they taste a little gritty and glutenous. The flowers and leaves of both plants can be made into strikingly coloured flower syrups and candies. Sweet Violets (*V. odorata*) are traditionally used for respiratory infections such as coughs, colds, and flu, where they soothe and help clear phlegm. They are used alongside some cancer treatments, to support healing, and can be used externally to speed healing of grazed or irritated skin.

Magical significance

Associated with modesty, emotional healing, protection, purification, and tranquillity. Dried flowers add colour and spark to incense blends and altars. Pansies are especially symbolic of thoughts and remembrance. They are well suited to love spells, divination, and rituals aimed at enhancing creativity and clarity of thought. The faces of fresh Pansies can also be used to represent individual targets, in symbolic magic.

Foraging notes

Find: Violets in shaded gardens and park woodlands. Pansies provide seasonal colour in gardens, parks and pots.

Harvest: Flowers on spring mornings after dew dries; handle gently. Young, pale-green leaves spring and summer. Avoid non-organic Pansies grown with pesticides.

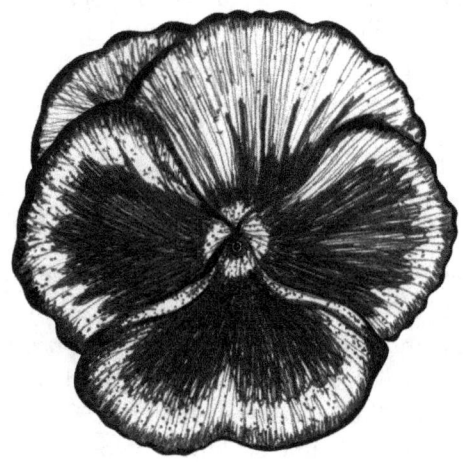

Wild Garlic/Ramsons (*Allium ursinum* L.)

French: *Ail des ours*; Dutch: *Daslook*
Family: Amaryllidaceae

Garlic-scented woodland perennial. Forms a lush carpet of bright green, lance-shaped leaves. The Garlic aroma intensifies through spring. Bulbs are white and ovoid. Flower stalks can reach 45 cm tall. They bear clusters of star-shaped white flowers. These develop into small, black seeds. It thrives before woodland trees are full of leaves.

Virtues

Wild Garlic has a mild Garlic flavour, with leaves, seeds, and flowers all being edible. The leaves can be used fresh in salads, cooked in soups, or made into pesto. The bulbs and seeds, though milder than cultivated Garlic, can be used similarly. The plant shares medicinal properties with Garlic, including diuretic, antiseptic, and respiratory benefits. It is used in traditional remedies for throat infections, skin inflammation, and high blood pressure. This plant is also an ingredient in Four Thieves Vinegar.

Magical significance

Associated with protection, cleansing, and aphrodisiac qualities. It has a playful fairy-like energy, tempting us into the woods. Traditionally, this plant was grown near homes for protective benefits and used in purification rituals. Use any part of Wild Garlic in magical work connected with protection.

Foraging notes

Find: In shaded, moist locations, including parks and gardens.

Harvest: Early spring when the leaves are tender and flavourful; bulbs, from paths in spring; flowers and seeds, late spring.

Look-alike: Toxic Lily of the Valley (*Convallaria majus*) and poisonous Dog's Mercury (*Mercurialis perennis*) often grow among Wild Garlic. When foraging, ensure accurate identification by its distinctive Garlic smell, and harvest carefully, leaf by leaf, to avoid damaging the environment.

Willow (*Salix* L.)

French: *Saule*; Dutch: *Wilg*
Family: Salicaceae

Fast-growing, water-loving trees. Slender stems grow from mature branches and deeply grooved, gnarled bark. Stems are yellow, red or green. Leaves are usually long and lanceolate, although Goat Willow (*Salix caprea*) leaves are oval. Soft female catkins attract pollinating insects. Some Willows have a weeping form, with narrow, trailing stems, while others are broad with upright stems. Willows are often pollarded (upper growth is pruned) or coppiced (ground-level pruning), regenerating with a mass of pliable stems in spring. Willows support a wide range of wildlife. Closely related to Poplar and Birch.

Virtues

The inner bark is astringent and analgesic, and can be used to soothe joints and reduce swelling. Externally, used as a poultice or compress to stop bleeding and relieve pain. Soothe headaches by chewing a thin stem. Willow tea (bark or catkins) can reduce fever and ease coughs, catarrh, and indigestion. The bark also helps cuttings of other plants to root; stand them in a cup of water containing chopped or living Willow and wait for new roots to form. Willow wood is used to make cricket bats. Young, flexible stems are woven into baskets, fences, and shelters.

Magical significance

Associated with the water element, whispering spirits, the Moon; you may notice that they have a shimmering energy. For the Celts, they were connected with the harp and the gentle soul of the poet. Try sitting beneath a Willow to write poetry or create spells. Supple Willow stems can be woven into headdresses or garlands in spring.

Foraging notes

Find: Near water.

Harvest: Pliable young stems, or catkins. Wash, cut fine stems, and use directly or peel bark from slightly thicker ones, with a knife or vegetable peeler.

Winter Purslane/Miner's Lettuce
(*Claytonia perfoliata; C. sibirica*)

French: *Pourpier d'hiver*; Dutch: *Winterpostelein*
Family: Montiaceae

Hardy annual, up to 30 cm tall and wide. Begins as a rosette of small, spade-shaped succulent leaves, maturing into dense clumps. Leaves are fleshy, round. Tiny white or mauve-streaked flowers grow above the fused leaves.

Virtues

With a mild, refreshing, crisp taste, Winter Purslane is possibly the best wild addition to salads. When adding to soups and casseroles, the leaves need brief cooking. Rich in vitamins, minerals, and chlorophyll. Winter Purslane can help support the immune system, detoxification, and overall health. It has a gentle laxative effect and may aid in removing heavy metals and toxins from the body. Easy to juice. A poultice can help speed the healing of cuts and sores, and soothe painful joints.

Magical significance

Associated with prosperity and good fortune. This is owing to its rapid growth and association with the California gold rush (hence the alternative name Miner's Lettuce). Discovering a mature Winter Purslane plant can be seen as a positive sign to seize and cultivate opportunities without delay. Use in spells and rituals related to wealth, sudden gains, and good health.

Foraging notes

Find: Below hedges and railings, occasionally in flower beds.

Harvest: Year round, especially in winter. If many are found, wait for dome-shaped plants to develop then twist off at the base of the rosette. Look-alikes include edible Chickweed (*Stellaria media*) and toxic Euphorbia species like Petty Spurge (*Euphorbia peplus*), which have irritating sap.

Witch Hazel (*Hamamelis Gronov. ex L.*)

French: *Hamamélis*; Dutch: *Toverhazelaar*
Family: Hamamelidaceae

Deciduous shrub, up to 5 m, with crooked, spreading branches. Its name probably derives from the Old English word *wice*, meaning bendable, owing to its pliable branches. It is an inconspicuous shrub until its shaggy yellow–red flowers erupt in winter. These are followed by explosive seedcases. Leaves, alternately arranged, similar to Elm.

Virtues

This potent herb should only be used externally, unless under expert supervision. It has an intense astringent action. Cooled infusion of Witch Hazel bark, twigs, or leaves makes a useful skin toner. It can relieve bruises, varicose veins, insect stings, and bites. The tea (externally) is a good alternative to Distilled Witch Hazel, which is sold by many pharmacists. Powdered Witch Hazel bark is used in creams or pastes for haemorrhoids.

Magical significance

Associated with fresh starts and renewal. Witch Hazel has a silver, shimmering energy, mystical and Moon-like. Its ability to dry and tighten can be woven into spellwork where the intention is to slow things down, or to prevent things from leaking away. Use Witch Hazel in Moon and water rituals. Traditionally, the forked branches have been used for water divination. The beautiful flowers are best left on the shrub, to provide winter colour, but they dry well and can be used in rituals. The empty seedcases are useful for altars, and as amulets.

Witch Hazel is a traditional medicine plant of Native Americans; taken to Europe from America by returning European settlers. I suggest you build your own relationship with this shrub.

Foraging notes

Find: In shrubberies of parks and gardens; thrives in urban environments and tolerates pollution.

Harvest: Leaves in spring/summer; bark from pruned branches in autumn. Avoid removing bark from live branches. This shrub is sensitive to harsh pruning. Flowers in midwinter.

Wood Avens/Herb Bennet (*Geum urbanum* L.)

French: *Benoîte commune*; Dutch: *Geel nagelkruid*
Rosaceae

Perennial with a basal rosette. Compound leaves, with large terminal lobe and smaller intermediate leaflets. Up to 60 cm height when flowering. Yellow, five-petalled flowers resemble Strawberry blossoms, with showy stamens and green sepals. Flowers from Beltane to midwinter, producing burr-like seedheads for effective dispersal.

Virtues

Wood Avens roots have a delicate, sweet, and spicy clove-like flavour owing to eugenol, a phytochemical also found in Clove (*Syzygium aromaticum*), making them suitable for seasoning biscuits, casseroles, broths, soups, syrups, and liqueurs. They don't dry well and should be used sparingly. Try preserving in oil, alcohol, or honey. The foliage has a mild flavour, useful in salads or as a cooked green. Medicinally, the analgesic roots can be chewed, or used in oil infusions, for toothache relief. Leaf and root poultices may also ease haemorrhoids. Wood Avens leaf tea is astringent and helps tighten gums, and soothe gastrointestinal issues.

Magical significance

Associated with protection from evil and negativity, and with easing pain, despair, and heartache. Wear an amulet and hang over doors. Look for it in ornate city architecture. Try incorporating the flower design into sigils. Use in spellwork to help heal from loss and sadness. It can also be used when breaking hexes and curses. Amulets and jars filled with the dried herb should be refreshed often, to maintain potency.

Foraging notes

Find: Shady edges of parks, gardens, and woodland. Easy to grow in pots, allowing plants to be lifted for gentle root harvest a few times a year.

Harvest: Roots (autumn equinox—Samhain). Take only 10% root growth each time, and replant carefully. Leaves: throughout the year, best spring/summer. The flowers are often confused with Cinquefoils (*Potentilla* species), so check the leaves, which are very different.

Wormwood (*Artemisia absinthium* L.)

French: *Absinthe*; Dutch: *Absintalsem*
Asteraceae

Woody, shrubby perennial. Up to 1 m tall and 80 cm wide. Soft, grey–green, deeply divided leaves, each with three main lobes. Wormwood leaves are covered on both sides with tiny downy hairs. Starts compact and bushy (late spring), developing tall, loose, flower stems. Flowers are tiny and wind-pollinated (yellow–green). All parts are highly aromatic. Tolerates dry, sandy soil and spreads efficiently by seed.

Virtues

Wormwood is bitter, aromatic, and antimicrobial. Used to flavour digestives, liqueurs like absinthe, and foods. Try adding a pinch to preparations where bitterness is required. Wormwood is used to treat gut inflammation, parasites, and depression. It contains a toxic phytochemical called thujone, which can cause adverse effects. Wormwood is also useful as an insecticide. It must be avoided by pregnant or breastfeeding women.

Magical significance

Associated with protection and divination, and is often used in saining rituals, creative endeavours, and to chase away pains and anguish. The plant is linked to Artemis, goddess of the Moon, and is believed to counteract poisoning. Wormwood is used in spells and charms for protection, love, and to lift melancholy. It is a powerful tool for exorcising negative energies and spirits. Place under doormats, over doors. Hide it away for quiet protection.

Foraging notes

Find: Gardens and streets (as escapes).

Harvest: Soft growing tips or individual woody stems from close to the base of the plant. Use sparingly owing to its potent effects and potential toxicity. Harvesting is best done during midsummer when the flowers are about to open. Look-alike Mugwort has hairs only on the underside of leaves.

Wormwood is endangered in many European countries so only harvest from cultivated plants.

Yarrow (*Achillea millefolium*)

French: *Achillée millefeuille*; Dutch: *Duizendblad*
Family: Asteraceae

Aromatic perennial up to 80 cm tall. Feathery, deeply divided leaves grow flat on the ground before becoming upright in summer. Strong, round, woody stems bear some leaves. Flat-top clusters of small flowers with five white to pale pink ray petals around a central disc. Some cultivars feature vibrant pink or red flowers. In lawns, Yarrow often appears as a miniature plant, rarely flowering.

Virtues

Yarrow has antiseptic, anti-inflammatory, and haemostatic properties. It is a useful bitter digestive wound herb, often known as the "Herb of Seven Cures". Yarrow leaf and flower tea are used to cleanse wounds, and soothe coughs, colds, and digestive issues. It can help regulate bleeding and blood pressure, and relieve rheumatism pain. Add small amounts of Yarrow to salads, or syrups, liqueurs, and baked goods, for a unique bitter–aromatic flavour. May cause contact allergy and nosebleeds.

Magical significance

Associated with love, protection, and divination, this herb is most potent at Samhain and Beltane. Include Yarrow sticks in fire-lighting bundles. Infuse in water for ritual cleansing and protection. For divination, wash crystal balls or scrying mirrors with Yarrow water. Cut seven Yarrow sticks of equal length and store in a special cloth; throw the sticks and interpret patterns, especially for matters of love and protection. Carry in protective charm bags, or sew into clothing hems. Use Yarrow in spells for love, fertility, and clairvoyance. Many Celtic love charms centred on Yarrow. Weave the flowers into wedding rituals and decorations.

Foraging notes

Find: Sunny lawns, verges, and parkland.

Harvest: Leaves, year round. Harvest for rituals at Beltane or Samhain.

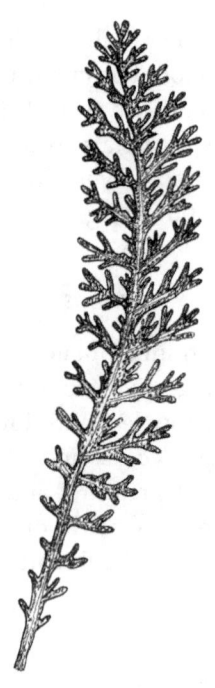

Yew (*Taxus* L.)

French: *If commun*; Dutch: *Venijnboom*
Family: Taxaceae

Evergreen conifer with shiny, dark green flat needles (new growth is light green). Females produce red (or yellow) berry-like fruits (arils), enclosing a tiny cone. Dense foliage creates deep shade. Long-lived and slow-growing, Yews can live thousands of years. They resist parasites and infections. As they age, new trees may emerge from within, forming a copse. Yews don't truly change sex but can temporarily express opposite-sex features, giving them a gender-fluid reputation.

Virtues

All parts are toxic except for the ripe aril. Taxol, a powerful anti-cancer compound used in chemotherapy, was first derived from the Pacific Yew (*Taxus brevifolia*). Today, Yew clippings from municipal gardens are periodically harvested for Taxol production. Some mammals eat tiny amounts of Yew foliage regularly, and build resistance. Historically, controlled doses of Yew leaves and bark treated respiratory ailments and were used as external skin washes. Even small doses can be lethal so do not experiment. Used in homoeopathy for skin, urinary, and rheumatic conditions. Yew wood, fine-grained and yellow, is prized for archery bows and wood carving.

Magical significance

Associated with long life, death, wisdom, judgement, and protection. Common in British graveyards, and closely associated with ancestral worship. Yew wood is suitable for making staffs or wands but not for kitchen tools, owing to its toxicity. Pictish warriors used Yew for poison-tipped arrows, and Druids washed their dead in Yew infusion. Religious relics were often kept safe in Yew boxes, until very recently. Yew is not suited to use in incense blends.

Foraging notes

Find: In hedges, graveyards, and parks. Yew is sometimes mistaken for Spruce.

Harvest: Only the red ripe aril is edible; do not consume the seed-like cone inside, or the foliage. Use extreme caution. Keep Yew safely away from pets and children, as even eating small amounts can be fatal.

Zebra Plant (*Tradescantia zebrina* Bosse)

French: *Zebrina pendula*; Dutch: *Vaderplant*
Family: Commelinaceae

Slightly succulent ground cover plant. Stems are jointed where the leaves emerge. Leaves are green or purple, with silvery stripes. Also known as the Inch Plant, it trails or creeps along the ground. This plant is native to Central America. Grows up to 60 cm tall, with stems trailing longer.

Virtues

Leaves and stems have antiseptic, painkilling, astringent, and haemostatic properties. In Costa Rica, an infusion is used to wash wounds or relieve facial nerve pain (as a compress). In some regions, it is used to help treat high blood pressure, though the plant is considered toxic to mammals if ingested, and the sap may irritate sensitive skin.

Magical significance

Associated with success in travel, relocation, expansion, and money. Spend time with Zebra Plants to help contemplate how to wisely use your energy. Include them in rituals to help find new directions in your life. Also consult their wisdom when dealing with takeovers, and invasions of space. Encourage the plant to grow upwards and outwards; if allowed to trail too much, downward energy may lower your mood. If you need better focus for challenging tasks, try pruning your Zebra Plant. This can keep you both growing in the right direction.

Harvest and care notes

Care: Zebra Plants prefer warm, bright conditions. They can tolerate shade and periods of neglect, but thrive with care. Water when the top soil feels dry, and avoid waterlogged roots. Tidy up and lightly prune when needed. Entire stems may drop off periodically; this is a natural attempt to spread and propagate. It is also a sign that your plant needs better soil or care. Zebra Plants can be easily grown from cuttings.

Harvest: Lightly and occasionally from healthy, vigorous plants.

ZZ-Plant (*Zamioculcas zamiifolia* (G. Lodd.) Engl.)

French: *Plante ZZ*; Dutch: *ZZ plant*
Family: Araceae

Glossy evergreen plant, 50–60 cm tall with tall succulent stems. Stems support oval leaves. The ZZ-Plant is a great choice for locations which don't receive much daylight, and for people who forget to water their plants. They look good too—with tall, glossy, dark green leaves.

Virtues

The ZZ-plant is an ancient medicinal plant from Africa. When snapped, the foliage releases a distinctive white chocolate aroma—a pleasure, but don't taste; the sap is said to contain calcium oxalate crystals. Calcium oxalate is toxic when ingested, and is found in other members of the notoriously toxic Araceae family. In Malawi and Tanzania ZZ-Plant leaf juice is used to treat earache, and a poultice of roots and leaves is used to relieve local inflammation and skin ulcers. It has been found by research to contain potent anti-inflammatory and antimicrobial plant chemicals, but it should not be used internally.

Magical significance

Associated with resilience, luck, fortune, style, perseverance, and tolerance. The upward-pointed leaves also bring protection by deflecting unwanted energy up and away. Grow at home and workplaces as a protective presence. Bring to indoor rituals linked with its magical associations, and when tending the plant whisper money and career charms.

Care notes

Care: This plant is drought-resistant so water occasionally, when the top centimetres of soil dry out and avoid standing the roots in water, as they will rot. If positioned in full Sun, daily watering may be needed, so be attentive to its appearance. Repot annually and create new plants by separating some of the rhizomes.

Harvesting: Although the toxicity of ZZ-Plant is unproven, it is wise to prevent people and pets from nibbling it.

Animal lore directory

Urban areas are home to a surprising diversity of wildlife, each playing a role in city ecosystems. Some of these animals are secretive, while others seem willing to form relationships with humans. Interactions with wildlife can feel magical, but it's important to avoid creating dependence, for their wellbeing and ours.

The Animal Lore entries that follow mention the key traits of commonly encountered city creatures. There is also a mix of modern and traditional symbolism. Let the information inspire, not dictate how you relate to your wild neighbours. Your own local observations will be more relevant than folklore based on rural creatures—which is where most traditional animal lore comes from. Also bear in mind that superstition has unfairly tarnished some animals' reputations. So observe the creatures in your own environment, and decide for yourself which magical associations resonate best with them.

Amphibians

Common European Newt (*Lissotriton vulgaris*)

French: *Triton commun*; Dutch: *Gewone salamander*

Small, nocturnal amphibian found in damp habitats. Able to regenerate lost limbs. Newts are well camouflaged and are secretive. They hide under rocks, logs, and vegetation when not swimming. Commonly found in parks, gardens, and near ponds During the spring and early summer breeding season, they are particularly active. May be found curled up under stones or logs.

Magical significance

Associated with transformation and regeneration owing to their ability to regrow limbs. They are symbolic of magic, healing, success through change, and cycles of life, death, and rebirth. Finding a Newt may indicate that a period of personal change is coming up. They were closely linked to witchcraft in medieval times, and perhaps used in potions and spells. But "Newt's eye", mentioned in various old texts, was more likely the seedpod of the Mustard plant (*Brassica nigra*).

Frog (*Rana* spp.)

French: *Grenouille*; Dutch: *Kikker*

Amphibians that must live in damp environments. They thrive in quiet areas of parks and gardens, usually near ponds. Frogs emerge from mud after rain. Their croaking, especially during spring and summer breeding seasons, is a sign of warmer weather. They have strong back legs, enabling them to jump relatively far.

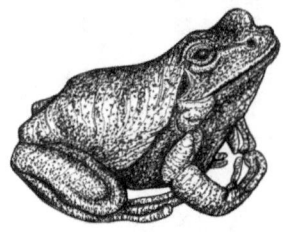

Magical significance

Symbols of fertility, rebirth, transformation, resurrection, and renewal. The Egyptian goddess Hekate is often depicted as a Frog or a woman with a Frog's head. Engage Frog energy when seeking abundance, prosperity, growth, and vitality through spells and charms.

Toad (Bufo bufo)

French: *Crapaud*; Dutch: *Pad*

These humble amphibians are better adapted to land-life than Frogs, thanks to their dry, bumpy skin. They can live many years, breed in water and hibernate through winter. Toads secrete a neurotoxin called bufotoxin, when threatened. They slowly wander damp, shady areas, sneaking up on prey (including Slugs, Worms, and Spiders) before catching them with their sticky tongues. They are most active at dusk and night; hiding under logs and long grass by day. Sadly, Toad populations have declined owing to superstitions and habitat loss.

Magical significance

Associated with transformation, fertility, healing, inner strength, patience, protection, and prosperity. However, medieval folklore linked them with bad luck and poisoning by witches; their venom was used in some potions. East Anglian horse whisperers (Toad Men) each carried a ritually prepared toad bone. This charm was used to encourage good connection between local ploughmen and their horses.[17] Like Frogs, Toads are associated with the goddess Hecate. Invoke Toad energy for earthy spells focused on self-reliance, potency, secrets, and change.

Birds

Birds are vitally important to urban ecosystems, as seed dispersers, pest controllers, and sometimes as pollinators. Their behaviours, migrations, and songs are fascinating. Birdwatching is an accessible way to connect

---

[17] A. Soth, The Toadmen, masters of equine magic. *JSTOR Daily* (2018). https://daily.jstor.org/the-toadmen-masters-of-equine-magic/

with nature, whether in city parks or on the street. Support urban birds by planting native trees, providing birdhouses, feeding stations, and fresh water, especially during harsh seasons. Offer safe foods like seeds or fruit, avoid bread and salty snacks, and keep feeding areas clean and Cat-safe to create a sanctuary for these feathered visitors.

In general, birds represent the soul, wisdom, freedom, fertility, prosperity, transformation, and communication. Their feathers can be placed on altars, added to charm bags, and stitched into the hems of cloaks to aid spirit flight. Use feathers in rituals to bring insight, healing, or change. Each species has different qualities; here are some of the most common city birds.

Blackbird (*Turdus merula*)

French: *Merle noir*; Dutch: *Zwarte merel*

Not a Corvid (Crow family), although the male has striking black plumage and a vibrant orange–yellow beak. The females are brown. Blackbirds are medium-sized garden birds, often seen in parks and streets. Highly territorial, they aggressively defend nests. Blackbirds have a melodious song, often heard at dusk. They forage in soil and leaf litter for invertebrates and also eat berries. Dense shrubs or low trees in quiet locations, are their favoured nesting spots.

Magical significance

Often associated with transformation, changing seasons, and wisdom. Blackbirds are messengers, announcing important transitions in life. In Celtic mythology, the Blackbird's song is thought to help communication between the realms. Work with Blackbird energy for personal reflection and decision-making.

Blue Tit (*Cyanistes caeruleus*)

French: *Mésange bleue*; Dutch: *Blauwe Mees*

Small, vibrant, blue and yellow bird, easily recognisable by the black line running down its face. Known for their intelligence, Blue Tits are skilled at extracting food from feeders and often hang upside down to reach seeds. They are energetic and common in gardens, woodlands, and parks. Mainly around mature trees and hedges. Blue Tits are social and form small flocks in late spring. They adapt to human activities, and teach each other new skills. Blue Tits are non-migratory. They frequent seed-filled feeders and nest in tree cavities or nesting boxes.

Magical significance

Blue Tits are symbols of intelligence, resourcefulness, and adaptability. They encourage us to think outside the box and find creative solutions to challenges. Tap into their energies to adapt quickly to new opportunities.

Chaffinch (*Fringilla coelebs*)

French: *Pinson des arbres*; Dutch: *Vink*

A small, colourful finch. Males have vibrant chestnut–brown plumage, grey–blue wings, and a white belly; females are well camouflaged in pale shades of brown. Energetic foragers of seeds and insects, often finding it while rooting around in soil. Chaffinches eat the crumbs dropped by larger birds from nut feeders. These cheerful garden birds thrive in areas with a mix of trees and open ground. They nest in branches, and have a high-pitched burbling song that is most energetic during the breeding season.

Magical significance

Symbolic of joy, renewal, positivity, harmony, good fortune, and the arrival of spring. In some cultures, their song is said to signal the arrival of good news, particularly in springtime. Let Chaffinch energy increase your sense of optimism and positivity.

Corvids (*Corvidae*)

The Crow family, or Corvids, includes a variety of strikingly intelligent birds, most with black feathers. All are known for their problem-solving abilities and complex social lives. They may use tools, mimic speech, and communicate in sophisticated ways. Resourceful and opportunistic feeders, Corvids are skilled urban scavengers; opening bins or using tools to access food. All Corvids are curious, many are mischievous, and some even collect shiny objects—a habit that has fuelled superstitions.

Corvids are highly social birds, forming lifelong bonds and close-knit communities. Their loud calls warn of danger, and help coordinate their activities. In cities, Corvids often thrive alongside humans. Their clever foraging antics keep municipalities busy redesigning litter bin lids to outsmart them. Here are some Corvids commonly found in European cities.

Carrion Crow (Corvus corone)

All-black, glossy plumage and larger than most other Corvids. These birds tend to be solitary or form small family groups. They are highly intelligent with remarkable memories. Individual Crows often return to places and recognise human faces. They are opportunistic feeders, frequently taking food waste from humans, and can slowly be trained through feeding. Their vocalisation is the loud and distinctive "caw" calls. Crows are associated with mystery, transformation, death, intelligence, and adaptability.

Jackdaw (Corvus monedula)

Smaller than Crows, with a greyish head, dark plumage, and pale blue eyes. Jackdaws are highly social, flock in large groups, and mate for life. They communicate by flashing their eyes, and noisy vocalisations. Like other Corvids, Jackdaws symbolise intelligence and adaptability. In some cultures they also represent death and bad luck.

Jay (Garrulus glandarius)

Brightly coloured with blue feathers on their wings and a black-and-white streaked head. Similar shape and plumage patterns as the Magpie. Jays often find and hide acorns for the winter. They are shy and hyper-alert when feeding but will visit apartment balconies for food. Their harsh, squawking calls are similar to Magpies but more muted. Jays are symbols of quick wittedness and resourcefulness, and are often seen as protectors or guardians.

Magpie (Pica pica)

Striking black-and-white plumage, iridescent feathers, and long tail. Magpies are highly social, intelligent, territorial, and notorious for collecting shiny objects (such as jewellery, coins, and canpulls). They communicate with harsh, chattering and squawking calls. In some cultures, Magpies are considered omens of good fortune, while in others, they symbolise bad luck. In British folklore, they are associated with mystery and trickery.

Raven (Corvus corax)

Large birds, all-black with a distinctive throat tuft and powerful bill. Ravens are playful, and fly in pairs or alone. They are excellent problem-solvers, can use tools, and mimic sounds, including human speech. Their vocalisations are deep, resonant, and often feature a "cronk" sound. In Norse mythology, Ravens are linked with the god Odin and are symbols of knowledge, foresight, and transformation. In the UK, Ravens were hunted to the point of extinction, owing to competition for food and superstition.

Rook (Corvus frugilegus)

Slightly smaller than Crows, with distinctive ragged plumage, and pale skin where their beak and face join. Rooks are highly social, living in large colonies (rookeries), often in tall trees. Their vocalisation is loud, harsh and constant, with "caw-caw" calls. Symbolically, Rooks represent resourcefulness and community, though in some cultures, they were seen as bad omens.

Other birds

Great Tit (Parus major)

French: *Mésange charbonnière*; Dutch: *Grote Mees*

Larger than the Blue Tits, with a clear black line down its yellow belly and a distinctive black and white head. The Great Tit is assertive, curious, and intelligent, capable of solving complex problems to reach food. They are fiercely territorial during the breeding season, and aggressively defend favourite food sources. Great Tits are found in woodlands, parks, and gardens, particularly near Oak and Beech trees. They nest in tree holes, birdhouses, or other suitable cavities. They do not migrate for winter and feed on seeds, insects, and peanuts from feeders.

Magical significance

Great Tits symbolise courage, resilience, intelligence, and strength in the face of challenge. They remind us to be bold and assertive when pursuing our goals and to protect what is valuable to us.

Heron (Ardea cinerea)

French: *Héron cendré*; Dutch: *Blauwe reiger*

Large, elegant grey and white bird with a long neck, sharp bill, and long legs. Often beside water, seeking out fish, amphibians, and small mammals. They remain motionless for long periods when hunting but can be aggressively territorial. They live in large nests, in trees close to freshwater. Many live in urban areas close to canals and reservoirs.

Magical significance

Herons symbolise patience, independence, grace, persistence, and solitude. In Celtic and Native American traditions, they are associated with wisdom, knowledge, and transition. A visit from a Heron may be a sign to reflect and look inward for answers, and prepare for the moment to strike.

House Sparrow (Passer domesticus)

French: *Moineau domestique*; Dutch: *Huismus*

Small social birds, often gathering in large shrubs or conifers. The male has a grey cap, streaky brown back, and chestnut wings with white wing bars. Females are plainer with brown feathers and a pale belly. These little birds thrive in urban areas, feeding on seeds, grains, and scraps.

They nest in buildings and old Swallow nests. Though their population has declined, especially in London, they are still common in cities. Most obvious in winter when they flock together to forage.

Magical significance

Sparrows symbolise community, cheerfulness, and the importance of social bonds. They are associated with homeliness and the simple joy of shared spaces, representing the everyday beauty of communal life. Call on their energy when seeking adaptability and community spirit.

Kestrel (*Falco tinnunculus*)

French: *Faucon crécerelle*; Dutch: *Torenvalk*

Small falcons, which hover in mid-air while hunting. Kestrels use their keen eyesight to spot prey such as small mammals, birds, and insects. In urban environments, they adapt well, nesting in tall structures. In Amsterdam, kestrels can be seen hunting Pigeons, from high in the Rijksmuseum bell tower.

Magical significance

Kestrels symbolise speed, precision, sharp focus, and the ability to see what others cannot. Call on their energy when seeking powers of observation and the ability to adapt to different environments. Kestrels also remind us of the importance of precision and patience in achieving our goals.

Pigeon (*Columba livia domestica*)

French: *Pigeon biset des villes*; Dutch: *Stadsduif*

Adaptable birds commonly found in urban areas around the world. City Pigeons are descendants of wild Rock Doves and thrive where there are food and nesting opportunities. They forage in parks, squares, and streets, and are known for their strong homing instincts and social behaviour. Pigeons pair for life and are able to mate year round. They often nest on balconies.

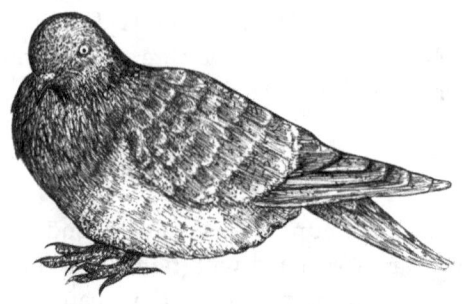

Magical significance

City Pigeons symbolise adaptability, resilience, and community. Their energy can help seeking a new home or meaningful connections with others. Pigeons also represent the value of home and family.

Robin (Erithacus rubecula)

French: *Rouge-gorge*; Dutch: *Roodborst*

Small birds with red breasts and cheerful songs. Male Robins fiercely defend their territory from other Robins, but will share food sources with other species. These birds are friendly and curious around humans. They often follow gardeners; feeding on Worms and grubs unearthed during gardening tasks. Commonly found in areas with dense undergrowth. They nest low in hedges or old structures. Robins are non-migratory birds.

Magical significance

Symbolise strong boundaries and clearly defined personal space. Robins know the importance of maintaining territory while also being open to the warmth and companionship of others.

Rose-ringed Parakeets (Psittacula krameri)

French: *Perruche à collier*; Dutch: *Halsbandparkiet*

Inquisitive birds, vibrant green with a distinctive neck ring. Probably released by accident in the 1960s, they now thrive in large populations within many European cities. They are highly social and noisy, and compete with smaller native birds for food and nest space. Rosering Parakeets feed on fruits, seeds, and nuts, and nest in tree cavities or old buildings. Adaptable and resilient but not so well adapted to cold European winters; their feet often show frost damage.

Magical significance

Parakeets symbolise community, inquisitiveness, domination, and the search for success. Their strength comes from social bonds and strong cooperation, encouraging us to support and protect one another. Their vibrant green feathers also symbolise growth, prosperity, and abundance.

Stork (*Ciconia ciconia*)

French: *Cigogne blanche*; Dutch: *Ooievaar*

Large birds (1 m tall) with white plumage, black wing tips, long red legs and beak. Live in wetlands but increasingly in European cities such as Den Haag and Amsterdam. They strut around urban parks, nest on tall solitary structures, and clatter their bills when excited or establishing territory. Storks are monogamous. They migrate to sub-Saharan Africa for the winter, and breed in Europe.

Magical significance

Symbols of renewal, fertility, new beginnings, loyalty, family, protection, and good fortune. European folklore often features Storks delivering new babies. In magic, use in relation to fertility, safe childbirth, and resilience through life changes.

Swan (*Cygnus olor*)

French: *Cygne tuberculé*; Dutch: *Knobbelzwaan*

Majestic freshwater bird, with graceful movements, long neck, striking white feathers, and piercing stare. Swans are monogamous, and fiercely protective of their nests and young. They eat aquatic plants, insects, and small fish, and are often found in urban waterways. Swans nest in secluded spots near water, using reeds and grasses to build their homes.

Magical significance

Swans symbolise beauty, grace, loyalty, protection, and eternal love. In Greek mythology, the story of Leda and the Swan represents transformation and seduction. In Celtic traditions, Swans are seen as guardians of the Otherworld. In Hinduism, Swans symbolise purity and divine knowledge. They are also linked to the idea of metamorphosis, representing change and spiritual growth.

Woodpecker (*Picidae*)

French: *Pic*; Dutch: *Specht*

These shy birds use their strong beaks to hammer trees in search of insects, as food. The red, black, and white Great Spotted Woodpecker is most likely to visit nut feeders in winter. Green Woodpeckers are less common. Woodpeckers nest in mature and dead trees, making cavities with their beaks. They also tap for insects. Woodpeckers occasionally swoop low over lawns but are more often high in trees.

Magical significance

Woodpeckers symbolise persistence, determination, uncovering secrets, pattern recognition, and hidden opportunities. They are also linked to communication with the spirit realm. Their energy encourages us to break through barriers and push forward despite challenges. Seeing a Woodpecker up close is a sign of good fortune.

Crustaceans

Crayfish (*Procambarus clarkii and other species*)

French: *Écrevisse de Louisiane*; Dutch: *Rivierkreeft*

Several invasive species, found in, and near urban waterways. Crayfish resemble small lobsters and were accidentally introduced to Europe in the 1970s. They have voracious appetites for aquatic plants and aggressively colonise new areas. This can destabilise river banks and upset freshwater ecosystems. Storks, Herons and large fish sometimes prey on Crayfish.

Magical significance

Symbolise adaptation, survival, boundary breaking, and resilience. Their shadowside reminds us of imbalance, and transformation through destruction or aggression. Engage Crayfish energy as a reminder to consider the long-term effects of change and to respect boundaries and balance.

Insects

Ant (*Formicidae*)

French: *Fourmis*; Dutch: *Mieren*

These highly social insects live in well-organised colonies, with each Ant playing a specific role. Ants breathe through spiracles, tiny holes in their exoskeleton. They communicate through pheromone trails, which guide nestmates to food, or warn of danger. They are industrious, and remarkably strong, able to carry objects many times their own weight. Ants prefer warm environments and are most active during the day. In urban areas, they build nests in soil, cracks, or under pavements, often foraging dropped food and small insects.

Magical significance

Ants symbolise strength in community, cooperation, resilience, and persistence. They help us consider alternative ways of being. Ant energy can be called on, when unity, determination, and resourcefulness are required.

Bed Bug (*Cimex lectularius*)

French: *Punaises de lit*; Dutch: *Bedwantsen*

Small, parasitic insects that feed on the blood of humans and other animals. They hide in cracks, crevices, and furniture during the day. Bed Bug bites cause itching, swelling, and allergic reactions. Infestations are common in urban areas, spreading through travel, second-hand furniture, or crowded living conditions. Bed Bugs are hard to eradicate, able to survive for months between feeds.

Magical significance

Usually symbols of irritation, Bed Bugs also represent our shadowside. This is the hidden or suppressed part of life that stays unnoticed until it becomes unavoidable. In magic, they can symbolise the need to confront underlying issues: psychological, emotional, or spiritual. Their resilience in harsh conditions also makes Bed Bugs symbols of persistence, adaptation, and strength. Try invoking their energy to help overcome persistent challenges, but don't welcome them into your home.

Bee (Apis)

French: *Abeilles*; Dutch: *Bijen*

Honey Bees live in colonies with a queen, workers, and drones; they pollinate flowers, supporting fruit and seed production. They transform nectar into honey, beeswax, propolis, and royal jelly. Bumble Bees and Solitary Bees may live in walls, soil and trees. They often pollinate single plant species and store just enough honey or nectar for their needs. Bees are gentle, hard-working creatures, usually only aggressive when under threat.

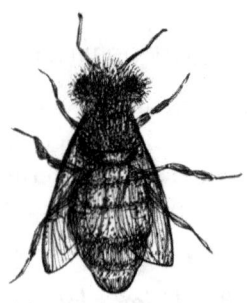

Magical significance

Bees symbolise hard work, fertility, abundance, sweetness, community, transformation, and immortality. They are associated with Druids, divine wisdom and guidance. Bees are believed to carry messages from the spirit world, making them important in divination and spiritual rituals. In magical practices, beeswax is used in candle-making, sealing spells, and creating talismans.

Butterfly (Papilionoidea)

French: *Papillons*; Dutch: *Vlinders*

Butterflies undergo metamorphosis from caterpillars to adults, with delicate wings and graceful flight. They are important pollinators; many species migrate huge distances, between breeding and feeding grounds. Butterfly wings are covered in specialised scales. Most feed on flower nectar or rotting fruit. Many lay eggs on Stinging Nettles. Butterflies are most active on warm, sunny days.

Magical significance

Symbols of transformation, beauty, freedom, transcendence, and hope. Often seen as messengers between the living and the dead. Butterflies remind us of the fleeting nature of life. Some cultures associate Butterflies with marriage and fertility. Try attracting Butterflies to summer rituals by wearing white clothing.

Dragonfly (Anisoptera)

French: *Libellules*; Dutch: *Libellen*

Fast-flying insects with colourful bodies and transparent wings. Found near water sources like ponds, lakes, and rivers, where they lay their eggs. These agile predators feed on smaller insects, including Mosquitoes. They metamorphose from water nymphs to flying adults. Dragonflies thrive in areas with stagnant or slow-moving water, and are often seen above city ponds, and waterways. Most active on warm summer days.

Magical significance

Dragonflies symbolise transformation, change, adaptability, self-realisation, and the ability to navigate obstacles with style. Their flight patterns are symbols of freedom, independence, spiritual awakening, and wisdom. In some cultures, Dragonflies are messengers of the spirit world, guiding individuals through life transitions. Their image is often found in graveyards.

Fly (Diptera)

French: *Mouches*; Dutch: *Vliegen*

Flies are known for rapid flight and adaptability. Many feed on decaying matter, while others are pollinators or parasites. They help decomposition and nutrient recycling. In urban areas, flies thrive around compost, and food waste, especially in warm, moist environments. They have specialised compound eyes, suction cup feet, and dissolve their food before swallowing it.

Magical significance

Flies symbolise degradation, decay, recycling, metamorphosis. and the cycle of life and death. Some traditions believe that they carry messages from the afterlife. They also represent secret observation (a Fly on the wall). Flies are used in protection spells, particularly against the evil eye.

Ladybird (Coccinellidae)

French: *Coccinelles*; Dutch: *Lieveheersbeestjes*

Small, round Beetles with bright red or orange bodies and black spots. Ladybirds are commonly found in cities. Their larvae are voracious predators of many plant pests, including Aphids. Some species defend themselves by secreting a yellow fluid. In cities, Ladybirds thrive in warm, sunny environments. They seek shelter in cracks or under leaves. During colder months, they often hibernate in crevices within human homes.

Magical significance

Ladybirds symbolise protection, good fortune, love, harmony, and happiness. In many cultures, spotting a Ladybird is believed to bring positive change, like a wish coming true or an improvement in life. In magical practices, they are invoked for good luck, fertility, and family protection. Ladybirds are popular in charms and talismans for positive energy.

Woodworm (Anobium punctatum)

French: *Ver de bois*; Dutch: *Houtworm*

These are the larvae of Beetles that eat wooden structures and furniture. The adult Beetles lay eggs in cracks, and the larvae burrow into the wood. They leave small exit holes, and dust, as they grow. This weakens the wood, a major problem in older buildings. Woodworms thrive in damp, poorly ventilated areas. Infested wood should not be taken inside homes. Wormwood and Elder oil is said to repel them (though this seems more symbolic than proven).

Magical significance

Woodworm symbolises decay and hidden forces that quietly weaken things over time. Their almost invisible energy can be called on when strong systems need to be overcome. And when long-standing beliefs need to be changed. Their presence is a reminder to stay alert to hidden dangers or weaknesses.

Mammals

Bat (Chiroptera)

French: *Chauve-souris*; Dutch: *Vleermuizen*

The only mammals capable of true flight, with wings formed by a thin membrane stretched over elongated fingers. Most Bats feed on insects like Mosquitoes and Moths. They are nocturnal but often seen at dusk or dawn in urban areas. They roost in cave-like spaces or trees. We can support these often-misunderstood creatures by installing Bat nesting boxes, protecting insect-rich habitats, and avoiding pesticides that reduce their food supply.

Magical significance

Symbolic of transformation, mystery, and adaptability. European folklore often links Bats to witches and the supernatural, mainly owing to their nocturnal habits. In some cultures, such as in Chinese and Mayan traditions, Bats are symbols of good fortune, vigilance, and protection. Engage the energy of Bats to help navigate in the dark, and for guidance through difficult times.

Cat (Felis catus)

French: *Chat*; Dutch: *Kat*

Cats have lived alongside humans for thousands of years, and were domesticated around 2000 BCE in Egypt. Known for their independence, intelligence, and curiosity, they are skilled hunters and highly territorial. In cities, they often roam at night, dodge traffic by day, and reproduce freely. Even well-fed House Cats prey on rodents, birds, and Bats. They tend to enjoy the chase and kill more than the food. Sharing space with a Cat can be life-affirming. They do develop strong bonds with humans but most Cat "owners" will readily say that their pet is really the one in charge.

Magical significance

Cats symbolise witchcraft, intuition, independence, mystery, feminine energy, and protection. Egyptian mythology linked Cats to Bastet, goddess of home, fertility, and protection. In Norse mythology, Freya, the goddess of love and beauty, travelled in a chariot pulled by Cats. Their abilities to see into our souls, move silently and slink into the shadows, are magical strengths. The intuitive behaviour of Cats has made them popular as witch familiars. Naturally shed Cat claws can be used in spells and rituals.

Dog (Canis lupus familiaris)

French: *Chien*; Dutch: *Hond*

Dogs were domesticated from wolves thousands of years ago. They are loyal companions and are bred to fulfil various roles such as hunting, herding, and guarding. Dogs can form strong bonds with humans and are highly social. They have keen senses, especially smell and hearing.

Magical significance

Symbols of loyalty, protection, and companionship across many cultures. In ancient Egypt, Dogs were associated with the god of the afterlife and protector of the dead, Anubis. In Norse mythology, Dogs were linked to the hunt, with the great hound, Garm, guarding the gates of Hell. In many cultures, Dogs are considered guardians of the home and are believed to have the ability to sense unseen spirits or danger. They are also seen as symbols of fidelity and unconditional love, providing comfort and protection to those in need.

Fox (Vulpes vulpes)

French: *Renard*; Dutch: *Vos*

Medium-sized carnivorous mammals with a bushy tail, sharp features, and reddish coat. The Fox is an opportunistic feeder, scavenging leftover food or hunting small mammals and birds. Urban Foxes may be seen in gardens, parks, and streets at night. They are elusive and solitary creatures, who rely on sharp intellect to find food and protect their offspring. They scent their territories and thrive in diverse habitats. Foxes help control Rabbit and rodent populations.

Magical significance

Associated with sharp intellect, survival, resourcefulness, transformation, and magic. The Fox is often seen as a trickster; able to navigate difficult situations and come out on top. In Norse mythology, it is linked to the goddess Freya, symbolising mystical and fiery femininity. In China and Japan, Fox spirits are believed to act as protectors or seducers. Foxes also embody the ability to move between the visible and hidden worlds.

Mole (Talpidae)

French: *Taupes*; Dutch: *Mol*

Small, underground mammals with streamlined velvet-covered bodies. With powerful front limbs, Moles tunnel in search of Earthworms, insects, and other invertebrates. This helps to keep soil aerated and balanced. Often seen as garden pests, but molehills are signs of healthy soil in parks and gardens. To support Moles, avoid disrupting their tunnels, and garden organically.

Magical significance

Moles symbolise hidden knowledge, intuition, transformation, adaptability, and breaking barriers. Engage Mole energy to help navigate through dark times, to detect hidden truths, or to bring awareness to things that are out of sight.

Rabbit (Leporidae)

French: *Lapin*; Dutch: *Konijn*

Small herbivores with long alert ears, flashing tails, and powerful hind legs. Rabbits live in warrens in grassy areas, which they graze. They are social animals and reproduce rapidly, and may upset humans by feeding on their plants. Rabbits are prey to Foxes, Cats, Owls and other predators in the urban food chain.

Magical significance

Symbolic with fertility, abundance, good fortune, vigilance, awareness, new beginnings, and the cyclic nature of life, Rabbits have deep cultural and magical significance. In Celtic and Norse traditions, they are symbols of the Earth and Moon. Their ability to live above and below ground represents the balance between worlds. Rabbits are often used synonymously with the Hare.

Rat (Rattus)

French: *Rat*; Dutch: *Rat*

Highly intelligent and adaptable rodents. Rats thrive in urban areas by scavenging from rubbish bins, sewers, and buildings. They play an important role in cleaning up city waste but their success can threaten biodiversity. A Rat pair can produce up to 500 offspring per year, so when food sources are scarce they will start eating birds, small mammals, and fish. Rats shelter where they can, dig tunnels, and chew through wood and wiring to find food or create nests. They are opportunists who like familiarity. Preventing Rat infestations helps the ecosystem and reduces the use of toxic pest control.

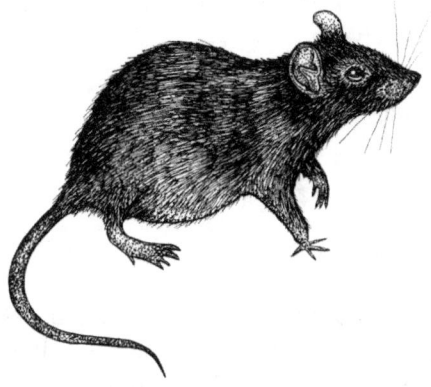

Magical significance

Urban Rats symbolise survival, intelligence, adaptability, wisdom, transformation, cooperation, and resourcefulness. From another perspective Rats symbolise decay and destruction. Rat energy is strong and powerful, whichever way we look at it. In magical work Rat energy is especially useful when trying to see both sides of a situation.

Molluscs

Slug and Snail

French: *Escargot*; Dutch: *Slakken*

Common in urban spaces, especially in wet weather, when these spiral-shelled creatures become more active. Snails eat plant matter, often preferring algae and dead material (including paper), to live plants. They thrive in damp, shady environments, and secrete antimicrobial slime to help glide around. Vineyard Snails can live ten years. Both Slugs and Snails chew their food using a flexible band of teeth, called a radula. The humble garden Snail has around 14,000 microscopic teeth. They can be heard rasping at food, if quietly observed.

Magical significance

Snails are symbolic of patience, persistence, shelter, and protection. Their shells also represent growth, renewal, and the spiral of life. Use found empty Snail shells in spells related to homes, protection, and growth. Or fill with protective berries and seeds, then bury them close to your home as a protective charm.

Reptiles

Lizard (*Lacertidae*)

French: *Lézard*; Dutch: *Hagedis*

Small to medium-sized reptiles, often seen basking in the Sun. They have long bodies, scaly skin, and four legs. Some Lizards can regenerate their tails if lost. They prefer sunny, warm spots on stone walls, and fences. Slow Worms are a type of legless Lizard. They also thrive in urban gardens, often found in compost heaps or tall grass.

Magical significance

Lizards are symbolic of regeneration, rebirth, change, adaptability, and resilience. They are also associated with the Sun, and in some traditions are seen as protectors, warding off evil spirits. The ancient Egyptians linked them with the gods of protection and healing.

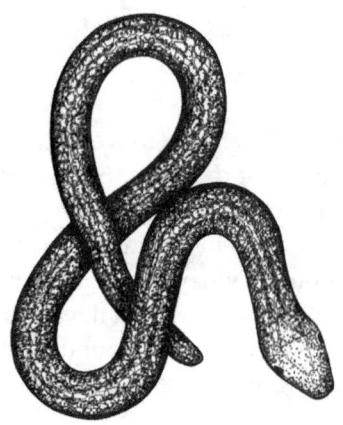

Snake (Serpentes)

French: *Serpent*; Dutch: *Slang*

Cold-blooded, legless reptiles with flexible jaws. Snakes can consume prey larger than their heads by dislocating their jaw. As they grow, they shed their skins. Grass Snakes (*Natrix natrix*) and the rarer European Adder (*Vipera berus*) are sometimes found in quiet green urban spaces.

Magical significance

Symbolic of wisdom, enlightenment, danger, transformation, cycles of life, renewal, and healing. Snakes feature in mythologies across the world, including the serpent in the Garden of Eden, tempting Eve to take forbidden fruit. Embrace Snake energy in magic related to shedding the past to make space for the new.

Other creatures

Spider (Araneae)

French: *Araignée*; Dutch: *Spin*

Spiders are remarkable creatures with eight legs, (usually) eight eyes, intricate webs, and the ability to thrive in quiet, undisturbed spaces. Their silk (which is stronger than steel) is used to catch prey, and create shelter and nests. Females lay egg sacs containing hundreds of Spiderlings. Most Spiders are solitary and feed on insects. Their silk has long been used in folk medicine to stop bleeding and promote wound healing.

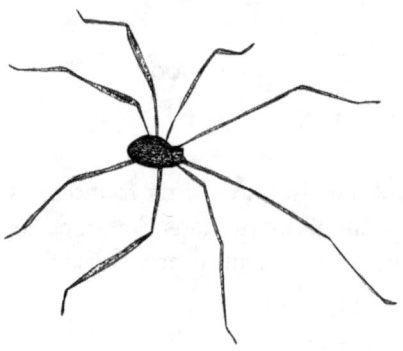

Magical significance

Associated with creativity, patience, fate, and interconnection. Many cultures see Spiders as guardians of ancient wisdom or language. In Celtic mythology, they are considered teachers, linked to the Ogham alphabet, with their webs reflecting the structure of this ancient script. Use their energy in magic involving language, nature, and destiny. Cobwebs symbolise how everything is woven together. Weave into rituals to trap and neutralise negative energy, to protect boundaries and heal energetic wounds.

Earthworm (*Lumbricus terrestris*)

French: *Ver de terre*; Dutch: *Regenworm*

These soil-dwelling invertebrates are essential for healthy soil. With their long, segmented bodies, they burrow through the earth, in urban green spaces. Earthworms are most active in moist, well-aerated soils and damp, cool weather. They often surface after rain, taking advantage of the wet conditions to move above ground, although this makes them more vulnerable to predators. Underground, they are a favourite food of Moles.

Magical significance

Earthworms symbolise humility, diligence, fertility, prosperity, growth, and renewal. In some cultures, they are seen as messengers between the physical and spiritual worlds. Engage their energy when seeking hidden knowledge beneath the surface, when there is a need to dig deep or look within.

Nematode

French: *Nématode*; Dutch: *Nematode*

Microscopic, thread-like Roundworms found in soil, water, and as parasites in plants, animals, or humans. Some species are helpful in pest control and nutrient cycling, while others cause disease. In urban areas, they help decompose organic matter and maintain soil fertility. Though largely unseen, Nematodes are vital for healthy ecosystems.

Magical significance

Symbolise hidden transformation. In spells, Nematode energy can be invoked to encourage personal growth, or reveal deeper truths beyond the immediately visible.

TOOLS AND TECHNIQUES

Tools

Witches are often pictured stirring cauldrons or standing at altars surrounded by beautiful tools and candles. This can give the impression that many physical items are necessary to practise magic, but that is far from the truth. The only essential tool for magic is the mind; additional paraphernalia can be helpful for focusing on tasks or making them easier, in a practical sense. But magic flows from intention, not physical objects. The tools we do use can be found in nature, repurposed from everyday items, or, at times, purchased new.

When buying tools, try to resist the pull of materialism. This is especially difficult early in our magical journeys when every tool looks tempting. But there is no need to buy much at all, and many turn out to be less useful than hoped. Over time, most witches find that a simple approach, with just a few books and favourite tools, is the most effective. These items often hold more value than a large collection of special objects that rarely get used.

Everyone is different, but adopting a minimalist approach can help keep your practice grounded in what matters to you while saving money and natural resources.

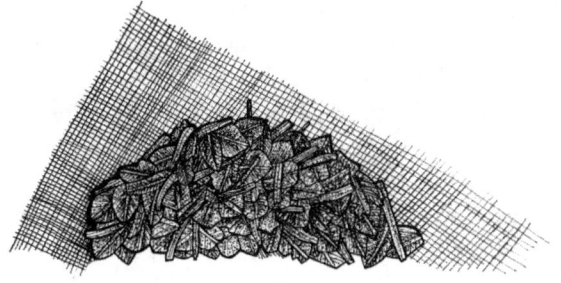

Sustainable tools

When you need new tools for your practice, make thoughtful choices. Opt for natural, sustainably crafted, second-hand, or recycled materials where possible. If not, go for high-quality, multipurpose items that are designed to last. Sharing some tools with friends can also help, and some witches take their old sterling silver jewellery to silversmiths to be crafted into new implements. This saves on resources and adds a personal touch to the items.

Although it is difficult to trace the origins of what we buy, steer away from trade that harms the environment or exploits communities. Sadly, several materials commonly used by magical practitioners do cause such harm. Palo Santo is the sacred wood (from several tree species) used in Indigenous South American traditions. It is often used in Europe to create smoke during rituals. Its popularity has led to overharvesting, deforestation, and cultural exploitation in its native habitat. White Sage (*Salvia apiana*) is similar; the herb from Native American smudging ceremonies has become so popular elsewhere that wild populations of the plant are now threatened. For both these herbs, there is the issue of cultural misappropriation, or at least using them without understanding or respect.

Abalone shells, often sold as heatproof holders for smudge bundles, are also surrounded by ethical and environmental concerns. These mother-of-pearl rich shells are the homes to molluscs, animals that can live for decades in the sea. They hold great cultural significance for groups like the Apache Nation and Māori. But sadly, poaching, overfishing, and pollution have pushed some Abalone to the brink of extinction. Farming Abalone has helped to meet the international demand, but that brings other problems including animal welfare as the creatures are treated as commodities. Lack of transparency in the Abalone industry means that very few esoteric vendors actually know where their shells have come from and how the animals were treated.[18]

The crystal trade raises other concerns; many mines rely on child labour and unsustainable practices. There is little transparency about how the crystals are extracted, and that secrecy means that most vendors have no way to verify the origins of the stones that they sell to us. Some crystals, such as tourmaline (a byproduct of the cobalt mining industry) and smoky quartz, are often mined by children and adults in tunnels without adequate safety procedures. Money-hungry practices lead to tunnel collapses and fatalities each year, but most crystal miners see little financial benefit for their precarious lives.

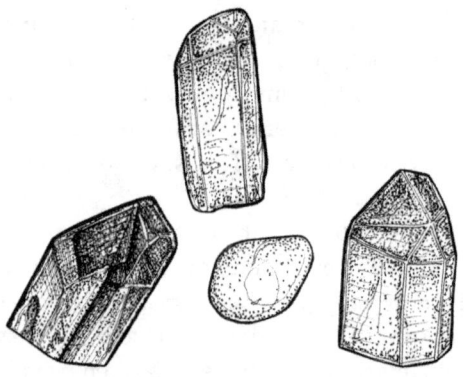

With some effort, it is possible to find ethically sourced crystals, but another option is to purchase crystals from old collections (pre-loved or second-hand). Purchasing these can help to reduce the efforts to take more crystals from the Earth. If you decide to use crystals in your practice, approach them as orphans, taken far from their home, and give them the care and respect they deserve for life.

Herbs also have sustainability issues. If you cannot harvest herbs yourself, seek out organic and sustainably sourced options. Overharvesting slow-growing plants such as Mandrake (*Mandragora officinalis*) or Frankincense (*Boswellia*) can endanger wild populations, while even commonly cultivated herbs like Lavender can harm ecosystems when grown in pesticide-heavy monocrops. So, whenever possible,

---

[18] O. Young, 10 Little-known facts about Abalone. *Tree Hugger* (2022). https://www.treehugger.com/abalone-facts-5180643

grow your own herbs or choose local organic, ethical suppliers to reduce environmental harm and deepen your connection to the plants you work with.

Some retailers demonstrate a commitment to ethical and sustainable trade, by refusing to sell items like Abalone and White Sage. But most don't, so as consumers we can help inspire meaningful change in the esoteric industry by telling vendors our concerns, and by supporting businesses that do prioritise sustainability.

If you are interested in using materials like herbs, crystals, and shells from other cultures, pay close attention to where they come from and all steps in the supply chain. Items obtained through pain and exploitation cannot add anything good to our magical work. Effective local alternatives are available for all of the exotic items that we sometimes want; if you can't find ethical and sustainable options, use something found and local instead. Local and pre-loved is not second best, as some shops may have you believe. Sustainability should take priority when we seek out new tools. Magic is not about the tools we use, it is about our intention. Choosing ethical and sustainable options can also encourage local suppliers to help improve the situation for crystal miners, herb growers, and creatures such as the Abalone.

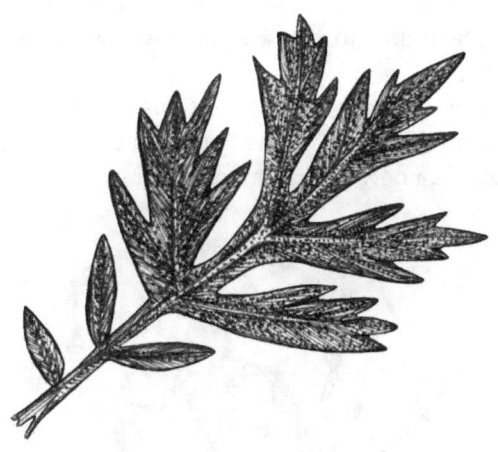

Alternatives

If you are looking for an alternative for an item, look at the core purpose the item was aiming to serve. Focus on the essence of a tool or ingredient; for instance, if Palo Santo smoke was to be used to clear a space, try a saining bundle of Mugwort or Lavender instead. Rather than using an Abalone shell to hold smouldering herbs, try a heatproof dish instead. If nothing is available as a substitute, look to the spiritual realm or visualisation. Try visualising the tools you need and use them in meditations or inner journeys. Or use something with the same symbolism. For instance, if a spell calls for a blade to be used to cut bonds, try using a stick or your hand instead. Most of our need to have tools is fuelled by the consumerist society we live in, rather than necessity.

Ultimately, the most important tool for magic is the mind, so prioritising simplicity and respect for nature creates the best environment for it to thrive.

Cleansing, charging, and caring for tools

Cleansing magical tools removes lingering energies and prepares them for use. There are many ways to do this, from exposing them to moonlight or sunlight, wafting incense smoke over them, placing them in a bowl of wholegrain rice, or a freshwater stream. This is especially important for second-hand or inherited tools. Charging fills tools with your intent and purpose. It can be done by grounding and centring your energy, then holding the object in your hands and channelling your energy into it. With wands, take time to practise channelling your energy not only into it, but through it.

You may like to use herbs and incantations when doing this, to ritual-cleanse and welcome the tool. Some like to place a few eggs, herbs, and light incense inside a new cauldron, for instance, to cleanse the tool.

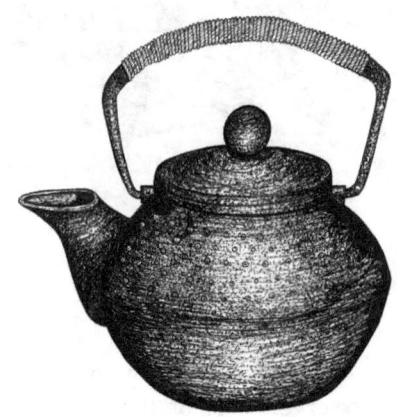

Over time, well-loved tools can develop their own personality. In Japan, the concept of *Tsukumogami* acknowledges how household objects develop helpful qualities through many years of careful use. Neglected tools, on the other hand, lose their effectiveness and may even work against their owner's intent. So take care of your magical tools and they will take care of you.

You may like to consider what you would like to happen to your special tools, when you no longer need them. Some cultures lay tools to rest with their owners, and others pass them on to friends with similar beliefs. Alternatively, you could bury or burn them. Magical tools often become extensions of our energy, and they deserve respect so do consider leaving instructions to ensure they are passed on to someone who will honour them when you are gone.

Frequently used tools

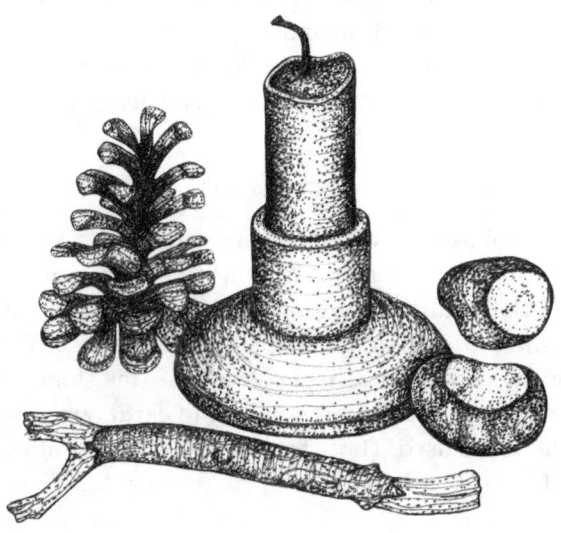

Altar

A personal space for magic, rituals, and inspiration. Altars should help to focus on magical intent. Fresh flowers, herbs, a candle, and a small bowl or cauldron are enough. You might also like to include stones, salt, divination tools, or symbols of the elements (like a feather for air, a seashell for water). But there are no rules with this, and you don't need to have an altar at all. If you do have one, arrange it in a way that feels useful to you, and avoid feeling any need to imitate any fancy setups that you may have seen online.

Some witches create permanent altar spaces at home, with books, plants, candles, crystals, and a few seasonal decorations. Others prefer temporary altars in nature, or portable ones such as a shoebox, that they can keep away from prying eyes. If space is limited, you may like to hang a Willow wreath on your wall, threaded with seasonal flowers. That can be a great focal point, which is the main purpose of an altar, after all. Another option is to visualise an altar, which can be called up during meditation.

Some years ago, I found an old wooden breadboard. It is small, round, and easy to find space for. It is rubbed with Elder-infused Olive oil, and charged. I arrange seasonal berries, leaves, or flowers on the board, around a tealight candle and incense stick. It creates a lovely focal point for my work, and is easy to clear away and store between use.

Keep your altar space clean and tidy. It is also wise to cleanse it by wafting incense smoke or wiping with Bay water decoction, or Elder infused oil, now and then, to remove stagnant energy.

Anchor stone

A grounding tool used to stabilise energy and connect with the physical realm during rituals or meditation. It helps the practitioner stay centred, especially during spiritual travel or emotional distress. They tend to be smooth, flat stones that fit comfortably in the hand, but they can be any convenient shape. Over time, the stone absorbs your energy, so rubbing it can bring you back to earth, when needed. Any type of stone can be used. Those found locally, while out walking, tend to work best.

Anointing water

Specially prepared or natural water used to anoint candles, tools, spaces, or the practitioner's body during rituals. Examples include Moon water, storm water, rain water, spring water, herb-infused water, and herbal distillates. To extend their shelf life, add a little vodka, but ideally use them fresh. Florida water, a commercial blend of aromatic herbs, is also used in this way.

Broom

Used to sweep away stagnant energy, bad luck, and even bad weather. In rituals, it may help in achieving spirit flight. Some witches anoint the handle with flying ointment and symbolically ride it. A broom (or besom) is often used to clear sacred space and altars before rituals.

To craft one, bundle twigs of similar length and secure tightly to a straight handle with string or a strong flexible stem. Hazel, Ash, and Willow are often used for the handle and Birch, symbolic of purification, is often used for the bristles. For a smaller version, Lavender seed stems can be tied together. After a year of use, a natural broom can be burned or buried to release any accumulated energy.

Candles

Choose candles for spellwork that are made from natural, sustainable, and non-toxic materials. Avoid paraffin wax (a petroleum byproduct) and be mindful of Soy wax, which can contribute to deforestation. Opt for eco-friendly materials like organic beeswax, which is naturally coloured and can be pressed into sheets. Rapeseed oil candles from local, organic sources are another possible choice. Look for candles free from harmful dyes or artificial scents, which can pollute the air. Beeswax tealights and small pillar candles are ideal for spellwork.

Rather than buying artificially coloured candles for rituals, try dressing a plain candle with herbs or a ribbon to match your intent. For lighting the wick, some witches use flints and natural kindling, like Rosebay Willowherb fluff or King Alfred's Cake fungi, but most use matches or lighters. Some practitioners let spell candles burn completely, while others extinguish them, often using a herbal infusion or thin sugar syrup to enhance the spell's effect.

Cards

Tarot cards most likely evolved from a 15th-century parlour game in Italy. They gained popularity after Pamela Colman Smith[19] designed the Rider-Waite deck in 1909. Those are richly illustrated cards, offering

---

[19] J. Palumbo, The woman behind the world's most famous tarot deck was nearly lost in history. CNN (2022). https://edition.cnn.com/style/article/pamela-colman-smith-tarot-art-whitney/index.html

layers of symbolism. Today, countless oracle decks are available, reflecting the diverse styles of magic. They include nature-inspired decks and the Round Motherpeace Cards. If nothing fits, try designing your own. Some believe that your first divination deck should be received as a gift, but this is not a rule. What does matter most is that you enjoy handling them.

Cauldron

A powerful symbol of transformation, creation, and renewal. Cauldrons are often associated with the womb, wisdom, and creativity, as in Welsh mythology, where Cerridwen's cauldron became the font of inspiration. For those who like symbols of the elements in their rituals, the different aspects of the cauldron embody fire, water, earth, and air. Used for alchemy, creating nourishment, and bringing community together, cauldrons also represent the heart of the home. In practical magic, they are used in potion brewing and scrying. Cast-iron cauldrons, or Dutch Oven-style saucepans are traditional but a pestle and mortar or ceramic bowl can work just as well.

Crystals and stones

These are versatile tools, each with unique properties, but often costly to the Earth. Clear quartz amplifies energy, aquamarine clears blockages tied to self-expression, and tourmaline is useful for protection. They may be arranged in "grids" to magnify their effects. Cleanse and charge them regularly to maintain their potency, and insist on ethically sourced crystals. Local sustainable alternatives include found stones and pebbles. Learning how specific types of stone were formed can add extra meaning to their use. Recycled glass crystal balls are now available, and Dorodango (highly polished, hand-crafted spheres—a Japanese craft) can be made from local mud.

Dressing oil

To add depth to spells and an excellent way to avoid artificially coloured candles. Choose herbs that reflect your intentions, infuse them in Olive oil, then apply a few drops to the surface of the spell candle. Some stroke the oil downwards (from wick to base) for attractive magic, and upwards for banishing work. Then perhaps roll the candle in complementary herbs or brick dust; briefly warming the candle surface beforehand with a flame will help these to stick.

Druid egg

A small stone, sometimes engraved with Celtic symbols, to bring clarity, protection, and decision-making to your practice. Hold or rub it when you seek guidance, inspiration, or reassurance. Used regularly, its presence can act as a reminder of your inner strength and ability to navigate challenges. Carry the egg in your pocket, so it is attuned to your energy.

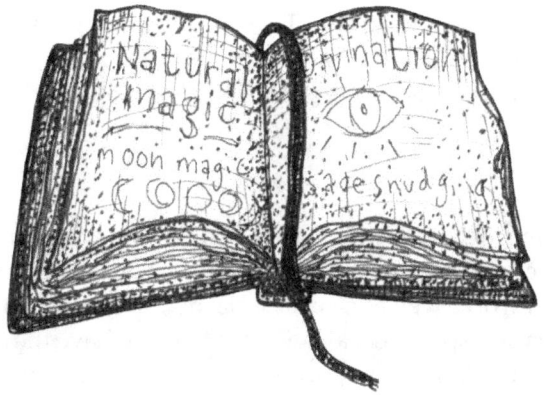

Grimoire

A magical journal in which to record aspects of your magical practice, such as rituals, spells, reflections, and results of experiments. Old grimoires, leech books, and herbals usually held a mix of records of magic, healing, and personal beliefs. They are fascinating historical records, which were usually quite personal and well worth exploring for inspiration.[20] Some, such as the Shams al-Ma'arif,[21] have quite a reputation and should be approached with caution.

---

[20] The oldest surviving herbal in Britain is the Pseudo-Apuleius (Oxford, Bodleian Library, 12th century): https://digital.bodleian.ox.ac.uk/objects/4ffa9d94-a1fb-495d-9deb-fcdccdec2c09/. An older version is held by the University of Leiden.

[21] Several English-language translations of this Arabic grimoire are now available. The title is sometimes translated as the Sun of Knowledge.

Today, formats vary, from bound sheets of Birch bark paper, to simple notebooks or digital files. To be valuable, a grimoire should be useful and meaningful to you, rather than beautiful. Entries might include materials used for certain intentions, pressed leaves, sketches, and poems. Protect the content of your grimoire in whichever way feels right, which could include hiding it and using coded language.

Hag stone (witch stone)

Stone with a hole, caused by weathering or use. They are carried as protective talismans, to ward off malevolent spirits and curses. Looking through a hag stone hole, or window, is believed to reveal hidden truths and glimpses of the spirit realm. They are often worn on a cord, placed in sacred spaces, or hung in homes to protect. Hag Stones are most powerful when found in nature; they occasionally emerge during gardening.

Herbs

Whether living, fresh-cut, dried, or crafted, herbs are used in most Green Witch practices. Many can be used for several purposes, such as Witch Hazel, which works well as a surface cleaner, skin toner, and protective ally in rituals and spells. Local herbs are likely to have the closest affinity to your work, because they grow in the same climate and conditions. So seek out local plants first, and you may find that the right herb for a task appears at the right time in a local street. The Plant Lore directory will help you to select and use locally growing herbs. Not all herbs are edible, or safe, for everyone, so approach with caution and respect.

Incense

Use incense smoke to cleanse tools and space, or to carry intentions to the spirit realm. Air that is gently scented with incense also helps us to enter the liminal space, so it is often used in rituals. Incense comes in many forms: sticks, cones, loose herbs, resins, or dried bundles. To work, all need to be warmed or smouldered.

Some commercial products contain synthetic fragrance and harmful chemicals like formaldehyde. Avoid those and also any containing endangered or unethically sourced ingredients. Some well-loved exotic ingredients, like Frankincense resin, are natural but are often sourced in ways that endanger the plants and harm communities. In such cases, look out for organic Fair Trade options or choose a local alternative.

Herbs like Mugwort, Spruce resin, Sage, and Clary Sage (*Salvia sclarea*) have been used as incense for millennia, and can be obtained from urban spaces.

Feathers are often used to waft incense smoke around, so find a local one. Any heatproof container can be used to hold smouldering incense bundles, so again opt for something local and sustainable. For burning loose incense, sustainably sourced charcoal blocks work best, perhaps placed on a bowl of white ash to insulate the heat.

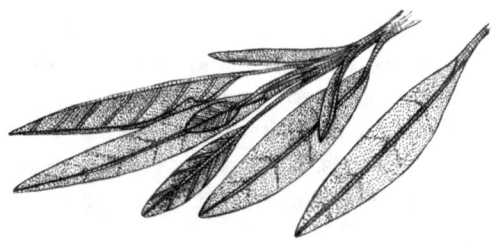

Knives

Used practically, to harvest and process herbs, and to symbolically cut, separate, or mark boundaries. The sharp edge also represents clarity, focus, and protection. Ceremonial knives and ritual harvesting blades can be beautiful and powerful, but a regular kitchen knife, wand, or even your own hand, can be used for the same effect.

Ogham sticks

Used for divination. A set of Ogham sticks is made from short lengths of wood from various trees. Each is marked with the corresponding Ogham symbol, from an ancient Celtic script. You can craft your own set by collecting sticks from local trees. The Techniques section below explains how to make and use them.

Ribbons, silks, and threads

Used for binding and protection work, and for colour symbolism. Many Green Witches collect ribbons from gifts and packaging. These can be used in charms, knot magic, or placed on the altar to invoke the energy of a specific colour. When wrapped around an unstained wax candle, a coloured ribbon lets it substitute for a coloured spell candle.

Robes

A cloak can be both practical and symbolic, offering warmth and comfort during outdoor rituals, and helping to connect with your inner power. Worn during ceremonies, it separates the witch from the mundane world and makes it easier to enter liminality. A long, hooded cloak that envelops you fully can enhance meditation, spirit travel, or simply create a private sacred space. The colour and fabric can reflect specific energies, such as black for protection, green for healing, or purple for intuition. Some witches stitch personal symbols into the cloak hem (feathers, dried herbs, crumbled bone…) to add layers of meaning and power. Those without a cloak often have preferred items of clothing that they wear during rituals. Whatever is chosen, these robes provide a sense of protection and familiarity during magical work.

Spoons

For mixing ingredients in a cauldron or saucepan, to combine and transform the materials for your spells, lotions, potions, and rituals. Chopsticks or porridge sticks (spurtles) make good alternatives. Crafting your own, from finding a fallen branch to anointing the finished spoon with a special oil, can be a very fulfilling project. The thick stems of aromatic herbs such as Rosemary and Lavender can be easily whittled into stirring implements, with a pocket knife. Whichever wood is used adds qualities to your creations, so be mindful of poisonous wood, like Yew. Only use non-toxic wood for food preparation tools. If you prefer a silver spoon, consider having old silver jewellery transformed into a small ritual stirring implement.

Staff

A long walking stick, almost as tall as the witch, crafted from a tree that resonates with their spirit. It represents wisdom and connection with nature and the spirit realm. The staff is a conduit for energy, used to direct energy, and to store energy. It also offers protection, and keeps the powers of the source tree close to the witch. They are taken on pilgrimages, harvesting walks, and used to aid spirit flight (much like a broom).

To make your own staff, take a straight branch from locally pruned wood; when finished it should reach somewhere between your waist and armpit. Whittle and sand to a fine smooth finish, perhaps engraving some personal symbols, then protect and polish. Do this by firmly rubbing herbs like Rosemary, Sage, and Elder leaf into the staff. Then finish with a natural beeswax polish. However it is used, the staff becomes an extension of your strength and intent.

Wands

For focusing and directing the energy and intention of the witch towards the chosen target. It is used during rituals, spells, and invocations. Each type of wand wood brings unique qualities: Ash is ideal for spells requiring quick action, Yew for protection, transformation, and healing, while Apple is favoured for love and intuition. The length of a wand is typically measured from middle fingertip to elbow crease, but other lengths work too.

Crafting your own is best; it yields a wand that is an extension of your spirit. Choose a branch that has recently fallen and appeals to you. It should be quite straight and tapered towards the point (this helps focus energy from your hand to the target). Whittle and sand until smooth. You may also like to add symbols or attach stones, with natural resin. Protect and polish the wand by firmly rubbing herbs like Rosemary, Sage, and Elder leaf into the wood, before finishing with a natural beeswax polish.

If you are gifted a wand, protect and polish it yourself, to align it with your personal energy. After cleansing and charging a new wand, spend time learning to channel your energy not only into it, but through it.

Techniques

This part of the book is about how to practise magic. It covers how to cast spells and charms, ask questions of the spirit world, design symbols that encapsulate intentions, how to protect yourself psychically, and how to deepen your relationship with the spirit world.

Firstly, we will consider what magic actually is and how we can enter the state of mind needed to perform it.

What is magic?

Magic is the act of causing change by altering one's state of mind to manipulate energy. Witches often use symbols, rituals, or call on unseen spirits to help achieve their aims. Since ancient times, magic has been a part of human culture, and still lingers in familiar religious and traditional practices. It can be used to attract, repel, bless, curse, protect, bind, liberate, and for some, serves as a path to enlightenment.

This ability to cause change is rooted in the idea that everything in the universe is interconnected. Chaos theory teaches us that small events in one place can have far-reaching consequences. This does not imply that every small action will lead to massive changes, but it shows the profound interconnectedness of everything. Similarly, quantum physics shows that even observing something can alter it, and that all matter and energy are linked at the most basic level. These scientific principles inspire the idea that intent and action can shape reality; an idea central to the practice of magic.

There are many ways to achieve this change, to work magic, and many reasons to do it. Esoteric traditions like alchemy and astrology employ magic to seek personal enlightenment whereas folk magic tends to focus on attracting qualities like love, wealth, and healing, to family and friends. Folk magic tends to take a very practical magical approach and often uses charms, herbs, and candles. In many NeoPagan practices, magic is used for personal empowerment and connection with nature, so is often aligned with cycles of the Sun and Moon. On a psychological level, magic can also be understood as focused realised intention, similar to visualisation, manifestation, or positive thinking, where our willpower helps to create change.

Magic, in all its forms, is a universal tool for connecting and improving our inner and outer worlds.

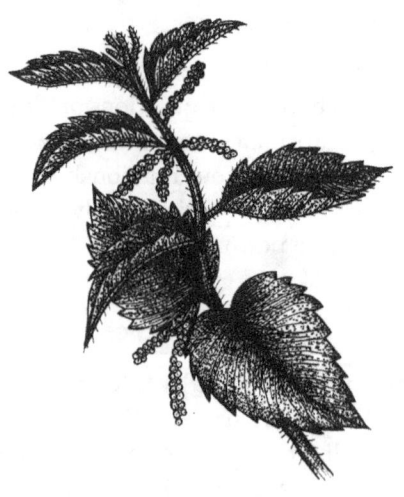

Which witch?

Most practitioners of contemporary witchcraft draw on knowledge and techniques from diverse sources to create an eclectic style. You may hear of specific types of witches, such as hedge-, hereditary-, and kitchen-witches, but in reality most embrace aspects of several styles and no two witches work in exactly the same way.

Then there are large organised groups, some of which are religions. Wicca is a NeoPagan, Earth-centric, twentieth-century religion, partly based on old practices. Some Wiccans are witches. Neo-druidry is a form of nature-based spirituality that draws upon natural elements and the folklore and history of Celtic lands. It is not a religion but welcomes members from different religions. Some Neo-druids are witches and some Neo-druid practices are deeply shamanic. Chaos magic is an attitude or philosophy that promotes experimentation, play, and creativity with magic. It emerged from the UK in the 1970s and encourages practitioners to find the core meaning in traditional practices. Chaos magic rejects dogma and hierarchy.

Magic in different forms

To help explain what Green City Witchcraft is, here is a summary of its components:

Folk and practical magic are centred on everyday needs like healing, protection, or good fortune. They involve charms, spells, and herbal healing, and are performed by mundane and magical folk. Such knowledge is passed down through generations in both town and country.

Natural magic works with the spirits and powers of nature. Herbs, stones, animals, and natural phenomena like the Moon, stars, or seasons, are often involved. It overlaps with folk magic and is commonly practised by Wiccans and Pagans.

Sympathetic magic is based on the belief that like affects like. Tokenistic objects with desired characteristics, or symbolic associations, are used to influence a target. For example, seeds may be used in a spell to represent a person's potential, in order to help them succeed. Or, a broom made of Lavender may be used to symbolically sweep and cleanse a space.

Contagious magic uses objects, once in contact with the target, as a means to influence it. For example, a target's hair, nail clippings, or clothing may be taken and used in rituals aimed at supporting them.

Shamanic magic involves communication with nature spirits, deities, and ancestors of place, time, and culture. Practitioners may enter lucid dreams, and trance states to heal, perform divination, and journey to other spiritual realms, to seek knowledge or to restore community balance.

Green City Magic is all of the above and more. It is an eclectic form of witchcraft, deeply rooted in nature and the environment, which is practised by people living in urban environments. Acknowledging that humans are part of nature, not separate from it, allows practitioners to respect and harness its power. Practitioners weave magical lives by building knowledge of their locality, magical techniques, and by living sustainably. They work closely with the seasons, Moon and weather. Local lifeforms support their work. Green City Witches seek harmony in nature so may forage, and craft simple tools for rituals, spells, and ceremonies.

They work ethically and sustainably; more likely to use a special pebble, seed, or flower, than the elaborate tools often associated with modern witchcraft. Green City Magic is for anyone seeking a deeper connection with nature while enjoying an urban life.

Guidelines for magic

There are **no rules** for Green City Witchery, but it's wise to consider a few guidelines:

Think it through

Consider your personal morals and the potential consequences of any magical work. Reframe negative intentions into responsible and positive versions. Send out energy that you would be happy to receive back, and aim to promote harmony and healthy transformation, not harm or control.

Respect nature

Show respect for all aspects of nature. Most Green Witches believe that humans are part of nature, not separate from it or superior to it.

Respect cultural practices

Acknowledge, respect, and protect indigenous cultures. Avoid cultural misappropriation. Use of plants and practices out of context causes ethical, social, and environmental problems.

Harm none

Ensure that your actions are rooted in fairness and respect for the greater good. Consider the ripple effect of all actions and use your words wisely.

Trust no one

Be cautious who you open up to. Find allies with open minds, but expect their values and interests to differ and perhaps change over time.

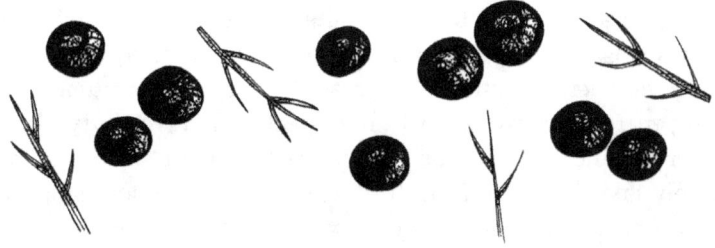

Core techniques

Several core techniques help witches to protect themselves, alight their energy appropriately and enter the state of mind where they can actually 'do magic'. These are:

- Grounding, centring, and shielding
- Engaging energy
- Entering the liminal state
- Using symbolism

Ground, centre, and shield

Some environments, people, and activities can drain our energy, while others nourish and leave us feeling vibrant and energised. It is important to balance exposure to these energies by listening to our gut instincts, taking rest when needed, and embracing excitement when it feels right. The following practices of grounding, centring, and shielding help to manage energetic shifts, restore balance, and protect against excess or depletion.

Grounding

This involves establishing an energetic connection between your body and the ground. It creates a feeling of balance and connection to the earth, improving wellbeing[22] and ability to work magic.

A popular way to ground is to visualise roots connecting your feet to the Earth. This can be challenging to visualise in tall buildings but it is possible. To try, place your feet flat on the floor wherever you are and feel roots growing from your soles. Visualise them rapidly growing through the floor, perhaps sideways at first, until they reach one of the weight-bearing walls of the building. Then picture those roots extending straight down to earth. Other methods, such as showering while visualising the water carrying away excess energy, can be just as effective. Glennie Kindred suggests this as a daily ritual to wash clinging energetic cobwebs away. It is effective and worth trying.

Other grounding methods use connection with earth and plants or simply taking time to rest, drink tea, or eat some nourishing food. Try immersing yourself in nature-based physical activities such as gardening, where skin contact with soil can quickly discharge excess energy. Walking barefoot, especially on Moss, or interacting with animals, which are natural energy grounders, can also work well. Tending to houseplants, foraging, or simply placing your hand on a tree trunk will also provide this earth connection and grounding effect.

Barefoot time

Connecting with the ground through barefoot walking or simply sitting outdoors without shoes and socks is a simple yet powerful practice. Often known as earthing, it allows us to reconnect with the calming, nurturing energies of the Earth. Whether it's a brief pause during lunch or a mindful stroll, barefoot time can awaken our senses and deepen our bond with the land.

Start gently—concrete paths can be harsh—and be mindful of hazards like broken glass or thorns. Over time, you'll cultivate the awareness needed for safe and mindful barefoot walks. Even in cold weather, baring your feet after a gardening session or during a crisp

---

[22] G. Chevalier et al. The effects of grounding (earthing) on bodyworkers' pain and overall quality of life: A randomized controlled trial. *Explore*, New York (2019) 15(3): 181–90.

walk can feel invigorating. Many people find it relieves any sense of disconnect from the Earth.

Palm stones

Holding stones can ground us instantly. It is so effective that this method is used during spiritual travel and shapeshifting work. Most stones can quickly bring us back to Earth, so find one that feels pleasant to handle and keep it handy. Hold or rub when you feel the need and imagine excess energy flowing into it from your body. When the stone starts to feel less effective, bury it in soil or sand for a day and night, to allow the stored energy to seep away and transform.

Grounding tea

Mugwort, Nettle, Chamomile, Dandelion root, and Oatstraw can all promote grounding. Choose a few herbs that align with your health and constitution. Mix equal parts by weight and store in a clean glass jar. Use 1 heaped teaspoon per cup of boiled water. Leave to infuse for 10 minutes before straining and drinking.

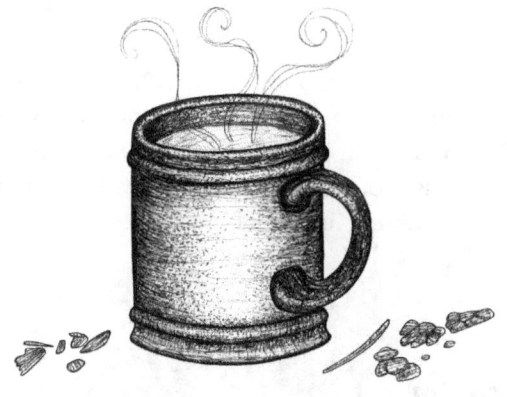

Centring

Centring focuses our energy towards the solar plexus, where it can be stored. It also aligns the energy inside of us with sources of energy in the wider universe. It helps clear feelings of being scattered or cloudy, and allows us to channel energy when needed.

Start by tuning into how your energy feels. Dream worker and witch Tree Carr recommends building awareness of your own energy by placing your hands in the prayer position, in front of your chest, keeping your palms about an inch apart. Then sense the energy between your fingertips or palms, and also in your solar plexus. This practice also makes it easier to direct your energy intentionally.

Another technique is to visualise roots extending from your feet into the earth (grounding), then sense energy being drawn upwards through your roots, towards your solar plexus. At the same time, imagine a silver thread connecting the crown of your head to the sky, channelling life force from above. As your solar plexus fills with light, allow the energy to spread through your body to strengthen you. When you feel fully charged, seal this energy in your body by mentally retracting your roots and the silver thread from your crown.

As with grounding, eating nutrient-dense foods can centre us effectively, because energy is needed in our core to help digestion. Meditation, particularly a body scan, can also be helpful. By focusing on different areas of your body, you become more aware of how your energy is flowing, and this allows you to direct it where needed for balance and grounding.

Centring tea

Rose, Lime blossom, Hawthorn and Lemon Balm can all bring a sense of calm, balance, and centredness. Select those that suit your health and constitution. Mix equal parts by weight and store in a clean glass jar. Use 1 heaped teaspoon per cup of boiled water. Leave to infuse for 10 minutes before straining and drinking.

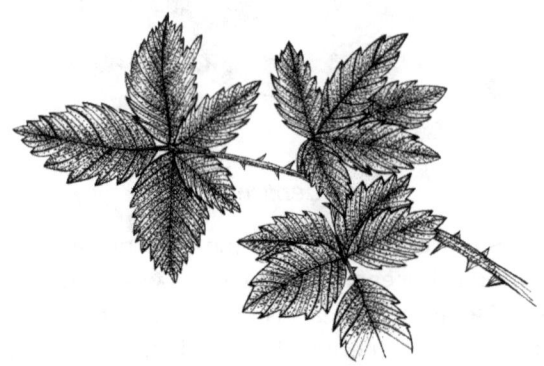

Shielding

This practice creates a protective energetic or psychic shield, and is key to maintaining psychic wellbeing. Shielding typically involves visualising a layer around your body, which prevents negative, harmful, or unwanted influences from entering. This shield acts like a filter, allowing positive energies in while keeping harmful energies away. Shielding can help us avoid feeling drained or manipulated by others, and is especially important for those who are emotionally sensitive, or who come in contact with extreme energy vibrations. Many practitioners combine shielding visualisations with protective affirmations.

It can help to develop a metaphorical "non-stick" coating, so that unwanted energy slips instantly away when it approaches us. This is especially useful when living in densely populated areas, but it doesn't mean you need to become tough or unfriendly. You can choose to soften your shield and let people in when you like. You may like to visualise a shield around you, perhaps with a non-stick coating, doing its work, all of the time.

Another shielding technique involves visualising a more complex protective forcefield, one with multiple layers. The layers can take the form of whatever you wish, perhaps a shimmering bubble, a golden egg, or a net of prickly Bramble stems. Play with the visualisation, choosing shield materials that suit you. Have fun experimenting with this during calm moments, so you can call up a shield easily.

Shielding is best done immediately after grounding, but it can be done quickly in times of sudden needs. And after creating them, watch how they deflect unwelcome energy back to its source. With practice, you will be able to use these visualised (or psychic) shields to help protect yourself, and others.

Other ways to shield are by using protective herbal infusions in foot baths, or as a final rinse after washing and showering. Rosemary and Bay are particularly effective, but choose herbs which suit your skin. Some witches also carry a small vial or pouch containing protective shielding herbs.

Shielding tea

Bay leaf, Mugwort, Peppermint, Rosemary, Nettle, and Lemon Balm are used to protect from psychic harm and to strengthen the body. Select those that align with your health and constitution, mix equal parts by weight (use only a pinch of Bay in your mix) and store in a clean glass jar. Use 1 teaspoon per cup of boiled water. Leave to infuse for 10 minutes before straining and drinking.

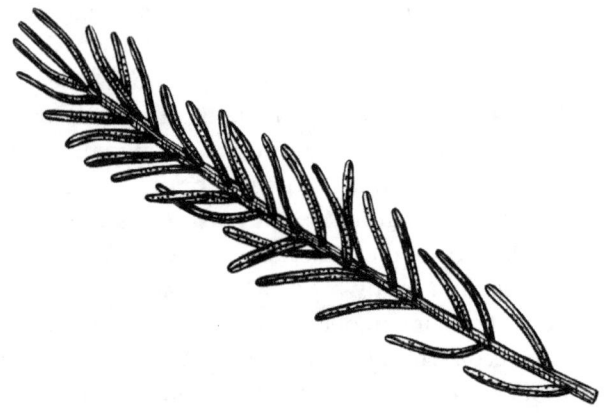

Engaging energy

After learning how to ground, centre. and shield, the next step is to develop skills in channelling energy, and controlling its flow. To get a feel for this, rub your hands together and then hold them slightly apart, with palms facing each other, and elbows against your body. You may feel a tingle or throb in your palms. Try moving them closer and further from each other, quite gently. You may feel a ball of energy building between your palms. If the feeling is clear, continue and see how big the ball of energy can grow. If you don't yet feel it, relax and come back to the exercise another day.

Different people have different sensations during energy work: they may describe them as buzzing, low, flat, irritable, itchy, and so on. Energy exercises can be a good barometer of how we are feeling, and to check if we are in fit enough energetic shape to perform magical tasks.

Once you are able to create the ball of energy from your palms with ease, you may like to work on directing it as a stream of energy into different objects and beings. With practice, it can be channelled into plants, animals, trees, and people when needed. This is often known as energy healing, laying on of hands, Reiki, or aura work. It is perhaps the simplest form of healing that we are capable of, and can have a wonderful effect on the receiver and channeller. You may like to try channelling energy into a glass of fresh water, to empower it, and then use it to water your plants—or yourself.

The liminal state

The state of mind where we can actually work magic is often called the liminal state or zone. This is the most effective state to be in to practise witchcraft.

Liminality is an altered state of consciousness. It is sometimes described as a waking dream or trance state, where we are conscious of what is happening but we perceive the world differently. When in this altered state, the right hemisphere of the brain is most active and it becomes possible to connect with both the spiritual and physical planes of this world. The right hemisphere governs intuition, imagination, and connection with the subconscious. It is essential for accessing altered awareness, creating mental imagery, and working with symbols and patterns in magical practice.[23] When we shift into this state spirits may be more accessible for guidance, identities are fluid, and it is easier for us to manipulate energy.

The liminal state is where personal and spiritual transformation happen most easily.

Some individuals can drop into the liminal state on demand. Others get there by touching a natural object, or gazing at reflections on water and letting their eyes go out of focus. It is not so easy for most of us, so many methods can be used to help. Here are some of the most common:

Yoga: An age-old system, which prepares the body and mind for meditation and connection with spirit. This is discussed further below.

Meditation: This naturally follows from Yoga but it can be practised alone. A regular practice trains how to control our thoughts, which makes entry into the liminal space easier. Zen meditation is an accessible form, which trains the mind while keeping the body still and eyes open. Movement meditations are also available, so if meditation appeals, find a style that suits you.

---

[23] The work of Iain McGilchrist, such as *The Master and His Emissary: The divided brain and the making of the Western world* (Yale UP, 2009), is central to our understanding of this.

Breathing: Controlled breathing can promote relaxation and reduce stress, making it easier to drop into the liminal state. Some breathing practices can overstimulate the mind, so progress gradually and stay within your limits.

Sound: Rhythmic repetition of mantras, chants, hymns, prayers, and invocations can create meditative and trance states. Regular practice improves breath control and produces vibrations that can affect the whole body. All forms of music can affect our state of mind. You may prefer sound baths, ritual music, trance, or dance but playing an instrument is one of the easiest ways to improve mental agility and enter the liminal state.

Herbs: Chamomile, Rosemary, Mugwort, and Tulsi, are among those that can help us prepare for magical work. Witches may drink herbal tea, apply infused oils, or burn dried herbs in saining rituals to help their minds change gear. Others use ceremonial Cacao, or strong psychoactive plants, such as Ayahuasca from indigenous communities in the Amazon Basin. Most quick-fix options do not train the body and mind to enter the liminal state at will. They carry serious physical and psychological risks, so should be approached with caution and professional guidance.

Dancing: Free or ecstatic dance forms can release physical and emotional tension while fully engaging the senses. This can help set the scene for entering the liminal state. Dervish Whirling, the ritual ecstatic dance of Sufi mystics, is increasingly popular with city mystics. Whatever form you choose, practice should feel safe, enjoyable, and helpful to you.

Recreational Drugs: Some turn to Psilocybin containing mushrooms, Cannabis, Peyote, *Salvia divinorum*, and other substances to access altered mental states. However, if seeking the liminal state to work magic, these substances need to be used with great care and preparation. Experiences with psychedelics are unpredictable and can trigger latent mental health issues such as anxiety, psychosis, or paranoia. They tend to offer an intense experience, with little chance to incorporate magical practice. Anyone considering this route should find an experienced and well-trained guide who sets use within a safe context. Legal and health implications must also be considered.

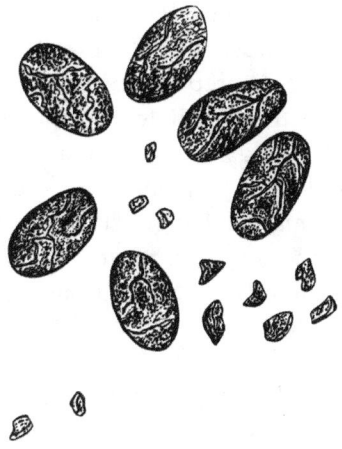

Yoga and the bliss state

The Eight Limbs of Yoga provide an ancient, structured path towards connection with the universal spirit. This purpose aligns with Green Witchcraft, and it can greatly support magical practices. The Eight Limbs of Yoga are as follows:

1. Yamas: Ethics for harmonious relationships through principles like right use of energy and non-greed.
2. Niyamas: Personal disciplines for inner growth, including study and contentment.
3. Asanas: Physical postures to build strength and concentration.
4. Pranayama: Breath control that balances emotions and sharpens focus.
5. Pratyahara: Withdrawing from external distractions, fostering deeper introspection.
6. Dharana: Concentrated focus on a single object or thought, training the mind to maintain attention.
7. Dhyana: A state of deep meditation where awareness flows continuously, allowing access to heightened states for consciousness for magical work.
8. Samadhi: The bliss state, where individual consciousness merges with the universal. This can happen during meditation, music, or time in nature. It is a transient state that comes and goes.

Dhyana and Samadhi may seem to be most relevant aspects for magical practitioners to explore, but we should remember that the other Limbs of Yoga are necessary steps to prepare the body and mind for meditation and eventual glimpses of the Bliss State. At its heart Yoga recognises that we humans are simply energy in a particular form; we are connected to both the earthly and spiritual planes, and use our minds to understand and react to information that our senses gather from each realm. The clarity of how we perceive that information, and the authenticity of how we react, depends upon how well various aspects of our brain and body function.[24]

Magical practitioners who practise Yoga find that their ability to enter the liminal state and work magic declines when they take breaks from their regular Yoga practice, and conversely see an improvement when they are in a good flow. If interested in exploring Yoga, find a style and teacher that suit you. There are many schools of Yoga, each with a slightly different approach, and some are more physically demanding than others. Just beware of the guru culture, which is sadly intertwined with some Yoga schools, and seek out a well-qualified teacher. Given the chance, Yoga can clear our bodies and minds of cobwebs and clutter that interfere with our perception of the world. Regular practice allows us to function in ways that allow human potential to be realised in both the physical and spiritual realms.

Gradually incorporate whichever practices you choose to try. Working on these skills is rather like training a muscle with exercise; regular practice is needed. Keep a balance between spiritual practices and the realities of urban living. Enjoy liminal moments when they come along; they certainly enrich magical experiences, but don't worry if you don't experience them. There are other ways to enhance your craft. Simply aim to keep your body and mind strong, and the rest will follow naturally. The better shape we are in mentally and physically, the easier it is to enter a magical state of mind.

A meditation practice

Here is a simple routine to try. If you prefer not to meditate, build your concentration by reading or crafting something that requires your full attention. Aim for 20-minute blocks of concentration, and build up to this gradually.

---

[24] Ranju Roy's book *Yoga as Pilgrimage: Sūtras for a modern age* (2024) offers a clear and accessible explanation of how the Yoga Sutras of Patanjali (the ancient text underpinning Yoga) are relevant to our lives today.

Do a few light stretches to settle your body. Aim to relieve tension in your back, neck, and shoulders. This helps remove physical distractions during meditation.

Set your intention for the practice. Choose something uncomplicated, perhaps "I am open to knowledge." As your skills develop, your intention may be to find answers or inspiration.

Sit or lie in a comfortable position. Take your time with this, to avoid any physical distractions as you meditate.

Breathe calmly, letting air flow in and out of your lungs as you simply observe the breath. Continue watching your breath, until it is calm and steady. Then gently control the length of your breath, making your exhalations slightly longer than your inhalations. Pause briefly between breaths, if that feels fine. Continue at a comfortable pace as your body and mind relax.

When your breathing has settled, close your eyes halfway so you are looking downwards. Focus on some small mark in front of you, perhaps a fleck on the floor or wall. Keep breathing at a comfortable pace and let your gaze soften. Allow your field of vision to soften so you can see but the image is wide and blurred. Keep this wide soft focus, and breathe.

If your attention drifts off, gently bring it back to the focal point, then soften and widen the focus again. Tell your mind to park up, or ignore, any intruding thoughts. You may need to do this repeatedly, as the mind brings more things to your attention. Keep the soft focus for as long as you can.

At times you may see images forming in front of you. This is partly the mind wandering, and partly your subconscious making sense of what it sees. This is how we begin interpreting patterns and shapes, such as clouds in the sky, swirls in inky water, flocks of birds, and so on. Try to keep your body settled and still throughout the exercise.

If you feel comfortable doing so, close your eyes. Focus on the intention, "I am open to knowledge," that was set at the start of the practice. Park up any distracting thoughts and let your breath move freely, at its own pace. Do this for several breaths. Then notice how your body feels.

Notice sounds within and outside of your body. Notice the feel of your tongue in your mouth and any tastes lingering there. Notice any scent travelling to your nose and pay attention to how your skin feels; notice where your clothes are touching your skin. Become more aware of the shapes and colours of light that reach your eyes through your closed eyelids.

Then return to focusing on your breath, and take a deeper breath. And let it out. Gradually move your fingers and your toes, then your legs and arms. Very gently move your neck to one side then the other. Continue moving your body as it wakes up. Then stretch or roll onto your side.

Come to a sitting position and then rub your hands briskly together. Place your palms over your eyes and feel the energy from your hands warming your eye sockets. Gradually lower your hands as you open your eyes. Take a deep breath in and out and settle your body. Then note down any observations or thoughts about your meditation practice.

Don't worry if you see little progress in shifting your state of mind; it gets easier with time. Likewise, don't become excited if you find entering the liminal state easy. We are on a personal journey; What we see through soft focus, and what we sense during meditation or spiritual travel is very personal, and it is invisible to others. Even those who seem able to slip effortlessly in and out of the liminal state can lose the knack at times. So keep practising if it suits you, be gentle with yourself, and don't let your ego feel dented or excited. It is what it is.

Symbolism

Witchcraft is rich in symbolism but so is the wider world. We humans attach meaning to everything from flowers and colours, to animals, crystals, logos, and days of the week. At their most simple, symbols are expressions of thoughts in our mind. Symbolism can be very personal and secret, or understood by communities. There are advantages to both. Seemingly endless combinations of symbols are used to share information with others, but to be understood both parties need to know the code.

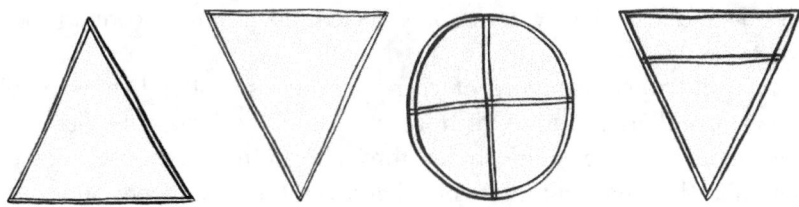

The earliest magical symbols probably were a dot or circle, and the line or serpent. These two simple markings are said to have led to all other symbols. Some magical symbols seem to be universal.

These are found cross-culturally in ancient art work so distant in time and space that they must have developed independently. These universal symbols include the swastika, spiral, pentagram, triangle, and inverted-Y (as found on the I Ching fire trigram). Many of them are considered archetypal, meaning that they represent fundamental human experiences and ideas.

Secret symbols

At times, it can be helpful for a magical practitioner to use language that the recipient or target cannot understand. This can help to keep secrets safe and give power to the practitioner. When someone hears words spoken in an unfamiliar dialect or language, or when they see symbols or script that they do not understand, they often place far more significance on them than is necessary. An air of mystery can amplify the power of symbols and deepen the impact of spells, charms, curses, or blessings that use them. It can have a significant emotional and psychological effect. So this is a good reason to experiment with symbols, and keep those you create and use secret, or shared only with a trusted few.

Shared symbols

When the meaning of symbols and codes is understood within a group, it can help the members to bond. For this reason some groups of magical practitioners create their own *lingua magica*, or secret magical language. As well as building camaraderie it can also prevent spells and rituals being understood or stolen by others. To share the meaning of such languages and symbols, a unique code or cipher is often used, to encode and decode privately. Many ancient magical texts contain code charts for this.

A well-known example of correspondences is the Language of Flowers, or Floriography, which was very popular during the Victorian era. Secret messages were shared through carefully composed flower bouquets, but even the best-considered combinations were only useful if the sender and receiver understood the same language; and with Floriography, many alternatives were available. A yellow Rose may have meant friendship to the sender but infidelity to the recipient—understanding depended upon which flower language they had learned.

Identical cipher wheels can be used to code messages and decipher them. There are many inspiring examples online, and they are fun to make. A simple option is to cut two concentric circles of card, join them in the centre with a split pin and then divide the circles into segments. When the wheels are lined up correctly, one shows the meaning, the other wheel shows the code, or cypher. Only those with the same cipher wheel, who understand how to line up the wheels correctly, will be able to decipher your messages.

Of course, cipher wheels, keys, and correspondence tables need to be kept safe, but they can be useful tools. If you don't wish to share personal codes with anyone else but want an added layer of protection for your spells and potions, you may like to create a private cipher wheel or correspondence table for your records.

Some old esoteric books make reference to unusual ingredients such as Toe of Frog. Some magicians did use unusual ingredients in their potions and charms, but most of these terms were encoded plant names. Just as with Floriography, there were different meanings for similar terms, but here are a few examples that may inspire your own work:

Bat's wings—Holly
Eye of Newt—Mustard seed
Toe of Frog—Buttercup
Graveyard dust—Mullein
Old man—Mugwort
Old woman—Wormwood
Witch bane—Rowan
Quickthorn—Hawthorn

Handwriting

Handwriting can reveal a person's state of mind, and their signature is a compressed version of that, a symbol representing the whole. Graphology, the study of handwriting, is a fascinating field that can also be valuable to magical practitioners. Graphotherapy uses the principles of graphology to help individuals change their mental patterns by altering their writing habits. Many texts on the subject are available, explaining how handwriting can enhance our lives.[25]

---

[25] Including Vimala Rogers, *Your Handwriting Can Change Your Life* (Touchstone Books, 2000).

The quality of our handwriting reflects our mental and emotional state—if we feel down, our handwriting shows it; if we feel optimistic and calm, that shows through too. By consciously changing our handwriting, we can influence our mood. Magical symbols can also benefit from this treatment, for example by using upward strokes and curves in symbols to promote positivity. You may like to experiment with this, working on your handwriting regularly for your own mental health and as a way to enhance your written symbols and spells.

Study of mystical symbols

Many mystical traditions encourage the use of symbols to alter consciousness or enable connections with spirits and deities. In Kabbalah, practitioners study symbols representing the *sephirot* (ten aspects of god) as a pathway to connect with the Infinite. Historically, this system was considered secret and was reserved for married men over the age of forty. Similarly, in Hinduism, yantras (geometrical diagrams) are used to focus the mind, support meditation, and elevate consciousness. In Sufism, certain practices involve the use of sacred symbols and patterns, such as Sufi mandalas, which help to deepen spiritual awareness.

Numerology is the mystical study of numbers. This is an accessible subject that can easily be woven into magical work. For instance, number 22 may help transform big dreams into reality, whereas number 21 could enhance conflict resolution spells. The relevant number could be used to inform the number of repetitions of a chant, the number of words in a spell, or become part of a symbol.

Nature-inspired symbols in cities

Exploring nature-inspired symbolism in urban environments can reveal interesting meanings too, especially in places like graveyards. When visiting these sites, take the time to uncover the messages that bereaved families intended to convey about their loved ones. Look for symbolic plants and animals on memorials, alongside written words and symbols. For instance, Laurel leaves may signify artistic achievement, while Roses usually represent love. Few gravestones have colour, so we can only guess at deeper Floriography meanings. Engraved symbols, such as craftsmen's tools, can indicate a vocation, and others reflect contributions to society. Specific plants are often grown to convey distinct meanings too, for example, Ivy for fidelity, and Cypress for mourning.

Nature-inspired symbols are also found in urban architecture, particularly in grand or historic buildings. Look for floral motifs, Vine patterns, and other natural elements incorporated into facades and interiors. These not only provide decoration but can also teach us about the cultural values from the times when these places were built. Nature elements are often used in architecture to promote feelings of harmony and connection to the natural world.

NeoPagan symbols and scripts

It can be useful to learn about ancient and modern scripts and symbols that are linked to our heritage. If interested in the Celts, a Neo-druidic emblem to explore is the Awen. This consists of three concentric circles around three dots, each with a ray below. This symbol represents inspiration, with the three drops and rays signifying the flow of creativity that emerged from Ceridwen's cauldron in the myth of Taliesin. This Awen symbol is quite modern and was designed by the Order of Bards, Ovates, and Druids (OBOD).

Another interesting Celtic symbol is the Triskelion, made from three interconnected spirals. It features in ancient Celtic artwork and often represents the concept of life, death, and rebirth, or the harmony of mind, body, and spirit.

If you have links to Scotland, you might like to learn more about Pictish Swirls. These are intricate designs, based on the art and beliefs of the ancient Picts. NeoPagans have created the modern script from historic examples. Pictish Swirls lend themselves well to writing out spells and rituals by hand.

The pentagram is perhaps the most well-known symbol among magical practitioners. When pointing upward, it signifies the triumph of spirit over matter, making it particularly useful in magical work. In contrast, a downward-pointing pentagram is often misinterpreted as a representation of evil, but it traditionally symbolises earthly gratification and the material realm, so is used to emphasise the need for balance between spiritual and earthly desires.

Adopted symbols

Symbols can carry whatever intent and meaning you give to them. But can they really be so flexible? Many symbols are used across various faiths for different purposes, illustrating how their meanings can shift dramatically depending on context. For example, the pentagram holds different significance in Wicca, where it represents the elements and the spirit; in Christianity, it has been associated with protection and the five wounds of Christ, while for Muslims, the five-pointed star represents the five pillars of Islam. Similarly, the Lotus flower symbolises purity and enlightenment in Buddhism, while it represents rebirth in Hinduism.

This mixed-use phenomenon often occurs when a new religion adopts symbols from an existing belief system. Familiar symbols seem to encourage acceptance of a new path, by those who may otherwise resist change. This is perhaps why in Ireland the Pagan Sun wheel symbol found its way into St Patrick's Celtic Cross, and why the sacred Pagan Shamrock symbol, with its three leaflets, was used to help Christians understand their holy trinity.

Sigils

Sigils are symbols that represent energy, words, or magical intent. When activated they can help manifest the things that they represent. Sigils often represent lots of information, such as the characteristics of a nature spirit. They compress the information into a symbol that can be replicated and understood.

Sigils are mentioned in ancient spiritual texts worldwide, and often relate to love, protection, exorcism or spiritual enlightenment. In medieval times, sigils were used to represent the angels and demons that a practitioner might summon up during rituals. Old grimoires often contained pages of these magical symbols. Brand logos are sigils, intended to attract success to their organisation. Some seem to take on a life of their own, often controlling our minds when we see them. Such powerful logos are sometimes known as Hyper Sigils. The logos of many contemporary global brands certainly satisfy this definition.

Some mystical groups, such as the Golden Dawn, have advised making sigils by combining letters, colours, and characteristics to symbolically represent the desired outcome of magical work. They can be created using tables or grids of correspondences, with numerology, invented patterns, a sigil maker grid or wheel. Or, make a code yourself from ancient and modern symbols such as alchemical symbols, Pictish Swirls, or the Welsh Barddas runes of Iolo Morgannwg. Another popular method arose with the Chaos Magic work of Austin Osman Spare.

To be effective our sigils don't need to be fancy, or be based on ancient symbols or strategies, but they do need to be created with clear intention because they are symbols of power.

How to create a sigil

Start by clarifying your intention or goal, and create a statement of intent, or affirmation. Words have power and energetic vibration, so avoid those that suggest a lack of what you need, such as I want, or I need. Instead, keep intentions positive, succinct, and in the present tense.

Write out your statement of intent, for instance:

I AM PROSPEROUS

Then encode the letters using a cipher or numerology, and arrange the outcome to your liking. Or, if you prefer the less complicated Chaos Magic approach, remove vowels from your statement of intent, and see what's left. The example above would become:

M PRSPRS

Remove any repeats:

MPRS

Now rearrange these letters, in your mind, on paper or a screen. Some sigil designers like to rotate or mirror symbols, letters, and numbers in their designs. All is possible. Arrange the shapes into a compact symbol. You may like to use the positive upward, expansive strokes of Graphology, to further empower the shapes, or you may prefer to leave some of the letters out of your design. Try not to overthink the process. Gazing at the sigil should make you feel like your intention has been realised.

Rather than using words and letters, some practitioners prefer to choose shapes, symbols, or images that represent a magical intention. These may be natural shapes, ancient symbols or something else that is personally symbolic. If necessary, simplify the images and shapes to make them easier to handle. Arrange them spatially on paper or a screen, in a way that makes you feel like your intention has been realised. Record your sigils so that you can later refer to them. Then when ready, it is time to activate them.

Activating sigils

After creating such special symbols, they must be activated to awaken their potential. This can be done in endless ways, such as:

Burn: Try writing the sigil on a Bay leaf, then burn it in a safe ventilated space. When fresh Bay leaves burn, they often fizzle, spark, and pop, adding extra magic to your work.

Paint or Make: Recreate your sigils with natural materials that are personally connected to you; perhaps a drop of spit, herb infused oil or ointment, or Nettle juice from local plants. Alternatively, craft 3D versions of your sigil, to keep on display.

Incense: Draw sigils with loose incense or dry herbs, sprinkled onto a metal plate (like a baking tray). Then heat from below for a short while with a candle flame, to allow the incense to release sigil energy into the air. If burning an incense stick, try drawing sigils in the air with the smoke.

Eat: Incorporate sigils into biscuits, bread, cakes, and fruit, either by shaping or decorating. Sprinkle herbs related to your magical intent over food and drink, in the sigil shape. Then stir in, eat, and enjoy them becoming part of your body.

Walk: Draw sigils on the soles of your shoes; each step you take will release their energy. This is a particularly good method for intentions linked to making progress.

Internal Circuit: Visualise the sigil moving around a circuit within your body, before being charged and released into the world from your solar plexus. Further details in Sigil Charging Ritual.

Personal sigils — lamen

This is a way to express your unique magical identity. Lamen are created from symbols with personal significance for you. They could indicate your strengths, ancestors, and purpose in life. The design could be your initials, entwined with a significant herb. Once made, your lamen can be used in many ways. Some practitioners incorporate theirs into jewellery, place it on their altar, or use it when writing spells, as a sort of magical signature. Signet rings, which were originally used to denote authority and personalise seals on documents, are another way to use a lamen.

Using sigils

After their initial activation, it is wise to keep your sigils alive until their work is done. Repeated exposure helps trigger your subconscious to remember the magic that these symbols are working, so engage with them regularly. Try marking magical tools and candles with them, arrange leaves and flowers in their shape, draw them in journals, clip them to the fridge door, and slip them inside of your phone case. However you choose to work with symbols and sigils, remember there are no rules; Use what works for you as a practitioner of magic.

Amulets and talismans

An amulet is an object used for protection, while a talisman is created to bring good luck or specific intentions into a person's life. We know they have been used since ancient times. The Leiden Magical papyrus of Ancient Egypt describes a special amulet worn to speed up a divination ritual:

> ... a band of linen of sixteen threads, four of white, four of [green], four of blue, four of red, and make them into one band and stain them with the blood of a Hoopoe, and you bind it with a scarab ...

Better-known examples include the Eye of Horus, Scarab Beetles, Kimpetbrivl, and the Hand of Fatima.

To charge your amulet or talisman, ground, centre, and shield. Then rub your hands together and feel your energy start to flow from your palms. Place them on or close to the amulet and let the object fill with energy until it can absorb no more. Once charged, programme it with your chosen intention, whether it's for protection, success, or healing. Do this by stating your intention aloud or saying it silently as your energy flows. Amulets can be carried, or secreted around your home.

Herbs can be used as protective amulets, alone or combined with symbolic elements such as sigils and stones. To make a herbal amulet select natural materials with properties that align with your intentions. You may like to mark symbols onto leaves, then crumble them to dust and pour them into a small vial, to be worn as a pendant. Or perhaps, add herbs to a small pouch and combine with a complementary stone or crystal. One protection combination could be three dried Black Nightshade berries, a Bay leaf inscribed with protective symbols, a found Cat claw or Rose thorn, and dried Rosemary leaves.

Witch Balls are powerful talismanic objects. These colourful glass balls are nautical floats, of the type once tied to open sea fishnets, to help fishermen find their catch. Old glass floats occasionally wash up on beaches around the world, and are thought to bring good luck, guard against hexes and other unwanted energies. They are often displayed in the windows of coastal houses, to keep watch for the owners.

Rituals

Rituals are structured actions with symbolic meaning, used to enter a heightened state of consciousness. They can be simple or complex, but always serve a deeper purpose, connecting us to something beyond the mundane. Familiar rituals can help us through challenging life events, seasonal changes, or crises. Whether done solo or in a group, rituals can elevate consciousness, ground us, and help us connect to ourselves, others, and spirit. Simple, everyday actions, like taking a shower, or opening windows to let in fresh air, can be transformed into rituals when done mindfully.

Rituals can also anchor us in the present and help us transition from the mundane world to the magical. They can guide us into the liminal state, so that we can work magic. Rituals do not need to be long, complicated or dramatic, but they can be if that pleases those taking part. Ceremonies used to mark special occasions often include rituals with symbolic meaning.

The core features of a ritual are:

- Intention—Have a clear purpose or reason for the ritual.
- Location—Choose a space conducive to the energy you're working with.

- Action/Words—Specific movements or incantations are prepared.
- Closure—Reflect on the intentions of the ritual, at the end.

Ethical considerations

Be mindful of cultural misappropriation in ritual practices. While candles, incense, and other tools are common in many spiritual practices, we must be aware of their origins and consider whether using them in the way we do is appropriate and safe. Some practices may seem universal, like lighting a candle, but others belong specifically to certain cultures or religions, like burning White Sage. Rather than borrowing these elements without respect, practitioners should aim to understand their deeper meanings and origins, so that local materials and traditions can be used in their place.

The elements

Many magical practitioners incorporate the four elements, Earth, Water, Air, and Fire, into their rituals, reflecting an ancient belief in these primal forces. These elements have been central to various spiritual traditions, from Eastern philosophies to Paganism, and medieval European medicine, which was based on the four humours.[26]

We are believed to be composed of these elements, and our energy can feel imbalanced when our connection with them is disturbed. Some magical practitioners meditate on each element individually, to develop a better understanding of its qualities and influence. In rituals, simple natural objects can symbolise the elements, such as a feather for Air, a pebble for Earth, Moon water for Water, and a candle or fiery crystal for Fire.

Incorporating elemental symbols can enhance magical practice but not everyone feels connected to this system, and that's fine; To be useful, rituals should feel authentic to the individual.

Ritual space

When a space is used repeatedly for spiritual or magical work, an inherent energy of place tends to build over time. Some locations, intended to be used long term for rituals, are consecrated or declared sacred, and

---

[26] Stephen Taylor, *The Humoral Herbal: A practical guide to the Western Energetic system of health, lifestyle and herbs* (Aeon, 2021) comprehensively covers this topic, and how different herbs relate to each humour.

only to be used for magical purposes. However, without the luxury of a dedicated space, most witches open and close ritual spaces as needed. These temporary spaces for magical work can be created anywhere. Perhaps the simplest way to do this is to raise a circle.

Raising a circle of energy provides protection from negative energy, and signifies that this is a place of connection with spirit, where magic is being worked. Circle raising can be done simply or with ceremony. A circle shape can be symbolically drawn with a pointed finger or wand around you. Or, dust, salt, herbs, stones, or whatever is appropriate to the setting, can be sprinkled or placed in a ring. At times, these circles feel like the centre-line of a protective shield that rises up and around, and below, enclosing the witch within a spherical forcefield, with the drawn circle at its equator.

At the end of the witch's work, the circle should be dissolved either by retracing it backwards, smudging the dust, or using focused intent to dissipate the energy field. Whether a circle is drawn or not, it is essential to establish and maintain clear boundaries for sacred space, at least to prevent mundane distractions, while you are working magic.

Planning rituals

Rituals can be simple and spontaneous. When creating your own, try to follow a logical, structured flow that helps you move through the phases of intention, action, and reflection. The more we practise, the deeper our engagement becomes and the better the results of our work. Most rituals follow this basic structure:

Cleansing

This initial step prepares the space and participants by shedding negative energies. Traditional methods include using fire, water, or smoke (with incense or saining bundles) for purification. Drawing or casting a circle around the ritual space is part of this. Space cleansing helps to clear mental clutter and create a sacred atmosphere.

State the purpose

Every ritual needs a clear intention. Whether it's to honour a seasonal transition, ask for guidance, or mark a significant life event, the intent should be communicated to all participants at the outset to focus energy.

Looking forward and back

Reflection is powerful. Acknowledge the past, whether personal experiences, ancient wisdom, or relevant events, and then look to the future. Setting intentions for growth, healing, or transformation can help with this.

Worship and gratitude

Expressing thanks to deities, nature spirits, ancestors, or the Universe helps to keep a humble tone. Gratitude often involves spoken words, offerings, or a quiet moment of reflection on the blessings of life.

Offering

Symbolic gestures include burning old items, offering food, or planting seeds, to show commitment to transformation. Ritual offerings are often seasonal and relate to the intent of the ritual.

Calling on spirits

Invoke the presence of spirits that you feel aligned with, or the Universal Spirit. Ask that they bless and witness the ritual. This step is an invitation for guidance and support, not a demand. It should be done respectfully.

Asking for healing or blessings

Request healing, protection, or specific blessings, whether for yourself, others, or the world. This part of the ritual often includes prayers.

Liminality

The liminal phase in rituals is the phase where transformation and true magic happen. This state can be reached through various means, such as dance, music, or chanting. Once in the liminal state, witches may engage in spellwork, shapeshifting, and spirit travel. This altered state of awareness allows for deep connection to the subconscious.

Return to the mundane

After the liminal phase, it's important to come back to everyday reality, the mundane. This can be done with grounding exercises, making a simple physical gesture, or touching something solid (like a palm stone).

Close the ritual

Formally end the ritual by thanking the spirits, deities, or energies invoked, and closing the sacred space. A clear ending further marks the return to normal life and ensures the spirits are respectfully released. The circle is closed, symbolically removing the boundary created at the start of the ritual. Any materials used to mark the circle are swept away, returning the space to its previous state and ensuring complete closure.

Feasting and social time

Food and drink help ground after the heightened energy of ritual.

Group rituals

Rituals can identify and strengthen our sense of community. Group rituals carry greater power owing to the collective energy of the participants. They encourage connection, discipline, and shared purpose, and often leave participants feeling more aligned. Group rituals often include drumming, chanting, and singing; all of which can greatly intensify energy. Group gatherings also open up options for using more impressive settings, and this is known to intensify the sense of engagement and magic. Sharing food, perhaps a pot luck supper or picnic, after closing the circle with a group, can be fun. Feasting together also gives time to reflect on the ritual, and help group members to bond.

It is vitally important that group rituals feel safe, familiar, logical, and inclusive. Not everyone enjoys working magic in groups, so we need to ensure that those attending are not pressured to participate in anything that makes them feel uncomfortable.

Ritual baths and showers

These can transform everyday cleansing into a sacred practice. Bathing in open water or adding herbal infusions, floating petals, oats, or honey to your bathtub can create a nurturing, womb-like environment.

Showertime can also become a ritual. You might start by skin brushing, then visualising the shower washing away negative energy. After drying off, oiling your skin with herb-infused oils can bring further grounding. Even shaking in the shower, a form of somatic release, can deepen the sense of grounding and rejuvenation—just avoid slipping.

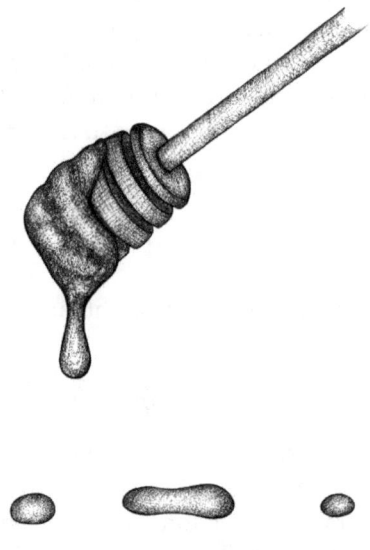

Ancient rituals

Ancient texts worldwide can help us understand the roots of modern ritual practices. The Leiden Magical Papyrus contains many spells, incantations, and charms from Ancient Egyptian times. It provides a peek into rituals from thousands of years ago.

It mentions an Oil Divination ritual, where a boy would gaze into a bowl of oil and seek guidance from the spirit world, on behalf of an adult. Anubis was kindly requested to intermediate between the boy and the spirits. A special amulet was worn by the boy, to speed up the process, and specific phrases and charms were used. These were repeated 7 times, some until the 7th hour of the day and offerings were provided; bread and wine were standard, although certain spirits required additional offerings. The Leiden Magical Papyrus also explains how to tell invoked spirits to leave:

> *If you wish to make (them) all depart, you put Ape's dung on the brazier, then they all depart to their place, and you utter their spell of dismissal also and some powder with alum on the brazier. ... Good dispatch, joyful dispatch!*

You may not have any Ape dung or alum powder to hand, but reading ancient texts like this can certainly inspire modern rituals. At its core, this Egyptian ritual involves adding certain things to the fire and using kind but firm words. This is possible today.

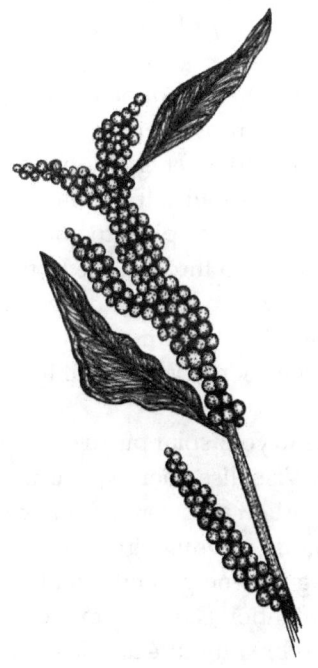

Example ritual—To charge a sigil

This technique, inspired by the late Stephen Russell, a Taoist practitioner (also known as the Barefoot Doctor), is designed to focus intense energy into your sigil before releasing it into the universe to manifest.

You will need a candle, lighter, pen, or pencil, a Bay leaf/Birch bark paper/recycled paper and the Sigil.

Light the candle and sit comfortably in a quiet, undisturbed area. Ground your energy and enter a calm, focused state. You can do this through deep, rhythmic breathing at a rate that you find comfortable (perhaps inhale for three seconds, exhale for five).

Then copy your sigil on a small piece of paper, bark, or leaf. You may like to use berry juice as ink. As you draw and then look at the sigil, focus on its meaning; what does it symbolise to you and what is the intention behind it? Place the sigil next to the candle, or beneath it.

Now visualise the outcome that you desire, as vividly as possible, in your mind. Imagine that what you want to achieve is already manifest. Engage all your senses: How does it feel to be in the situation you seek? What do you see, smell, and hear at that time? What can you touch or hold? Experience the reality of your intention, in as much detail as possible.

Once fully immersed in the intention of the sigil, see the sigil inside of your head. Visualise it there as clearly as you can, feel all it represents, then send the symbol around an energy loop in your body, slowly and smoothly as you breathe. Visualise it moving up to the crown of your head, then down your neck and spine, to your tailbone. From there, in a continuous loop, move it up through the front of your body, through your belly, solar plexus, heart, neck, face, then crown. Then again, move it down the spine. Repeat this twice more, breathing and visualising the sigil moving through the energy loop, until it has completed three full circuits.

Now send the image to your solar plexus and let it sit there, becoming brighter and stronger. Visualise energy pouring into the sigil from all directions until it is so bright and charged that it explodes into a trillion particles, each a hologram of your sigil. These spread out through the universe, each carrying the energy and intent of the sigil, enabling the magic to work. Your intention is now in motion.

Take time to let your breath settle and feel your connection with the earth. Gently centre yourself. Feel yourself calm and energised. Finally, take a moment to visualise yourself shielded from harm. Keep the sigil paper under the candle, or on your altar—somewhere safe.

The sigil only needs to be charged in this way once. From now it can be kept alive by any of the other techniques mentioned in the sigils section.

Nature spirits

Many Green City Witches work with nature spirits, calling on them for inspiration, guidance, and support during rituals. They may honour and communicate with these spirits through offerings, meditations, or rituals.

Nature spirits are entities that inhabit and protect the natural world. They may be associated with specific elements such as fire, water, earth, and air, with specific places (often called genius loci), or they may reside in rocks, plants, rivers, mountains, mushrooms, trees, and animals. Some are quite fluid, such as river and air spirits, or they may live in one type of tree, animal, or even a specific street. In different cultures, it is common for nature spirits to be called upon to support, in both magical and mundane life. Green Witches tend to view them as guardians of the land and allies in their magical and spiritual work.

Nature spirits from different cultures

Nature spirits are mentioned in the folklore and mythology of most cultures. At least some impression of Fairies, Brownies, or Elves can usually be visualised by even the least spiritually inclined Brits. We often grow up with tales about them, images in story books, customs, and superstitious warnings. We may even recall personal experiences of spiritual encounters with them when we were young and more open to otherworldly possibilities.

Some cultures have favourites that they associate with different purposes and places. For instance, the house Brownies of Scotland and the Kobolds of German mines, homes, and ships. Certain elements of nature are protected by spirits that have specific personalities, like Hyldemoer, who resides within the Elder. There may be guidance, passed on through folklore, to help humans working with them avoid misfortune. Whether we perceive them as benevolent towards us or not, nature spirits should be respected.

Finding out about local nature spirits (at home or away) can help to connect with them, avoid accidentally disrespecting them, and also explain how local customs, names, and traditions came to be. The Welsh Tylwyth Teg, the Irish Aos Sí, Cornish Knockers, Scottish Wee folk, tree-dwelling Dryads, Encantados of Galicia and Kabouters of the Netherlands, are just a few of these, and all are fascinating to learn about.

Some magical practitioners work with deities (gods and goddesses), and may think of them having higher status than nature spirits. Deities tend to be formally worshipped and may be part of a structured pantheon, such as the ancient Egyptian pantheon, with deities such as Isis, Osiris, and Thoth. The ancient Celtic pantheon includes deities associated with all aspects of life and includes fascinating characters such as Brigid, Cernunnos and Morrigan.

Building a relationship with deity is certainly not a necessity for the Green City Witch but it can be fulfilling. One witch described:

> *I don't really work with particular deities, but perhaps I do. My pantheon is all of nature—I need to take care not to neglect any part of it.*

Many of us have international lifestyles that put us in contact with deities from diverse cultures. My travels to India brought me awareness of the Hindu deities Ganesh, Lakshmi, and Saraswati. I do not have the same relationship that a Hindu might have with them, but I have developed a quiet respectful connection of my own. I show them respect, and when their strengths are required, I might reach out to them for support. We each weave a unique life, and this is reflected in the spirits that we work with.

Respect for nature spirits

In general, nature spirits around the world tend to be benevolent—when we humans respect the aspects of nature that they protect. However, they tend to turn against us when we abuse what they care for. This is not difficult to understand. In Japanese folklore, Kodama are nature spirits believed to inhabit and protect ancient trees of dense forests. They can bring great misfortune to a person responsible for cutting down one of these trees. Kodama are sometimes depicted as small, ghostly figures or simply as the voices or sounds people hear in the forest. In some regions of Japan, those trees believed to be inhabited by Kodama are marked with sacred ropes to protect them and appease the spirits.

Spirit form

In folklore, nature spirits are often depicted human-like, with a face, and physical features linked to their characters. But nature spirits are not restricted by human form, and the older the cultures we examine, the further from human form the entities are shown to have. It seems that over time, we humans have anthropomorphised nature spirits. Perhaps this is because spirits are energy and energy is difficult to see or describe, until it changes something.

When we think of the Celtic and Norse Green Man, the usual image of this spirit is a masculine face, leaf-framed, symbolising power and virility. This is how the Green Man energy has been considered for generations. We could try instead to envision a swirl of green energy, playing through tree leaves—everything it touches bursts to life. Green Man energy is fresh, fertile, and abundant; found inside every cell of every tree and every herb of every forest, and also your local park. Green Man energy is playful, wise, and kind, and yet also scary and sometimes cruel. This is harder to show in an image, but it can help us understand what the Green Man is.

Building relationships with nature spirits

Nature spirits are often requested to help in the magical work of Green City WItches. We are among them often so this is logical, but it is important to build relationships with spirits during good times, so that we can call in them when in need. There are many ways to do this.

Spending quiet time where they live is a fine start. Visiting water, a woodland corner of a park, an old building, or sitting next to a plant can also work. Clearing litter and taking care of an area they protect is often better than leaving physical offerings, but some nature spirits are known to value specific offerings. Perhaps dribble a little organic milk or cream into the ground, or leave a small amount of oatcake, bread, or seeds.

If leaving anything, be certain it is completely biodegradable and suitable for local wildlife. The salt in regular peanut butter, for instance, can harm garden birds. Also consider asking the spirits what they need. If you spend enough time in areas rich in nature spirits, they will find ways to tell you. Nature spirits often like music, especially when played on simple instruments such as the wooden flute, lyre, or voice. Play to them kindly and gently, as if recreating the sounds of a soft breeze through reeds.

When we have built up a relationship with nature spirits, we can choose to communicate with them at relevant times. Nature spirits can also be asked to guide us during spiritual travels, and shapeshifting. Before attempting to engage them, remember to ground, centre, and shield yourself from harm. If you have time to prepare, consider using something symbolic of your relationship with them (perhaps music, a leaf) when asking for their support and guidance. But they can also be called by a simple evocation such as:

> *I call on the spirits of air, to support me in my work today.*

Don't forget to thank them, and just as in the papyrus ritual, remember to say goodbye to them at the end.

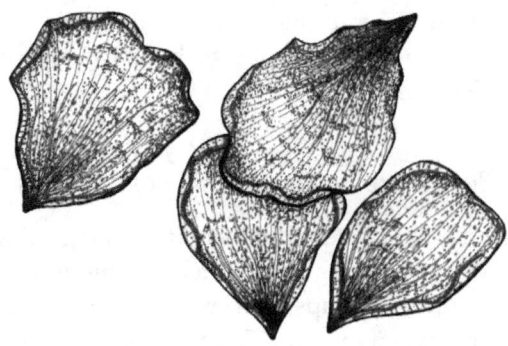

Divination and special senses

We all need to seek guidance at times, and many witches do this through divination. This skill can take many forms of interpreting signs or employing tools such as herb sticks, cloud patterns, or cards. The insights gained from divination are intended to help navigate life's path, rather than predict specific outcomes. Techniques vary widely but typically involve the seeker asking a question, receiving signs, and then interpreting their meaning. These signs may come directly, or through the use of tools. Divination methods have been practised in all cultures throughout history. They are ways to access knowledge from the unconscious.

We all have the potential to sense subtle energies, and to interpret signs. With practice, we can develop these abilities. Below are some techniques used by Green City Witches who draw upon natural materials or signs from the environment. Whichever you try, be playful, because when we feel relaxed, our subconscious is free to work. But when we feel stressed, the mind has other things to worry about and is unlikely to give a useful reading. Likewise, don't cling to what comes to you through divination or be bothered by it, just interpret what you can.

There are many places where the power of nature is palpable. You may have noticed that some places you visit have a special energy, perhaps a corner of a park or woodland. These could become places where you would like to practise divination techniques outdoors. But anywhere is a possibility for this, and your apartment can be perfectly suitable, especially if you are able to find quiet time there. Nature spirits are everywhere, and what matters most for divination is having an open mind.

Gut instinct or intuition

Your gut instinct is the knot in your stomach telling you to find a new job, or the uneasy feeling warning against walking in a certain direction. When we learn to trust our gut instinct or intuition there is less need to use divination tools. The role of these feelings is to guide us and keep us safe; the more we listen to and act on them, the stronger they become. You may like to make a habit of tuning into your intuition each day, perhaps during your morning routine. Pay attention to the subtle messages it's giving you, and note down anything significant. Then, as you go about your business, reflect on whether your instincts held much truth.

Science has now confirmed that many of our emotions and instincts do actually come from the gut. Some 400–600 million nerve cells are found in this enteric or second brain, which pass messages to and from the brain.[27] So our state of mind affects how the gut works, and gut function affects our mood. We should take our gut feelings seriously, but we must also realise that its messages are quite raw, unfiltered, and affected by our diet. Gut instinct is there to protect us but it lacks the logic of the conscious mind, so we may need to balance the feelings it gives with reason before acting on them. However, if we constantly suppress our intuition, eventually it will stop sending us the messages we need to stay safe and well.

Some people pick up on information in extra, special ways. Some forms of this clarity (clairs) are well known. They include clairvoyance (clear seeing), where without using any tools, images appear in the mind's eye. Clairaudience is where voices or sounds are heard, although other people can't hear them. Clairsentience is where the emotions or energies from other people or places can be felt, and claircognisance is a sudden, unexplainable knowing that seems to arrive without previous thinking.

Many people have moments of these clairs, but we can all learn to develop our intuition with divination techniques. Some divination

---

[27] M.A. Fleming et al. The enteric nervous system and Its emerging role as a therapeutic target. *Gastroenterol Res Pract.* (2020): 8024171.

techniques attempt to make sense of patterns (scrying), others use tools such as divination sticks, and others try to interpret signs in nature. Divination helps us because although it may appear completely random at first, our selection, placement, and interpretation of the tools is influenced by our subconscious and gut instinct. So to allow ourselves to open up to divination, we must begin by taking time to relax. This allows our enteric brain and mind to communicate calmly, and allows us to enter the receptive liminal state. Here are examples of the three groups of divination technique.

Scrying

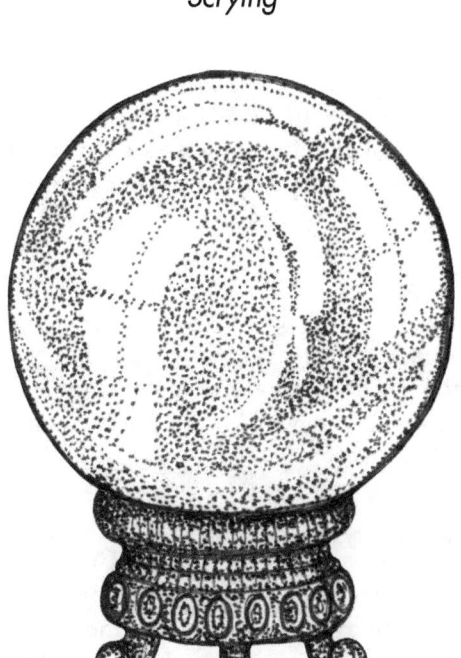

Scrying (or gazing) reveals images that are reflected from surfaces like crystal balls, or candle flames. It involves allowing the seer's focus to soften and the field of vision to widen, so that images may arise from the subconscious. The process is similar to daydreaming. Thoughts, images, and sounds emerge as the mind processes light patterns from the eyes. The impressions that follow are then interpreted for meaning. Various surfaces can be used for scrying. When developing this skill, begin by asking yourself what guidance you seek. Choose a calm, uninterrupted space, and reflect on the meanings that surface for you. Focus on how they resonate with you personally, rather than relying on traditional interpretations. Here are some nature-based scrying techniques:

Water scrying

Gaze at the surface of water, perhaps a pond, lake, or even a dark bowl filled with water. Some practitioners focus on the images produced when light is reflected from water onto another surface. Water scrying by Moon- or candlelight is popular.

Fire gazing

Scry by softly gazing into a fire or candle flame. Some prefer the flicker of flames, others gaze at glowing embers as a fire dies down. Gaze from a safe distance and don't fall asleep with an unattended flame.

Cloud scrying

Clouds constantly shift in shape and pattern. This is another relaxing form of divination. Lie near a window or, better yet, outdoors, and let yourself daydream as you gaze at the changing cloud formations. Your subconscious will often make a sort of movie in the sky from cloud shapes.

Bird murmurations

In certain seasons, large flocks of birds (often Sparrows or Starlings) create stunning, transient patterns in the sky as they move together. These fluid shapes and sounds can offer insights to the seeker. Again, let your gaze drift out of focus and see what comes to mind. Relax, daydream, and scry.

Patterns in nature

Other natural patterns, like the shifting shapes of tree leaves, can be used for scrying. Try lying on a park bench beneath trees, to interpret patterns of light and shadow dancing in the leaves above.

Some forms of scrying use physical tools, two popular examples being:

Tea leaf reading

Often known as Tasseography, the art of interpreting patterns in sediment left at the bottom of a cup after drinking tea (or other beverages), is another natural option. Try gazing at coffee grounds, wine dregs, and the patterns left after juice, or herb tea. Let your gaze soften and see what your subconscious makes of them.

Crystal balls and dorodango

To do this you will need a sphere with a shiny surface, such as a crystal ball or a dorodango. The material you work with does not need to be transparent to work; they are an aid to softening the gaze, so that the scryer can look for shapes within or on the surface of the ball.

Place your shiny sphere stably on a dark surface (some use a black cloth for this). Sit comfortably, perhaps light some incense, or sprinkle some local herbs linked to divination around the ball (e.g. Yarrow or Mugwort). Settle your breathing and then consider your question. Either hold the sphere for a short while or place your hands over it, so that some of your energy can merge easily with the ball. Then return the ball to the stable surface and gaze softly at it.

Let your eyes float over it, into it, focus near and far, but always on the ball. Let your focus soften, widen, and drift. Become almost dreamlike, enter a state where you no longer see sharp images but see patterns and shifting light. Do this for as long as it entertains you and feels comfortable. Allow your subconscious and gut instinct to work. Let any thoughts, images, and patterns bubble up and fade away as they will. When finished, focus clearly on the ball, so you again see its edges and form. Hold the ball, and thank it for its help. Spend a few moments interpreting what you have seen. Then polish the ball and tuck it safely away. You may like to keep a Bayleaf with the crystal ball, to help protect it.

Geomancy

Geomancy is an earthy form of divination that asks questions of stones or earth. Feel free to make up your own rules, but a useful medieval method, mentioned in Agrippa's 1532 book *De Occulta Philosophia*, is as follows.

Draw a circle in the ground with a stick. Then ask your question and throw a number of stones at the circle. Count how many of these actually land within it. If the number landing within is odd, the outcome counts as 1. If the number falling within is even, the outcome counts as 2. This throwing and recording is repeated four times, for the same question. Each result, 1 or 2, is recorded as a list going downward, as either one or two dots. The dots become arranged as a symbol. A table of correspondences[28] could then be used to help the seeker interpret the geomantic symbols.

A simpler stone divination method involves a collection of nine small pebbles. These may be different colours, patterned with quartz veins, or quite plain. Each stone is examined, and what it is thought to represent is recorded, either on the stone as a symbol, or in a book. The seeker's question is asked while they handle the bag of stones. They select three stones at random, and place them on the ground from left to right, in that order representing the past, present, and future. The meaning is interpreted by referring to the list showing what each stone is felt to represent.

Alternatively, a circle could be drawn in the ground, with two lines to cut the circle into four quadrants. Each quadrant represents a different element of Earth, Water, Air, and Fire. Drop the stones into the centre of the circle. Interpret the meaning by considering where the stones fall. This system also works well with Horse Chestnut tree conkers, rather than stones.

Oracle cards

Many Green Witches use tarot cards, or oracle decks of cards with nature-inspired artwork. Originally, playing cards were used for divination so feel free to use whatever you have available. Witches use them in various ways, with some shuffling the cards and drawing one at random to provide spiritual focus for the day, while others ask a specific question and perform more complex readings, laying cards in traditional spreads to gain deeper insights.

Card decks usually come with an interpretation book, or you can find them online. They explain the meaning of the card if pulled upright, upside down, or in certain combinations. They are helpful guides, but learn to respect your own interpretations.

---

[28] Shown in Fred Gettings, *Secret Symbolism in Occult Art* (1987).

Divination sticks

Wormwood and Yarrow have wonderfully strong flower stems, which can be cut into manageable lengths when fresh, then dried and marked with meaningful symbols for use in divination. Some like to keep a set of sticks in a pouch, consult an oracle to interpret stick patterns, or use them spontaneously.

I Ching

The Chinese I Ching, or *Book of Changes*,[29] is said to be the world's oldest oracle. It is used to interpret arrangements of sticks, which are counted and arranged in a meditative way. Exactly fifty Yarrow sticks, each about 14 cm long, are required.

Short straws

Collect a number of sticks and cut them to different lengths; perhaps also mark one end with ink. You may like to cut half short and leave the other half long. Shuffle the sticks in your hands as you ask your sticks a question, preferably where a yes/no answer is sought. Decide whether a short stick means yes, or no. Then hold the sticks so that the length cannot be seen, just allow the level tops to be visible. Close your eyes and pull a stick from the bundle at random. Interpret the response.

Ogham sticks

Ogham Sticks are short sticks, each marked with a symbol from the ancient Ogham alphabet, traditionally associated with trees. These sticks are used for divination by randomly drawing one or more from a pouch, or casting them onto the ground, then interpreting their positions and symbols. Each tree has symbolism, which guides the interpretation. The Ogham alphabet is based on the ancient Celtic tree alphabet. Modern Green Witches often create sets using trees with personal or local significance. For example, a Lime tree stick could symbolise tranquillity and transformation. Even though Lime is not part of the traditional Ogham, it is common in urban landscapes and offers much to the urban witch.

---

[29] R. Wilhelm, *I Ching or Book of Changes* (Routledge & Kegan Paul, 1950). This well-respected translation is worth locating.

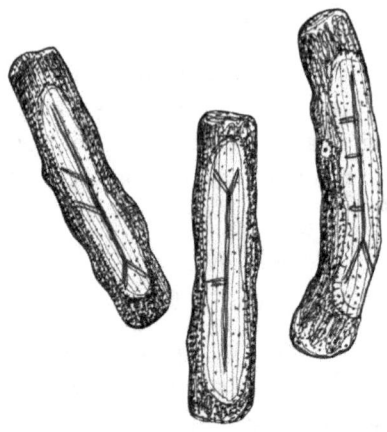

How to make ogham sticks

To craft your own Ogham sticks, collect small, finger-thick sticks from trees that are significant to you. Ideally use fallen or pruned branches to avoid damaging the trees. Remove the bark with a knife or vegetable peeler, to prevent the sticks rotting, and allow the wood to dry slowly, preferably outdoors, over several weeks. Once dried, mark each stick with its corresponding Ogham symbol or a symbol that reflects the tree's character. These symbols could be carved, branded, or painted. Keep a written key or cipher for your symbols to help you to remember them. Consult your Ogham sticks when you have challenging questions to answer.

Dreams

Dream journaling and interpretation can teach us much about ourselves. Dreams are often thought to be glimpses of the collective unconscious that binds all spirits in the universe together. Some dreams are prophetic, some provide comfort, others are processing events from the day. Whatever their purpose, dreams are a wonderful gift in our lives and worth learning more about.

Love divination often involves dreams and simple charms. One method, from the Middle Ages, required the seeker to place Thyme in one shoe, Rosemary in the other, and lay them either side of their bed. The hope was to dream of the identity of their future partner.

Signs in nature

We can ask questions to nature, set parameters for what the response will mean, and then wait for something to happen. Ash uses the following method:

> At a place where you can see some sky through a sort of window, a gap formed from trees or buildings, settle yourself and ask a question. It should be one that you really want answered. Then decide what the response Yes or No will be shown as. Perhaps a bird flying across the window from the left will mean Yes, and one flying from the right, will mean No. Keep it simple and clear ...

Weather lore

Reading signs in the weather is as old as the hills, because being able to predict approaching weather was important to people living on the land. Although we city folk may not have the same concerns as farming communities, weatherlore can help us to plan our daily activities, and help us to better understand the environment.

Signs which predict rain

Many flowers close to protect their pollen.
Bumblebees shelter inside cave-like flowers, such as Himalayan Balsam.
Frogs croak more frequently.
Aching joints.
Swallows fly low.
Birds are unusually noisy.
Crows flock together.
A halo around the Moon.
"Curds and whey" clouds.
Vapour trails from aircraft are long, and smoke curls back on itself from chimneys, rather than drifting upwards.
Huge sunbeams under the Sun, mist creeping up hills, and wind moaning in keyholes.
Thunderbugs swarm when storms are approaching.

The season ahead

If Oaks trees come into leaf before Ash trees, dry weather will follow.
If Ash comes into leaf first, wet weather will follow.

The day ahead

Red sky at night signals fine weather the next day, while a red sunrise predicts rain.
Soft, green Moss in the morning predicts a wet day. Dry Moss in the morning, predicts a dry day.
Cloudy skies in cold months reduce the chance of frost.
Many pollinating insects flying around indicate fine weather.

Snow

Fine hairs on some animals, including humans, become static and stand up, as snow is approaching.
Skin feels dry.

Wind

Anxious, agitated mental states and migraines worsen when air pressure fluctuates and conditions are windy.
Animals become agitated.

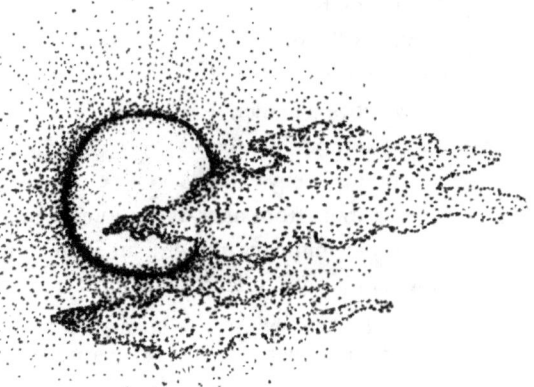

Prayer

Prayer is not exclusive to organised religions like Christianity; it is a practice relevant to anyone who believes in spirit. For magical practitioners, prayer may feel similar to spellwork or ritual, being a time to send thoughts to the universe and our spirit guides. It can be a conversation with spirit, not just one-way communication. Prayer is central to many healing traditions, such as that of the Maya.[30] It is often used to clarify our needs, and ask for guidance and assistance for ourselves, others, or the natural world. Prayer is a way to connect with spirit, and the more we engage in it, the more natural and healing it becomes.[31]

As we build relationships with the spirits that we pray to, our sense of wellbeing can improve. Faith, regardless of its form, is linked to optimism, health, and longevity. In fact studies show that faith-based activities, such as prayer, can reduce rates of depression.

As Western society moves away from organised religion, many people find themselves without faith or a practice of prayer. While this shift brings freedom, it also leaves some of us feeling uncertain about

---

[30] Rosita Arvigo & Nadine Epstein, *Rainforest Home Remedies: The Maya way to heal your body & replenish your soul* (Harper One, 2021) is a very accessible guide.

[31] E. Bendien et al. A Dutch study of remarkable recoveries after prayer: How to deal with uncertainties of explanation. *J Relig Health* (2023) 62(3): 1731–55.

how to seek spiritual help in times of need. Those who have experienced the benefits of prayer often return to it during hard times; it can be a lifeline to help face serious challenges.

For prayers to be effective, they need both a clear recipient and intention. Whether you pray to ancestors, deities, or nature spirits, specifying who you're addressing and what you're asking for increases the likelihood of success. Prayers sent without a specific recipient become scattered. The entity you pray to is also more likely to respond if you've already established a relationship with them. It may help to have a physical token to hand, as you pray, something symbolic to enhance the connection.

Gratitude plays a vital role in any relationship. Without it, recipients may feel neglected. With prayer, sending requests to spirits that we have never shown appreciation for is not a recipe for success; even the most heartfelt prayers will fall on deaf ears in these situations. Learning to express gratitude, even when we are in a place of sadness or great need, can shift our perspective and help us cultivate a sense of abundance and positivity. Sending gratitude to spirits strengthens our bond with them, just as it would in any friendship where support and goodwill are exchanged.

How do green witches pray?

For Green City Witches, prayer is a humble and heartfelt practice that connects us to the spirits of nature and any deities we choose to honour. Whether spoken aloud or silently, prayer is an act of gratitude, trust, and request. There is no one right way to pray; what matters most is sincerity.

Below are steps to guide your prayer practice. Use them as a suggestion, and adapt to your needs.

1. Preparation and invocation

Find a quiet, private space. You may like to have something symbolic to focus on, perhaps a flower or leaf, to help you to feel close to nature spirits.

Ground and centre your energy, then call for the attention of the spirit or deity you're praying to. Address them by name if you can. Speak aloud or in your mind. You might use words like:

Dear Spirits of the Universe, Mother Earth, Father Sky ...

Personalise this as you wish, and introduce yourself. Some may use a private or spiritual name, or simply say:

> *I am* [your name], *part of nature on this Earth.*

2. Gratitude

After this invocation, offer gratitude for the gifts you've received from nature. Express thanks for both the large and small blessings in your life, and remember that with practice, this gratitude will flow more easily and deeply. You might say something like:

> *Thank you for the nourishing food, the connections I have with others, and the lessons that life has provided. I thank you for these gifts, and for enabling me to be part of this world.*

3. Intention

Now, share the reason for your prayer. Be clear about what you're asking for, whether it's healing, guidance, or support. Your prayer should align with the greater good of the universe; asking for personal gain without considering the bigger picture will not be effective in the long term. So, frame your request in a way that respects others or the natural world. Depending on your needs, you might use words like:

> *I ask that your strength, kindness, and healing energy be shared with me so that I may help* [person's name] *to feel better. I trust that you know the best way to bring healing to them and that it will be for the good of all.*

Or

> *I seek your guidance and inspiration as I search for a new job/home/ friends/etc where I can use my strengths to better the world, and where I will feel safe and valued ...*

If you're uncertain about the outcome, allow the spirits or deities to guide the process. Perhaps simply ask, *"Help!"* That also works. Surrendering control to the wisdom of nature shows trust in its ability to help you.

4. Closure

Finally, close your prayer with a heartfelt thank you. Feel gratitude within you as you thank the spirits or deities for hearing your prayer. Trust that your message has been received, and express your appreciation once more. Perhaps:

> *Thank you for hearing my prayer. I trust in your wisdom and the love you have for the world. ... I am grateful for your support, and will continue to honour you the spirits of nature.*

With practice it becomes easier to pray using words and feelings that resonate with you; words that feel positive, heart-felt and in line with your beliefs and values. The suggestions above are for inspiration; there is no need to follow anyone else's script. What matters is that you aim for genuine connection with spirit.

Group prayer

Prayer can be practised alone or with others. Private prayer is a great way to build your own connection with spirit, but it may help to join a circle of trusted practitioners who share prayers as part of their gatherings. Whatever route you choose, the more you practise, the better your connection to spirit will become. Remember that prayer is about trust, gratitude, and respect for the spirits that guide us.

Sound

Sound can be used in many ways to focus magical intent, purify space, and help us to work magic. Many options are available to us.

Chants and incantations

These are forms of vocalised sound. Incantations are spoken, muttered, or whispered phrases that work through the meaning of their words. The quality of their sound is secondary. When used in spells and charms, incantations tend to be concise, and may be spoken just once or a few times, to invoke power.

Chants, however, work through both the meaning of their words and their vibrations. Chants are usually repeated many times and can profoundly affect our consciousness and spiritual awareness. Vocalising sounds also tones the vagus nerve, which in turn can reduce stress. So if we take opportunities to hum, sing, and chant, whenever we can, it can deepen connection with spirit and improve our state of health.

Sounds in nature

Simple instruments can be made and used during magical work. Crafting your own from local materials is usually more fun and eco-friendly than purchasing imported instruments from esoteric stores. Drums can be made from wood and local animal hides. Rattles and wind chimes made with found materials can be used to break up and disperse stagnant energy. We can also welcome the natural sounds of rain, wind, rustling leaves, and birdsong into our magical work.

Ideas to Try:

Vocalise: Hum, sing, or chant whenever you can. Start quietly if you like, but exercise your vagus nerve and notice how it feels. As your confidence grows, get louder and embrace the sensations that self-made sounds can bring. Consider joining a local choir or singing group.

Drumming: Create your own drum or rhythm sticks, using natural materials. Try to mimic the rhythm of your pulse and the sound of waves, and welcome the sunrise with your drum.

Homemade Rattles: Try placing different natural materials inside of a hollowed-out piece of wood, or tubes made from Birch bark. Seal up the ends and shake. Try tiny stones, acorn caps, conkers, or other seeds. Use it to cleanse space, shaking it to disperse stagnant energy.

Wind Chimes: String natural found objects together and hang from a piece of wood to create a wind chime. The element of air can then make its own music, inside or outside of your home.

Protection techniques

Just as clothes protect us from severe weather, psychic protection protects us from unwanted energies. But we should not rely on magic alone for this. Psychic protection needs to be matched by practical actions in the physical plane; actions like using good door locks, checking that friends get home safely, and trying to avoid dangerous situations. Alongside using protection magic, anyone who feels vulnerable should reach out for support. Protection spells and techniques are designed to awaken and strengthen your inner power. That can help us navigate city life and become brave enough to seek help when needed.

There are many ways to use green magic to strengthen the defences in your life. The following techniques focus on deflecting and clearing away unwanted energies, defining boundaries, and building strength.

House spirits

The feeling we get when entering a home reflects a lot more than the people who live there. Homes are filled with different energies. Some are spirits of place—nature spirits who are as old as the land that supports the building. Other spiritual energies linger in fabrics, furniture, and appliances. Some seem to hold memories of where their raw materials originate, how they were crafted, or how the building was previously used. Plants growing within or around a home also add to the energetic whole. Even components like plumbing, electrics, and door hinges can have associated spirits. All appreciate being valued and cared for, and may become cranky and mischievous when neglected. But, when respected, house spirits can be tasked with protecting your home.

In some regions house spirits are well recognised and named, such as the Brownies of Scotland. These house spirits appreciate being treated kindly. In return, they care for the home. To keep your house spirits happy, treat your home and possessions with care. A simple ritual, like lighting incense regularly, or saying *"Goodbye, lovely home. Stay safe,"* when leaving for the day, can help to maintain a strong bond with these spirits. Of course, remember to lock the door and close windows before leaving as house spirits can rarely manage that. When you return home, greet the house spirits warmly and thank them for their protection.

Protective herbs

Traditionally, many herbs are valued for their protective qualities. Some that grow in towns and cities are Houseleek, Elder, Yarrow, Acanthus, Rosemary, Rue, Garlic, Bramble, Feverfew, and Sage. These herbs are among those recommended in the Spells and Charms section of this book.

Aside from spells and charms, there are endless ways to use herbs protectively. Some simple ways are: Placing sprigs of Tansy, Mugwort, or Wormwood under doormats to deter negative energy (and Flies); pressing Rue or Mugwort leaves between pages as protective bookmarks to keep away prying eyes; hanging Clove-scented Wood Avens roots above doorways to repel the evil eye; and tucking a Bay leaf inside clothing, to promote safe travels.

Try planting protective herbs near your home entrances or boundaries. Some popular options for city homes are: Rosemary (which repels negativity), Hollyhock (distracts attention), Ivy (conceals), Rose (fiercely protective), Fig (deflects the evil eye), and Yew (repels evil). Some plants also seem particularly watchful, such as Pansy and Asters. Both are easy to grow and have flowers that resemble watchful faces or eyes. Choose protective plants that suit your location. There are more examples in the Herblore section of this book.

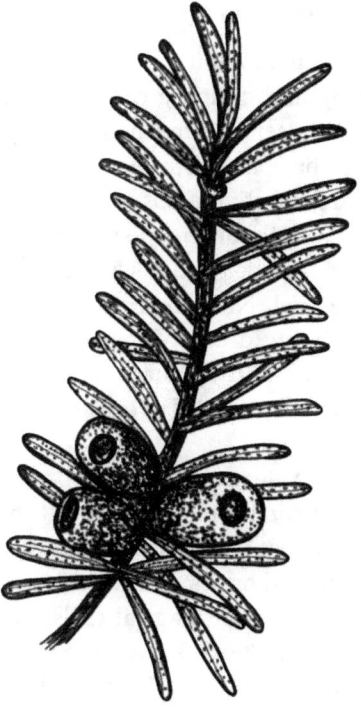

Spiky plants

To repel unwanted energy from your workstation or home, grow plants with spiky characteristics, like Cacti, Aloe Vera, or Rosemary. Position them near vulnerable places, where they can move energy upwards and away, helping to deter intruders. They are quite easy to care for and could be grown on a sunny windowsill. Away from windows, Snake Plant (*Sansevieria*) prefers indoor semi-shade and the ZZ-Plant (*Zamioculcas*) can manage with little to no natural light. Both can efficiently deflect negativity.

You can also make protective herb bundles to hang over entry points: simply cut a prickly plant stem, such as Rose or Bramble, into convenient lengths, then tie into a bundle with some Rosemary and Sage. Rosemary deflects negativity and encourages warm relationships, Sage promotes wise decisions, while prickly stems are fiercely protective. Refresh herb bundles when you notice they have lost their vitality.

Cleansing homes and tools

Regularly clean your home, even if it's not your favourite activity. Short periods of decluttering and cleaning can help keep a home free from negative energy. Less clutter also means more space for growth. After basic cleaning, sweep the space clear of unwanted spirits with a magical broom, made from protective herbs (details are in the Tools section).

Wipe surfaces with a cloth that has been slightly dampened with Bay or Holly leaf decoction. But be cautious: if too much is used, Bay water can stain pale surfaces red. Natural room sprays are very convenient to use. To make, add a few drops of Lavender or Rosemary essential oil to a water-filled spray bottle. Spray to clear the space of stagnant air and bring a sense of calm (with Lavender) or mental alertness (with Rosemary).

Incense can be used to cleanse tools and spaces. The smoke binds to unwanted energies and carries them away, but this must be done in a well-ventilated space; unless the incense can travel outside, any energies it carries cannot be removed or transformed. To use this method, simply waft a little smoke around your magical tools. Before using incense to clear spaces, many practitioners break up the stagnant energy by shaking a rattle or chimes around the area. The fast, high-frequency vibrations are thought to pierce the air, making it easier to disperse stale energy.

Cleansing people and companion animals with smoke can trigger respiratory issues, so it is not advised. Whatever you smoke-cleanse, use natural non-toxic products and avoid using misappropriated tools such as White Sage and Abalone shells.

Cobwebs

Not all homes have Spiders, but if yours does, remember to leave a few of their cobwebs intact after cleaning. Spiders are helpful housemates whose webs trap negative energy and help control Fly and Mosquito populations. Dusty cobwebs are no longer being used by Spiders so can be cleared away to make space for fresh webs.

Property boundaries

Maintain the physical boundaries of your home. Regularly check for damage or gaps and repair them promptly. Fungal issues may be dealt with using natural cleaning products and antifungal herbs like Bay and Calendula. If you rent, make sure your landlord corrects any issues that could compromise your safety.

Sprinkle brick dust, salt, or a mixture of both over the thresholds of your home for protection. Red brick dust is particularly effective for boundary protection, though it can be hard to come by unless you're willing to find and scrape the bricks yourself. As an alternative, clay-rich soil can be used. After finding a lump of clayey soil, let it dry completely before crumbling or grinding to a fine dust. A pestle and mortar works well for this. Ensure the dust is so finely ground that when sprinkled it will be unnoticeable to others.

Setting the wards

Periodically reinforce the protection around your home by walking along its boundaries, both inside and out if possible. Visualise the wards (guardians) of your home as strong, powerful spirits, rather like nightclub bouncers. They are steadfast protectors: firm, fair, and fierce. Be respectful when asking for their help, and ensure they understand their role and where your boundaries are, especially if living in shared space. As you walk your boundary, notice the areas requiring the most protection and communicate this with the wards. These guardian spirits are part of your home's spiritual team, working to safeguard your space.

Stone and crystals

Quartz, Tourmaline, and crystal grids are popular spiritual protection tools. If you use them, remember to cleanse and clear your crystals regularly and obtain ethical crystals. Stones found locally can also be placed around the home for protection purposes and may align better with eco-friendly magic. Try placing a shallow bowl of found pebbles on a windowsill, or place found stones with personal meaning on your altar. They can absorb or deflect negative energy very effectively and should be cleansed as for crystals. Pocket stones and Druid eggs can also be carried for personal protection. More information about these in the Tools section.

Strengthen your health

We become vulnerable to negative energy when our physical health is not strong. Eat well, move regularly, and pay attention to your body's signals, especially when feeling susceptible to psychic or physical attacks. Whether through daily walking, yoga, swimming or self-defence, building physical strength will enhance your life force and protective energy.

Mental health is equally important, so be clear about your emotional and social boundaries and fiercely protect them. Prevent burnout by balancing work, rest, and play. Protect your financial situation too by taking action to control and build your assets. This is a way to protect the future-you.

Vital Energy (Nwyfre, Prana, Chi, Ch'ulel)

This subtle energy is known across cultures to enter the body through our senses, diet, and skin. Build up this life force by spending time in environments rich in green energy. Beaches, woodlands, and windy hillsides are usually full of it, but urban gardens, especially organic ones, usually are too. It is important to refill energy reserves when we can, as it is used by everything we do, and especially by stress. This subtle energy is a major part of our psychic protection shield, so keeping a good reserve is vital. Deep breathing practices in clean air can also help recharge your vital energy, as can many Yoga practices.

Jiva Bandha is a simple Yoga technique that can be used to help enhance mental focus and control the loss of our life force. Jiva Bandha involves placing the tongue on the roof (upper palette) of the mouth. It is traditionally done during meditation but any moments of concentration will do, making this a useful yet subtle protection technique that anyone can try.

City-specific protection

Urban life presents many challenges for those who are sensitive to energy. Even if we have a peaceful home, in the city we inevitably need to interact with people who could challenge us energetically and perhaps physically. Each time we step outside, we may even feel exposed to a barrage of negativity, so we need ways to protect from this. This is also true to everyone who consumes a lot of current affairs, or negative content on screens. Sometimes it can be difficult to manage the energy that we are exposed to.

Cities sometimes face problems such as sudden peaks in Mice, Rat, and Scabies populations and even Bed bug infestations. Infestations highlight vulnerabilities in your protective shields, so if they occur, we need to address the root cause rather than reacting impulsively. Many precautions can protect against infestations. These include practical measures like maintaining good hygiene, repairing holes in walls and floors, and storing food in airtight containers.

While Green City Witches generally respect the presence of all creatures, House Mice shouldn't be encouraged to breed. So please avoid leaving food around that could encourage them and certainly don't treat them as pets. When visiting parks, we can help control the Rat population naturally by removing litter. And consider freezing any suspicious clothing or food items like flour or herbs, in closed bags, to eliminate Bed bugs, Moth larvae, and other bugs. Clean your bedclothes often, and seek treatment promptly if you are affected by an infestation.

Shielding

Sadly, an instinct for some humans is to pick on weak or different individuals. As well as the shielding methods mentioned in the Ground, Centre, and Shield chapter, we can use our body language to help against this. Presenting ourselves confidently can attract positivity and can help to shield against negativity. Practise projecting an air of confidence and strength when you go about your day. Try to find a balance that shows others that you can take care of yourself while also being approachable enough when needed.

Guard your solar plexus

We all encounter extreme energy at times, but some of us are regularly exposed to it. Shop workers and healers in Glastonbury, Somerset, are often confronted by individuals with different energy levels. Some can be quite draining, so their presence can have quite an impact on the staff. Several esoteric shop assistants have found ways to manage this. Some place their hands gently against their solar plexus (between breastbone and navel) when faced by strongly energetic people. It doesn't look at all strange, in fact it gives the demeanour of strength and controlled power. Others wear energy-absorbing stones on wristbands, or small tourmaline pendants to absorb negativity. They find it effective, and feeling protected increases their enjoyment of the work.

Evil eye amulets

The *evil eye* is the belief, in many Indo-European cultures, that a person can curse another by looking at them with a malevolent gaze. This act can be intentional or accidental. To ward off any misfortune from such gazes, many options have been developed and passed on through the generations. The most popular is the use of an amulet, worn in jewellery or displayed in cars, homes, and workplaces. It resembles a blue eye made from four concentric circles. These *Mati* or *Nasir* amulets are used to reflect the evil eye back to its sender.

Some Balkan cultures use house dolls or *Motanka* to deflect the evil eye. They are placed around property to reflect jealous gazes back to the sender. The Hand of Fatima, or *Hamsa* is also used to protect from the evil eye in several cultures. Other amulets are common too, such as carrying or displaying cloves of Garlic, or wearing silver medals. All of these amulets are used to help keep evil away.

Psychic hygiene

Regularly clearing away any psychic debris or negative energy that has attached to you is an important protection practice. There are many simple ways to do this, from letting incense waft around you, bathing or soaking with infused herbs, to showering it off. As you stand in the shower, try visualising yourself rinsing away spiritual cobwebs. Let them disappear through the drain, to be transformed into useful energy by the sea. Clean the shower tray strainer to prevent any of the cobwebs settling there. After this a final rinse with diluted Bay decoction or Rowan leaf infused water will prevent further cobwebs from attaching for some time. Dry yourself gently before lightly oiling your skin with Olive oil or a herb-infused oil.

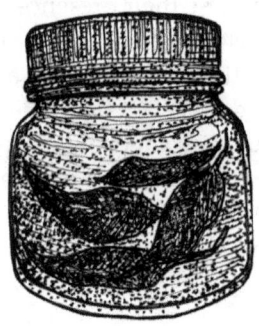

Nature spirits

It is also possible to call on nature spirits for protection. Saying a simple affirmation such as "Tree spirits protect me," in times of need, can increase our alertness, and bring strength. Clearly, we need to continue taking practical steps to protect, but building skills in communicating with the spirits of nature is worthwhile. Try practising at calm times like when you are out walking. If you notice birds in nearby trees, silently ask them to alert you when something interesting happens out of your sight. Continue your walk and stay alert for any message that they may send you. Messages could be a sudden rustling of leaves, birds shrieking, or even birds falling silent. With regular practice, our ability to be aware of these signs improves so we will notice what these creatures do when they actually want to warn us of potential harm.

Identify what you value

With so many ways to consider protecting what you value, it is useful to reflect on what is most important to you. Whether your health, wealth, family, or environment, knowing what you really value in life can help to channel your protective efforts in the right directions.

Spells and charms

Spells are carefully considered words, used to achieve a specific purpose. To cast a spell you will need to clarify your intention, gather any materials, create sacred space, perform the spell, and then follow up with some action. This can all happen quickly and spontaneously, or could involve some planning.

Spell Casting involves three steps:

1. Intention
2. Invocation
3. Action

Intention

Clarify what your spell needs to do. Spells are used to feel safe, loved, healthy, wealthy, wear nice clothes, get a new job, date or new home, breathe clean air, and many other things. The intention may be targeted towards yourself, others, or the planet as a whole.

The way we phrase our intention will determine the type of spell we cast: curses or hexes have negative intent because they intend to cause harm; blessings have positive intent and intend good things to happen; bindings intend on keeping certain things together.

Intentions need to be well considered and concise. They should focus on the qualities needed to get the results we want, or they should describe how it feels when we get there. For example, when planning a spell to help us move into a new, more clean, and spacious home, our intention will focus on the qualities that new situation will bring; how it will feel to live there. Or it could focus on what we need to embody in order to get the new home. So, being a considerate housemate, smart with our finances, attracting certain home decor, and so on. We then shape some of these into an incantation of well-considered words to use during invocation.

The words used in spells need to be carefully considered. Words hold immense power: they can soothe, inspire, trigger war, bring peace, unite, or separate. They must be used with care. When spell crafting, use positive phrases, even when a spell's aim is to keep something away. For instance, if you want a Dog to stop barking so much, it would be wise to create a spell to bring quiet and calm to your environment and contentment to the Dog, rather than to focus on reducing irritation. The slightest mention of negative qualities in manifestations, affirmations, and spells will attract those qualities towards us. So visualise a haven of calm, rather than the removal of noise.

Invocation

This is the use of ritualised words and actions, such as incantations and specific body movements. These channel and focus energy, and are an invitation for spirits to bring your intentions to life.

Ground and centre

Before you begin spellcasting take a moment to ground and centre yourself. If convenient, connect yourself to nature somehow—perhaps place your hands on a tree or stone. Take some time to top up your vital energy reserves by channelling it through your roots and crown. Spell casting releases energy, so try to top up your reserves before you start. Shield yourself, perhaps by drawing a circle around your workspace, with your finger or wand. A simple request is made to invoke your preferred spirits, like:

I call on the spirits of this place to support my work.

It is best to invite spirits rather than demand their presence, and approach ones that you have already built a relationship with (through prayer and kind actions). If you have not had a chance to do that, just be polite and request support from the universe.

Incantation

Use an incantation of whatever length you like to request what you want. It can be phrased in the present tense, as if all your wishes have already come true (an affirmation), or it could be stated as a request, rather like a prayer. It may be a rhyming incantation or not. It could be in your home language or another, such as Latin, to add more mystique. Some witches like to end their incantations with a phrase such as *So mote it be*, or *It is done*. This is optional, its purpose being to announce that the intention of the spell is realised, it brings it into the present tense, and can add some extra energy to the spell.

However it is done, an incantation should be delivered with the strong belief that your intention will be realised. Depending upon the mood, it may be called aloud, spoken softly, or muttered under the breath. Some Green City Witches prefer to cast spells when outdoors, perhaps in a place where the sky and earth are somewhat visible, but that is not essential.

Gestures

Movements or gestures can help add passion to spellcasting. Any gesture that feels good to you will work. Some clap their hands as they send their spell out into the world, others hold their arms out in front, with palms up or down, as they speak their incantation. You may like to raise your arms skyward, or perhaps place your palms on the ground to send out your intention through tree roots and fungi. Whatever the hand placement, it helps to direct your energy away—above, below, sideways, or through the trunk of a tree, whatever you prefer.

Wands

To focus the energy even more, some Green Witches point a wand, or their index finger, and draw a symbol in the air in front of them such as a circle, star, or the infinity sign. If trying this, direct your intention and energy into the wand or finger while repeatedly drawing the symbol in the air until you feel it is sufficiently charged. At that moment you may feel it quickening, about to burst from being so full. Point it up to the sky while visualising a stream of energy flowing from the wand or fingertip into the universe, carrying your intent. Depending upon the purpose of the spell, you may prefer to point the wand or finger at a part of your body that needs healing, a plant, the ground, water—wherever the energy will have the greatest effect.

Natural materials such as herbs, stones, bones, and seeds can also be incorporated into spells. Depending on your choice and the nature of the spell, these could be arranged around a candle, used to dress a candle, eaten, burned, used to anoint. There are endless options. Use what is available to you and feels connected to the intention of your spell.

Action

This is the part where we take physical steps to bring the intention to life. It could be making a phone call to a housing agent, greeting your neighbour and their dog when you see them in the street, dressing like people who already have your dream job, and so on. It also involves being open to the universe sending you the answers to your prayers.

These answers may come in unexpected ways, such as finding an old doll house at the garbage collection point (when asking for a new home), finding small coins on pavements (when asking for financial wealth), or perhaps a Squirrel finding you in the park (when requesting friendship). These are not exactly what you were asking for but perhaps they were. However obscure the signs, smile and give a thankful nod to the universe to acknowledge that the process has begun—the spirits are working for you, and desires are coming your way. Keep your faith, keep taking physical steps in the direction of your intentions too. Both are needed.

After some time you may want to go back to your spell book and rework your spell with a more refined intention or incantation. Actions may also include repeating the original spell regularly, or repeating the incantation as a mantra or affirmation each day. You decide, but without action on the physical plane, magic on the spirit plane cannot be realised.

Charms

Depending on the purpose and setting, a charm may be a physical item like an amulet or talisman, or could be spoken words or rituals. Charming is mostly used for protection against evil or illness. Because charms are quicker to perform and less complex than spells, they are very popular among urban witches.

Spoken charms are incantations, usually short phrases or chants, and are often linked to a specific herb and purpose. They can be used to invoke deities, nature spirits, or elements. They often have a rhythmic or repetitive structure, more often than spells, although this is not essential.

Because spells also consist of well-considered words, it is quite easy to transform a charm into a spell by adding layers of ritual. But these additional layers do not necessarily upgrade them, as charms are powerful magical tools in their own right. Uttering a charm effectively involves saying the incantation aloud and with great intent. Its effectiveness is amplified by the practitioner's focus and belief that it will work.

The best charms are quick and memorable, although some are quite long. Charms often serve as magical tools and memory aids, to help communities remember the characteristics of plants and animals. For example, this charm about Rosemary: you may like to say it when touching the plant or dried herb:

Evergreen Rosemary, keep me safe,
Protect from evil and make me brave.

This mentions an identifying feature of Rosemary (being evergreen) and the three requests (safety, protection, and bravery), which all link to its medicinal properties. These days we tend not to think of evil as a medicinal term, but charm writing allows for poetic licence and should be fun. You could also experiment with more mysterious languages, just as when creating incantations for spells. When you create charms, play with words, language and symbology; try to make them rhyme and keep a record of your creations.

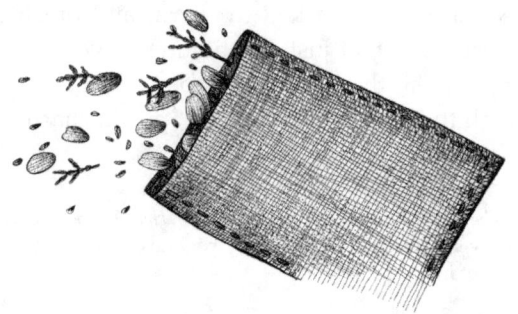

How to charm

No specific preparation or materials are needed for uttering charms: simply speak, whisper, mutter, or silently think of your charm. Charm at special moments or not. This is often a spontaneous form of magic, so try not to overthink or restrict yourself with ideas of what would be ideal. Charms also work well with repeated use; the more we use them, the more they come to life, rather like the hyper sigils mentioned earlier in this book. Charms are a convenient form of magic; try saying them whenever you get the chance, including as you go about your daily activities. The money charm later in this section is well suited for that.

Historical charms

Several historic charms are still in use today.[32] Two favourites are the traditional children's song "Ring a ring of Roses a pocket full of posies," which may have been used to ward off the plague, or the Daisy divination charm "She loves me, she loves me not," still popular while plucking petals.

Studies of old European manuscripts, such as the Danish Urebog, show that charms used in medieval times tended to focus on several things. These were healing physical problems in humans, protection from evil, exertion of control (through fear in your enemy, to get whatever you wanted etc), treating animals and soil (animal behaviour and disease, improve farming land), and for discovery or divination (to help find a thief, learn the gender of an unborn child etc).

Until quite recently many so-called Pellars and Charmers would be consulted in the English West Country, to help with various problems. Perhaps some are still working there, in quiet corners of that region. The best Pellars and Charmers would attract seekers from far and wide, for help with issues related to health, relationships, property, protection, and career. They were asked to charm and break curses. Often they were so respected that just mentioning in your community that you were going to visit the Pellar (perhaps to find out who stole from you) was enough to resolve the problem. Spoken charms were uttered

---

[32] Roger J. Horne, *The Witches Art of Incantation: Spoken charms, spells, & curses in folk magic* (2nd edn, Moon Over Mountain Press, 2023) contains many historical and adapted charms that may be of interest.

in English, Welsh, Cornish, or local dialects.[33] As we know from considering symbolism, using language that the listener doesn't understand can add great power to the work.

Alongside incantations, some Pellars and Charmers used charm bags or pouches, filled with symbolic items, such as a nut, flower, or stone. These were given to the seeker, sometimes also with a simple charm to incant or act out, at home. These additions would amplify the magic. In Albania, and other Baltic countries, this practice continues today, quite openly, through Pëllars or Mjeks. They utter charms and often create personal amulets and symbols for seekers.

The issues that humans are concerned about have changed little over the years. Modern charms may incorporate different details but they all work the same.

Signs that magic is working

Witches are often asked how to tell if spells are working. Results rarely come instantaneously in a flash, although that is possible, but there are signs that things are going well. Manifesting magic may show itself as serendipitous events, strange coincidences, animals acting differently, or by finding exactly what you need at just the right moment. These are indications that your spell or charm is taking effect. Stay open to these subtle signs as you continue to take actions in the physical world.

There's a belief that if you ask the universe for something and ignore its offerings three times, the universe may stop "playing the game" with you. For example, you may put out a request for financial help and then see a copper coin on the street. Instead of seeing this as a positive sign, you ignore it and leave the coin because it feels insignificant or it's awkward to stop. Later you see another coin but don't stop. You may be dismissing the universe's answer to your prayers, and the third opportunity, of greater wealth, may not come at all.

At times like this, turning back, picking up the coin, and thanking the universe, can be a small but significant act—remember to show gratitude for small blessings. Universal energy, or spirit, flows freely, but it doesn't respond well to stagnation and negativity. If you can flow with it, you'll find that your spellwork will thrive.

---

[33] G. Macdonald & J. Penberth, *West Country Witchcraft* (Green Magic, 2007).

Record keeping

Keep a record of your spells somewhere, using whatever media works best for you. We may think that all witches use a magical journal or grimoire for this, but they don't, so avoid feeling restricted by that ideal. Use something that works for you and try to keep your spells private, to increase their power; when spells slip into the hands or minds of others, their potency is decreased.

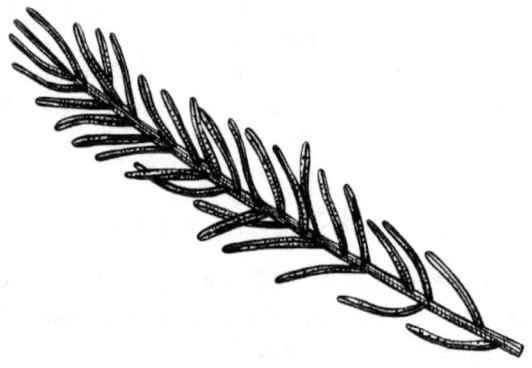

Weaving nature into spells and charms

Perhaps the easiest way to weave nature into an existing spell or charm is to look at the tools you already use and find more natural and local replacements where needed. This doesn't mean that your well-loved non-sustainable tools and ingredients should be thrown out, just look out for natural, ethical alternatives when next replacing your supplies. Everything we use from ink, paper, candles, herbs to pots and pans, has an impact on nature. If each is aligned with nature, eventually your magical toolkit will feel completely in line with your values.

Checking your incense is a good start. When you next choose incense sticks or cones, check the ingredients carefully; many contain unsustainable ingredients as well as toxic chemicals that pollute the air. Quick-light charcoal discs or briquettes, often used in rituals, may be loaded with toxic ingredients too. The charcoal itself is often manufactured and traded unethically, using wood taken from wild, or poorly managed forests, then plastic-packed and transported around the world.

So choose carefully, work within your budget, ethics and what is available to you. There are always options, but be gentle on yourself;

do your best, but don't try to change everything at once. And don't feel like you are failing if you can't find a local natural alternative for a favourite spell ingredient. It shouldn't become a pressure. Magic works better when we are lighthearted, so rather than trying to do all of the things, aim to do something that helps, and gradually build on that.

Timing spellwork

It doesn't matter when we conduct our magical work, but we may have preferences. Perhaps early morning is best for you, when your housemates are asleep. That time is associated with growth and expansion. Or evening may be the time when you feel most relaxed and in tune with your spiritual side. That time is associated with quiet and reduction. Twilight (dawn and dusk) can be a powerful time to work. These are daily moments when the veil between physical and spirit realms is thought to be thin, and our prayers are heard more easily.

Phases of the Moon also offer opportunities to enhance spell and charm work. The Moon Magic section offers further suggestions about how to embrace Moon energy, such as casting spells linked to expansion, increase, development, gathering, and abundance during the Waxing (growing) Moon phase. The Waning Moon is more associated with reduction, cutting ties, minimising damage, loss, and separation.

Likewise, each season has a different energy, and these can be woven into your work. Sunny midsummer days could be helpful in abundance spells, although when conducted at midwinter, they may work even better as from that time until midsummer, day length will expand—and that can encourage growth. Work with what is possible for you, and respect your own judgement about when it is best to cast spells.

Adapting spells and charms

Each of the spells and charms listed below can be adapted to your location and season, simply by using local seasonal natural items. The examples suggest simple natural materials, which can be substituted if needed. For example, Sycamore seeds and Clover flowers can be used in place of sugar or honey, to symbolise sweetness. If you want to use a herb but can't find one that seems relevant, use Rosemary instead. Rosemary is so multi-talented that it can be used for any spells and charms. Alternatively, simply write the names of any missing ingredients on a piece of paper and hold it as you cast the spell. Or try to visualise it, and imagine it there with you. Always work with the resources you have available to you, and remember that your greatest magical resource is your mind.

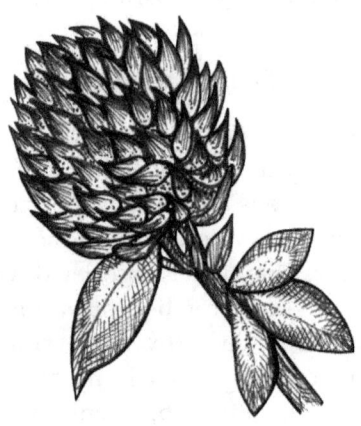

Curses, hexes, and bindings

A Hex or a curse is a spell intended to cause harm. They are cast with the same clear intent as benevolent spells, but we must ask ourselves if it's wise to use our magic in this way. When we feel anger or hurt, it is tempting to seek revenge, but we must remember that all magic has consequences. Harmful magic comes at a price, so it is better to focus on prevention and protection, and any actions we take against others should be done with respect for all involved.

Techniques that can creatively deal with difficult problems without causing harm include cleansing rituals, protective spells, karmic spells, reflecting negative energy to its source, or transforming it into something neutral or positive. You may also like to use charms that invoke the assistance of plants. For instance, you might ask a female Ash tree to counteract the influence of a troublesome male witch, or vice versa.

The following incantation reminds us that when we are angry we may want revenge but it will solve nothing. Saying it can help keep our integrity when we are thinking of working magic from a place of anger:

> *When blood is shed, dark seeds take root,*
> *Shield my spirit; let Viriditas fruit.*

Most Green Witches stay away from curses or hexes due to the amount of negativity it involves. As Mana states:

> *If someone deserves to be hexed then they will bring about their own problems anyway.*

Bindings

Something of a grey area in magic, falling somewhere between curses and blessings, bindings can take many forms depending on their intent. A binding might intend to protect someone or prevent harm, but it could also be used to control, like intending to prevent a partner from leaving you.

It's important to avoid binding yourself to another person or place, especially without their consent, as unwanted consequences can follow. Bindings can be used to protect belongings, such as ensuring your travel bags stay with you, but they must be matched by commonsense actions.

Knot Magic is sometimes used to enhance bindings. It involves tying threads of various colours—red for those related to love and protection, white for healing, and black for darker purposes. Including symbolic plant material with these colours can add another layer to your work.

When performing any kind of binding spell, your intention should be pure and harmless, to ensure the spell has positive outcomes. Including phrases such as "If this is for the good of all" can prevent a binding working in a way that causes harm.

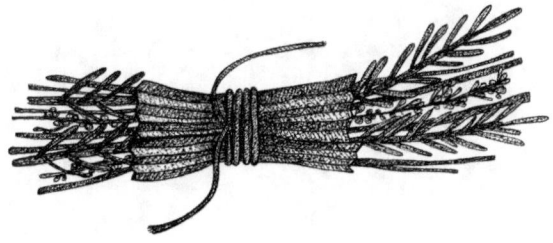

Metaphysical scissors

This sounds better than curse breaking, but that is in fact what metaphysical scissors do. Use for breaking hexes, curses, and any form of malevolent magic or energy. They are also used for symbolically cutting out disease, to set boundaries, to cut unhealthy ties, and to break binding spells when they no longer serve their purpose. They effectively sever connections that may be causing harm. This practice involves visualising the negative energy or unwanted ties and using the visualised (or physical) scissors to symbolically cut through them.

When using metaphysical scissors, it's important to set a clear intention. Focus on what you wish to cut or be free from, and ensure that you are grounded and centred. Some practitioners also recommend following this action with a cleansing ritual, such as burning a Bay leaf or using saltwater, to clear any residual energy.

Charm directory

Charms can be used to help protect anything that you value, from the local street Cat, to your kettle, or family. See them as a way of showing your appreciation and respect, helping them to lead a charmed life, rather than an attempt to bind yourself with your charm targets. Of course, you will need to take action in the physical realm too, such as maintaining your possessions and looking after your health.

Gadgets charm

Why would a kettle, alarm clock, mobile phone, or washing machine keep serving you well for many years, if not shown care and respect? Help your devices to work well, long beyond their expected lifespan, with this simple charm. You may like to perform it at the spring and autumn equinox, or any day at twilight—these are times of perfect balance, and that is what your devices need. But any time will do. Face your palms in the direction of the appliance and say:

> *I hold you dear, long to serve,*
> *Without fear, never losing verve.*

When cleaning or maintaining the appliances, consider brushing the air around them with a Lavender broom, to purify them.

Safe travels charm

This charm for safe travels can be used whatever your mode of transport and however far you plan on going.

> *I travel well, enjoy the ride, and reach the end point safely.*

Bay leaf charm for safe travels

Unless you have especially sensitive skin, try slipping a Bay leaf against your skin somewhere inside your clothing. City witch favourites are inside a bra or waistband. A trouser pocket, where the Bay will become warm but not directly against the skin, is also suitable. Keep it there for the duration of travel. The charm can be boosted by muttering:

May the power of nature protect me!

Say this inwardly or aloud whenever you feel insecure during travels. And, of course back up the charm with sensible protective actions. Bay leaves can be reused many times, if clean.

Good food charm

This charm is suitable for when seeking food, whether through foraging, grocery shopping, looking for a restaurant in a new town, and so on.

Good food I seek, with ease it flows,
Nourishment found, wherever I go.

Enhance the charm by either placing a hand on your abdomen or touching a few seeds in your pocket.

Healing charm

To be said just before ingesting nourishing food or drink. Place your hands lightly above the items as you chant, to focus your intent.

Each sip I drink makes me well,
Each bite I eat, in health I dwell

Or more simply:

Heal me, please.

Plants health charm

Bringing the vital energy of green plants into a sick person's home is a form of magic. You may like to take time to clean houseplants of dust (wiping gently with a damp cloth usually works) and bring in some greenery, such as Holly or Ivy, indoors, to help freshen the living space. As you do this speak the following charm:

> *Come green spirits, do your best,*
> *Bring good health through love and rest.*
>
> *Fill this home fresh and green*
> *That once again we feel pristine.*

Health charm

This is inspired by an entry about how to cure fevers in the medieval herbal, *Physica*, by Hildegard von Bingen. If a person has a raised temperature, from the common cold or flu perhaps, use a clean and sharp crystal or polished stone to carve out three trenches in a generous doorstep of soft bread. Place the bread in a waterproof container, to prevent wine seeping everywhere. Pour wine in the bread trenches until they are filled like rockpools. Gaze at the surface of the wine pools, as if looking in a mirror and say:

> *I look at my image in this mirror with love and kindness.*
> *May these fevers be cast from me.*

Follow this by sipping a generous mugfull of warm honey, Lemon and Ginger (and perhaps some appropriate medicine). Relax, watch some comfort TV or read a good book and have an early night. Donate the wine-soaked bread to a compost heap the next morning.

> *The charm is done.*

Negativity clearing charm

While washing or showering utter:

> *Cobwebs and clingons, down the drain.*
> *Transform in the sea and make me clean!*

Visualise any stagnant energies entering the water and flowing away down the drain. You may like to extend the visualisation until the cobwebs and clingons reach the local sewage treatment works, and are transformed into brilliant white light by the wonderful microbes living there.

Protection charm

Say this charm to make any protective plants in or around your home tingle with pride at the good job they are doing for you and yours:

Spirits of green, I welcome thee,
Your watchful eyes, protecting me.

Keep intruders far away,
Let all within be safe today.

Boundary charm

Tie an odd number of red strings or fabric strips to both hidden and conspicuous places along important boundaries. The boundary could be the entrance to your room, home, community garden, work area, etc. As you tie the strips or string, say aloud:

With this string, I set my will,
Boundaries strong, no contents spill.

I tie this knot and raise my guard,
Unwelcome energies are now barred.

Pocket charm

Be sure to close any holes in your purse, pocket, and bank account because holes in these are symbolic of money slipping away. Here is a simple charm to say as you sew up holes in pockets, or place a shiny coin in each of your pockets. This can easily be adapted to charm a purse or wallet, by substituting the word *pocket* for another money holder:

I charm my pockets to keep things safe
And draw great wealth into my space.

As coins and notes flow my way
My pockets keep them from harm's way!

Money charm

This works particularly well with plants that you meet each day, such as a houseplant or one just outside of your home. Plants with plenty of healthy foliage, and even better, with coin-shaped or papery leaves, are highly symbolic of money and good fortune. It also helps to nod your head respectfully towards the plant as you say hello, and be happy around it. Depending on your current needs, say one of the following as you check on the plant and tend to its needs.

Money loves me and flows my way,
Help me catch it, my bills to pay.

or

Money she loves me and flows my way,
Bills all paid, plenty left to save and play.

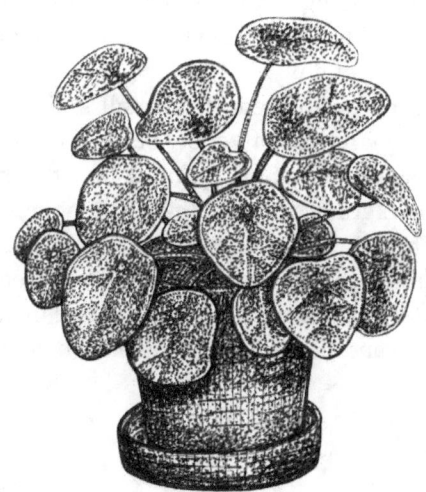

Love binding charm

Tie white or red ribbon or string to the springs or slats beneath your bed, if you can access them. Otherwise tie to the bed frame or mattress handles. This is a form of binding, so be playful with it and consider asking your partner to take part in the charm, so it is done with their knowledge. The knots should be tight enough to keep the strings in place for a long time, but loose enough to be unpicked if healthy separation is needed. As each knot is tied, speak these words:

These knots hold us together, so long as love's in sight.
Contentment reigns forever, if we find it just and right.

Then place a small pouch containing some Agrimony, Rose, and Chamomile flowers under the bed, perhaps between the mattress and bedframe. It should be small so that it doesn't disturb sleep. Refresh the herbs in the charm bag and repeat the charm each time you feel that harmonious energies in your relationship need a boost.

Gossip charm with spring snow

The Elm tree is traditionally thought able to stop people spreading gossip. An old charm, mentioned by Lucy Jones, in *A Working Herbal Dispensary*, involves tossing a knotted yellow cord into an Elm wood fire. Symbolically, the knot binds the tongues of the gossips, while the colour yellow symbolises envy.

This charm can be performed on a small scale using papery Elm seeds (Samaras) and a length of yellow silk or cotton thread. Samaras are known, in Amsterdam, as Spring Snow. Take the thread and tie one knot for each known gossip; if you are unsure how many are at work, tie seven knots. Then light a candle and carefully catch a few Samaras alight with the flame. Place them directly onto a heatproof container and as they burn, let their flames catch the knotted thread alight. As you do this, recite the incantation. Say it once for each knot.

Elm of old, hear my plea,
Bind the tongues that gossip free.

With Spring Snow, I cast this light,
Let silence reign and peace unite.

When it is done, and the seed and thread ash is cold, bury it outdoors in soil, so that it can be transformed.

Wart charm

Warts can hang around on our skin for a long time, so many old charms are concerned with trying to cure them quickly. Several of these involve rubbing the warts with a specific natural item, such as best beefsteak or half of cut apple, and then burying the item in the ground as words were muttered. These charms have remained in use because they certainly have worked for many seekers.

Here is how to do it: Depending on your preference, obtain a delicious-looking apple or a piece of raw prime beefsteak, cut a chunk off to use in this charm, save the rest to cook. If using an apple, slice it in half witchwise, across its equator, so that the six-pointed star is visible. If using steak, you will also need a small tin, large enough for the piece of steak to fit into.

Rub the apple or steak on the warts just once but thoroughly. Then bury the apple half in soil outdoors, or place the chunk of steak in the tin and bury it deep enough in soil that it will not be found by animals. Leave it there and don't return to it. To amplify the charm, speak these words as you rub the warts with the apple or steak:

> *Wart, wart, you will depart,*
> *As I bury this steak (or apple) in the earth so dark.*

After this symbolic death of the wart, eat the rest of the apple or steak (prepared to your liking, of course). When that is complete, the charm is done. Wait as long as possible that day, to wash the affected skin.

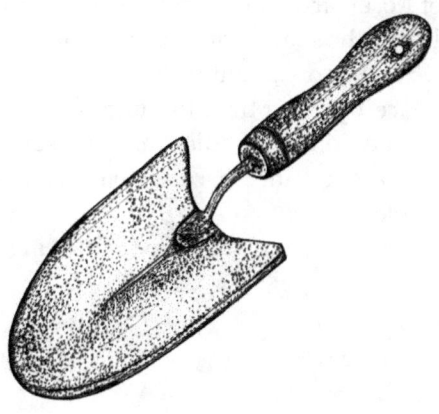

Love divination charm

Yarrow is one of the most magical herbs, and many divination charms use it. If possible harvest ten leaves, or stems (ideally at the New Moon) and keep nine. The extra leaf or stem should be thrown over your shoulder while reciting an incantation such as:

I pluck the Yarrow to ease my mind,
Will my lover be faithful?

Am fair of skin and rich of mind,
I pray, tell me their virtues.

Then chop the nine retained pieces of Yarrow and tuck them into a cotton charm bag. Place this under your pillow and enjoy dreaming of your lover's true character.

Pest control charm

Many old grimoires and leechbooks contain spells and charms aimed at clearing living spaces or vermin. They often create noxious fumes, by burning certain herbs, keeping windows and doors closed, to effectively fumigate the property. But smoke, trapped in a building, is always unhealthy and could seriously harm humans and pets. Here is a safer fumigation charm, inspired by old ones. Take care and work safely.

You will need a saining bundle, made from the root of one Geranium, a hand's length of Rosemary, and a hand's length of Cedar.

Thoroughly cleanse the space, with a brush, vacuum, cloth, etc. Then open the windows and doors. Light the saining bundle, and announce to the spirits of place that it is time to purge this space of unwanted energies. Blow out the saining bundle, and let it smoulder. On a heatproof surface, walk around the space so that herbal smoke can drift throughout the whole area.

Say the words below before safely extinguishing and storing the saining bundle:

With smoke, This space I cleanse.
With smoke, Unwelcome spirits I purge.
With smoke, Fresh space I create.

Hail to the spirits of air that carry the smoke far away from this place.
Hail to all spirits of nature.
Out with the old and in with fresh new possibilities!
It is done.

Also take practical steps, such as storing food in glass containers.

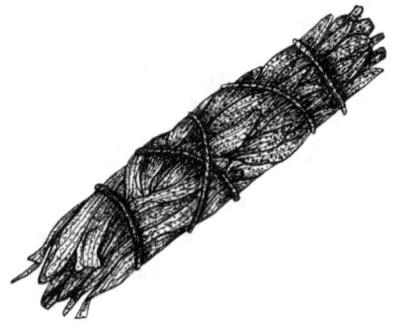

Meadowsweet charm

This charm was written for a Neo-druid gathering, as a lighthearted way to remember some of the characteristics of the plant. It can be spoken while harvesting the herb, or making tea.

Sweet Meadow Queen stands tall and fair,
In low lands of plenty.

Her leaves green–white split 3,2,2,
Ease pain from joints and bellies.

Bees and bugs adore her flowers,
Which sends them into frenzy.

At Midsummer, her mead and ale,
Can't fail to make us merry.

Filipendula ulmaria,
Meadow sweetheart of the Druids,

I'm grateful for your fragrant drifts,
And hope to taste your honey.

Spell directory

For each spell start by grounding, centring, and shielding. This may include drawing a circle. Spell candles are mentioned; these are optional but very useful as the flame is transformative. If you would like to use one, choose a small pillar candle or a tealight, made from natural sustainably sourced wax, rather than paraffin wax.

Love spell

This spell is based on a heart health recipe from medieval abbess Hildegard von Bingen. She used Herb Robert (*Geranium robertianum*), Tansy (*Tanacetum vulgare*), and Nutmeg (*Myristica fragrans*) or Wood Avens (*Geum urbanum*). Tansy should not be used internally. This spell can be used to attract the qualities of a lover that you desire, to heal a broken heart, or for self-love.

Materials

Herb Robert

Nutmeg or Wood Avens root

Tansy flowers

Spell candle and lighter

Paper and pen

Make some Herb Robert tea, add a pinch of grated Nutmeg or Wood Avens root. Place a few yellow button Tansy flowers around the spell candle (or you may prefer to dress the spell candle with dried herbs). Light the candle then focus on the qualities you seek in love, rather than a specific person. Write these on a small piece of paper. Be careful with the wording; you don't want to attract someone who smothers your ability to develop, or leave! Tuck the paper under the candle and drink from the tea.

Let the candle burn down as you incant the following charm. I include a French version of the spell, as that language is often associated with love. Use whichever version you prefer.

> *Robertianum, feed my heart,*
> *Make it ready for love's art.*

With Myristica or Geum, sweet warmth grows,
Attracting virtues, I wish to know.
In your powers, I place my trust,
Grant me love that's true and just.

Beside the candle, I drink your tea.
Love is here. So mote it be.

Sortilège d'Amour (French version)

Robertianum, nourris mon cœur,
Prépare-le à l'art du bonheur.

Avec Myristica ou Geum, douce chaleur,
Attirant vertus, que je veux en cœur.
En tes pouvoirs, j'ai toute foi,
Accorde-moi un amour loyal et droit.

Près de la bougie, je bois ton thé,
L'amour est là. Qu'il en soit ainsi.

Prosperity spell

When you want to increase your wealth (in whatever way you define it), the first step is to identify where your wealth might be slipping away and clear space for great things to come to you. Before trying to attract more, it's important to clear out cobwebs, and clutter and stop any losses. That's why spells for wealth and abundance should begin by cleansing and then closing the gaps in your finances. Rosemary, Yarrow, and Comfrey are great herbs for helping to protect and strengthen your financial situation, but others that you are drawn to will help too.

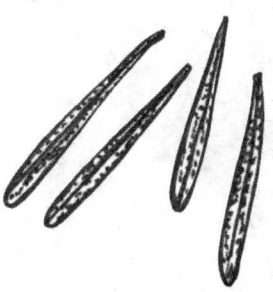

Herbs for prosperity are those with abundant leaves, flowers, fruits, or seeds. Mint, Chickweed, Pine needles, Rosemary, Rowan berries, Mustard seeds, acorns and Yarrow are popular options. Also those with sweet qualities, because they are able to attract prosperity in a positive and gentle way. Grapes (or raisins), Dandelion flowers, sprigs of Heather, Sweet chestnuts, and Clover are all sweet. But don't be limited by what you read: go out and see what's abundant in your area when you want to work abundance and prosperity magic.

Arrange some of your chosen herbs around the candle, and smear a little honey or syrup around it. If you have access to it, wind a flexible stem of Grapevine around the candle. Then gather a small handful of your chosen herbs.

Now energetically clear the space. Make space mentally and physically for wealth and abundance. Then light the candle, hold the herbs, and say the following charm three times:

> *From (leaf/nut/mint etc) to hand, great riches flow,*
> *Now my wealth and fortune grow.*
> *Wealth and plenty, come to me,*
> *With harm to none, so mote it be.*

Another way is to make a charm from this by carrying a little of the herb in a pocket. As you walk, say the charm silently as you hold the herb. This works particularly well with Rosemary as it reminds us to stay alert to opportunities that provide what we need.

You may want to set a clear intention to meet your wealth goal by a certain time. This could be written on a Bay leaf, or Birch bark paper, or similar. Place this under your spell candle and light it each night, as in the Moon Magic section.

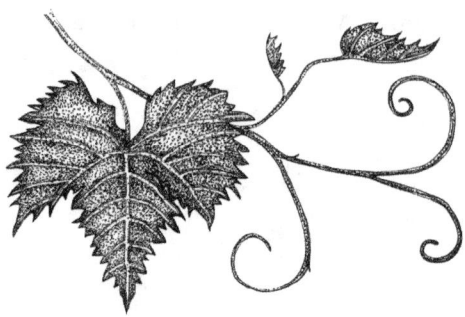

Invisibility spell

Ivy (*Hedera helix*) is very useful for this, but other cloaking, creeping plants will work too. Find either an Ivy leaf or a whole length of it to weave into a circle. Place it around your spell candle. This spell is partly in Latin; use whichever part you prefer.

> *Hedera helix, grant me grace,*
> *Cloak my body, hide my face.*
> *Hold me in shadows, keep me concealed,*
> *Keep my voice, invisibly sealed.*
> *It is done.*
> *Hedera helix, gratiam da,*
> *Corpus tege, faciem ne ostenda.*
> *In umbris tene me, abscondito,*
> *Vocem meam custodi, invisibilis sigillo.*
> *Factum est.*

Say the words calmly, with determination, over the Ivy leaves. Repeat three times as you visualise the Ivy gently but safely surrounding you. Sense it concealing you when needed. Let the candle burn for as long as feels right and is possible for you. Once you feel the spell is complete, extinguish the candle, and thank the Ivy for its assistance. Carry an Ivy leaf with you, to act as an amulet and extend your connection with the spell.

Banishing spell

This spell is for when you have unwanted attention, or obstacles of any kind. Perhaps someone is trying to control you, or wants more of your attention than you are happy to give. Or perhaps something is getting in your way. Banishing spells can also help you to build the strength to take appropriate action in the physical plane, to keep yourself safe and deal with problems.

This spell is particularly potent during a Waning Moon when energies to remove blockages, eliminate negativity, or bring something to a close, are particularly strong.

Materials

Candle

Lighter

Bay leaf

Pen/pencil

Rose thorn

Bay water (optional)

Write your own name or sigil on the Bay leaf. Draw three circles around it, representing physical, spiritual, and energetic protection. Visualise yourself enclosed and protected by a golden shield, some distance from your physical body. Its purpose is to allow only positive energy to reach you. Within the shield, see a red–green layer, prickly and dynamic, as if you are surrounded by a rambling Rose that reacts and repels anything that might harm you. Then within that, a deep green smooth shield. This layer absorbs any tiny remnants of energy that manage to get through, perhaps because the sender has good intentions for you. The red layer is Rose-scented, the green layer is Bay-scented. See these shields deflecting unwanted attention and energy.
Say:

> *With Rose and Bay, I'm safe from harm,*
> *By scent and thorn, avoid alarm.*

Burn the leaf to release the energy of the spell. Now dip the thorn in Bay water, then hold it, pointing away from you, close to your solar plexus. Close your eyes and feel your solar plexus completely protected from unwanted attention and attempts to control you. The thorn can be left in a safe place and reused, or carried with a Bay leaf in a small charm pouch.
Say again:

> *With Rose and Bay, I'm safe from harm,*
> *By scent and thorn, avoid alarm.*
> *It is done.*

Protection spell

This can be used to help ensure a safe journey, whether by foot, bike, or vehicle, and to protect property or loved ones. Remember to follow protection magic with practical steps in the physical realm. Any three strongly protective aromatic or prickly herbs will work for this spell.

Materials

Bay leaf

Rosemary

Bramble (any prickly parts)

Small bowl of water

Spell candle

Lighter

Find a quiet area where you won't be disturbed. Set up your altar or workspace. Infuse a bowl of water with the Bay and Rosemary. Let it steep for at least a few minutes (ideally overnight), allowing the energies of the herbs to infuse the water. Use a little of the water to rinse your hands, or anoint parts of your body. Envision the water creating a strong layer of protection around you, at skin level.

Then light the candle and focus on its flame. Imagine a net-like barrier of protection surrounding you. Visualise it being eggshaped and impossible for negative energy to pass through. As you visualise, chant:

> *Bay, Blade and Thorn, I call to thee,*
> *Protect from harm, hold safe the key.*
> *Gold filigree egg to build my shield,*
> *Guard my soul, from harm concealed.*

Place the Bay leaves, Rosemary, and Bramble around the candle, creating a circle. This forms a protective barrier that amplifies your intention. Spend a few moments in meditation, feeling the protection around you. When you feel ready, thank the herbs for their support and say aloud:

> *It is done.*

Allow the candle to burn down safely or extinguish it when you are ready. The herbs can be composted or returned to the earth elsewhere.

Study success spell

Materials

Spell candle

Lighter

Seeds (tiny ones work best)

Light the candle. Sprinkle a few pinches of seeds around the candle, and let some fall through the lit flame. Gaze quietly at the flame. Visualise yourself working calmly on your project, pulling on your resources, digging deep to build your knowledge and to pull your work together. See it coming together, and then see the work complete. See yourself handing the work in, with a feeling of satisfaction at a job well done.

Visualise the sprinkled seeds gathering together at the base of the candle, as if it were a group of Bees coming together to swarm. Then see them forming a trail up the candles to the flame, where you visualise them sparkling in the heat, combusting, and spreading their essence throughout the universe.

Let the candle burn down if safe to do so. Visualise everything coming together for you, and then take some practical steps towards your tasks, right there, as you sit quietly near the flame. Gather the seeds and plant outdoors.

Karma spell

This is an alternative to a curse. It invokes the principle of karma, ensuring that someone receives the consequences of their actions, good or bad. It focuses on justice, balance, and returning the energy they've put out into the world, without causing harm or ill will.

Enchanter's Nightshade is the herb of choice for this spell, it really is the one to use. It is strongly associated with ancient witchcraft, the balance of energies, and ensuring that the recipient gets back what they have put out into the world. Herbs that are strongly protective and defensive, such as Nettle or Sage, would be suitable alternatives but Enchanter's Nightshade is ideal for karmic spells.

Materials

Dried or fresh Enchanter's Nightshade (*Circaea lutetiana*)

Spell candle, perhaps with a black ribbon

Mirror or other shiny reflective surface, to reflect energy back

Small piece of paper

Birch bark or Bay leaf

Pen/pencil

Fireproof container

Choose a quiet place where you won't be disturbed. Set the mirror on your altar or table, positioning it to reflect the person's actions symbolically back towards them. Place the candle in front of the mirror.

On the paper, bark or leaf, write the name of the person you want to direct this karmic energy towards. If the name is not known, use a symbol to represent their energy. Focus on their actions and how they affect others, rather on them as an individual.

Take a pinch of Enchanter's Nightshade and sprinkle it over the paper. As you do, say:

> *Enchanter's Nightshade, herb of fate,*
> *Bring what's due, swift and straight.*
> *Energy given, returned in kind,*
> *Actions mirrored, justice find.*

Light the candle and focus on the flame. Visualise a colourful wind blowing from the person or source of the problems. See it hitting the mirror and blowing straight back to them. Picture this happening without judgement. Witness the recipient change for the better, learn from their actions, and do good things.

If safe to do so, light the paper using the candle's flame and place it in the fireproof dish to burn. As the paper burns, say:

> *What flows returns, a circle found,*
> *Deeds reflected, justice bound.*
> *With this flame, I set things straight.*

Karma's balance is never too late.
So mote it be.

Once the paper has burned completely, extinguish the candle. Place any remaining ash or unused Enchanter's Nightshade outside, to compost.

Good health spells

Weaving magic into food preparation is a great way to work healing magic. Even if you won't be creating something for them to eat, select safe herbs with qualities suited to the spell target's health needs. If you don't know which to select, try popular healing kitchen herbs such as Parsley, Sage, Rosemary, and Thyme. Honey, Self-heal and edible plants of the Rose family are useful too. Blackberry, Apple, Rose, and Cherry are all in that family.

Try adding medicinal herbs to soups and smoothies, or sprinkle dried Nettle seeds or Rose petals, in the shape of a sigil or the target's initials, over food. Channel healing energy from your hands into whatever you prepare. Visualise your target being strong, healthy, and happy as you craft food and drink for them. Stir your intention into it, or visualise white healing light empowering it.

Consuming the food or drink completes the spell, so be sure that whatever you make is tasty and safe. Also tell the recipient that it has been prepared to bring them health. Try lighting a candle in your kitchen and saying this incantation as you prepare the food:

Food so bright, full of wealth
Bring my friend, strength and health.

As they eat, magic flows.
From my fingers, to their toes!
So mote it be.

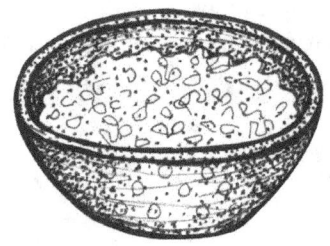

Career spell

For this spell, you will need to be clear about what you wish to achieve in your professional life. Be specific about what you want to manifest. Condense these into short but clear goals and record them in your journal. You will write an abbreviated version or a sigil to represent this during the spell. Basil is used because it brings clarity and strongly attracts success and prosperity. It also protects from negativity. Mint and Parsley are useful alternatives.

This spell is particularly potent during a Waxing Moon when energies for growth and new beginnings are strong.

Materials

Fresh potted Basil plant in a plant pot holder

Spell candle

Green thread

Bay leaf, Birch paper, or paper

Pen/pencil

Small cup of water

Write your career goal sigil or abbreviation on the Bay leaf, bark, or paper. Light the candle. While gazing at the flame, visualise yourself having achieved your career goals, being in your dream job—as if your goals have already come to fruition. See yourself in the situation, feel it, smell it, and hear the sounds you will enjoy when you step into your professional wishes. Look at your career goal sigil again, or see it in your mind's eye.

Rub your hands briskly together. Place them either side of the Basil plant. Feel the plant's energy travel into your palms as your energy flows into it. Feel your career success as you do this. Take a few deep breaths then say to the Basil plant:

> *Basil bright, bring forth my aim,*
> *Help me rise in fortune and fame.*

Now slip your career sigil either under the pot or between the pot and holder—somewhere that it will stay hidden but in good condition.

Pick one vibrant Basil leaf, roll it, and eat it. Maintain your visualisation throughout. Take a sip of water and then use the rest to water the Basil plant.

Sit quietly, considering the practical steps you need to take to achieve your career goals. Decide which you will take first and make notes in your journal to help you remember. Work on one of these steps while the candle burns down, or plan a time to do it.

Extinguish the candle and keep the Basil in a safe place. Revisit it regularly, eat from it as you would usually, each time feeling your spell being reinforced. Repeat the spell weekly if possible. If the Basil plant fades, replace it with a new one, and try growing Basil from seed.

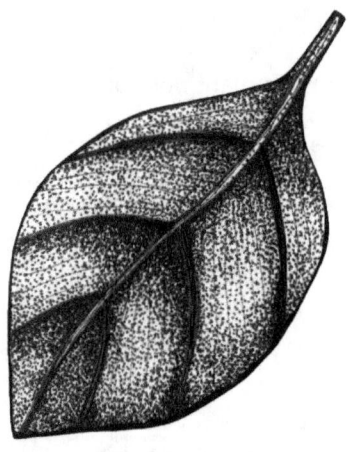

Binding to prevent harm

Materials

Spell candle

Sharp point

Lighter

Trailing herb (such as Ivy, Bramble, or Ground Ivy)

To prevent something from causing harm, use a sharp point to mark a symbol or initial, to represent the cause of the harm. Then bind a length of a trailing, clinging plant around a spell candle. Whisper the following words as the candle burns down:

> *By vine and flame, I bind this ill,*
> *To harm no more, I set my will.*
>
> *It is done.*

The intention of this binding is to prevent harmful energy from being sent from some source. Remember to avoid binding in ways that could make problems worse. Also, combine binding with practical protective actions, and refresh your energetic shields.

Moon Magic

Quiet and mysterious, the Moon has long fascinated those seeking deeper understanding of the natural world. Whether we see it in the sky or not, day and night, the Moon's circuit around the Earth affects our personal growth, communities, ecosystems, and the planet. Understanding and working with lunar energy cycles can enhance our spellwork and affirmations, and help us to harmonise with natural cycles.

Lunar cycles

The Moon is in constant predicable motion around the Earth. It passes through eight phases, from New Moon to Full Moon to New Moon, each lunar month. The Moon's phases are the different shapes that we see as the Moon orbits the Earth. They are caused by the way sunlight illuminates it.

The New Moon (or Dark Moon) is when the Moon is directly between Earth and the Sun; the side facing us is in shadow, making it almost invisible. As it moves around Earth, a thin crescent of light begins to appear, growing larger each night during the waxing phase. It reaches the first quarter phase when half of the Waxing Moon is illuminated, and then the Full Moon when Earth is between the Moon and the Sun, so that the side we see is fully lit.

After the Full Moon, the Moon appears to shrink in what's called the waning phase. The illuminated portion decreases each night, moving through the last quarter, when it is half-lit again. Then a waning crescent is seen until it disappears to the new Moon. This cycle takes about 29.5 days and is called a lunar month.

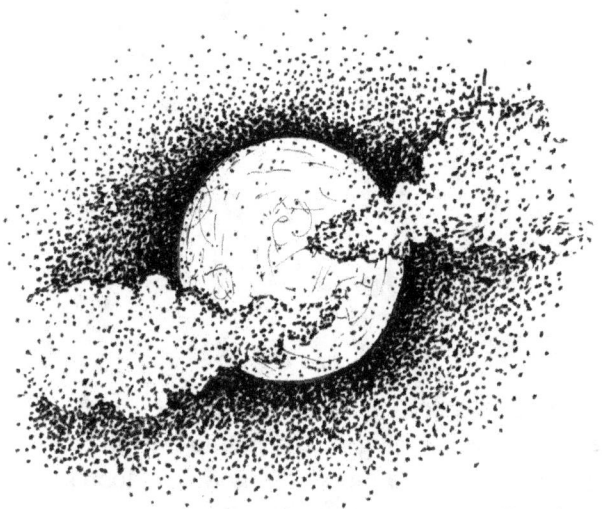

All objects have gravity, and pull other objects towards them. The Moon's gravitational pull creates tides by drawing water towards itself, affecting the oceans and other bodies of water. The Moon also attracts the Earth towards itself, but less so than water. And the Earth pulls the Moon towards itself. This gravitational interplay between the two huge spheres causes the tides.

There are two high tides and two low tides every 24 hours. These are caused by the Earth's rotation; the side of the Earth closest to the Moon has a high tide, the side furthest away, also. The areas between have low tides. As the Earth rotates each day, every body of water will pass through two high and two low tides each day.

The tides also follow a monthly rhythm linked to the Moon's phases. During the New and Full Moon phases when the gravitational forces of the Moon and Sun align, we experience spring tides, with more extreme high and low tides around that day. However, during the first and third quarters, when the Moon and Sun form a right angle, their gravitational pulls are least aligned, milder neap tides occur. So each lunar month sees two spring tides and two neap tides, although each day has a high and low tide. This cycle repeats each lunar month.

Even if we don't live near a coastline, estuary, or large body of water, we can often see that the Moon's cycle has significant effects on nature. Lunar cycles often mirror shifts in our physical bodies, emotions, and spiritual states; many people find connections between the Moon's phases and their own emotional "tides". Menstrual cycles are often naturally synchronised to the lunar calendar. Plants are also known to respond differently to the energies of Waxing and Waning Moons, and understanding how can help with gardening. The additional night light at Full Moon, even in cities, encourages animals to be more active. The lunar calendar also guides many mainstream religious events, such as the Christian festival of Easter, which takes place on the first Sunday after the first Full Moon after the spring equinox.

Moon and mind

We know that strong intent and emotional release are required for our magic to work. By following the Moon and our emotions month by month, we can get to know when we are most likely to be able to work magic effectively. Everyone is different, of course, but in general we may feel more energetic and ambitious when the Moon is waxing. And, we may find it easier to let things go, when the Moon wanes. So this can guide when to cast different types of spell.

In previous years, it was widely accepted that our emotions become more erratic at the Full Moon. Risky, uninhibited, and manic behaviour were thought most common then, and the now-outdated word lunatic came from this. If you notice such changes in your emotions at Full Moon, you could plan to harness them to make brave choices at that time. People tend to become more introspective, quiet, and thoughtful at the New Moon. We are more likely to feel down, or *Moony*. If this is true for you, it can help to plan to do less and nourish yourself at the New Moon. In spellwork, the New Moon is a potent time for beginnings, fresh starts, and growing ideas. Many witches also notice that the New Moon is a time of heightened intuition, and they prefer it for divination.

The following practices can help you to work with lunar cycles.

Lunar spells, charms, and activities

The Waxing Moon is best for casting spells focused on growth, attraction, and abundance, whereas the Waning Moon is best for spells aimed at releasing whatever doesn't serve you, banishing negativity, and reducing obstacles.

Lunar journaling

Keeping a Moon Journal can track how lunar phases influence your emotions, productivity, and health. Over time, this can help you to plan for and work with these shifts. Try to regularly note the Moon's phase, along with any corresponding mood changes, dreams, or shifts in energy. You could also add simple Moon phase symbols to notes in your grimoire or spell book, to show the lunar phase when different techniques were used.

Moon gazing

Observing the Moon, whenever you get the chance, is quite calming and will help you align with the lunar phases. Gazing at the Moon can also work as a spontaneous scrying tool—try gazing softly at it, at any phase of the cycle, and interpret any patterns, thoughts, or images that come to you.

Full Moon rituals

Many coastal communities ritually purify themselves, by bathing in the sea at Full Moon. Others use rivers or waterfalls. Many city witches take a ritual bath or shower at Full Moon. Try to bare some of your skin to the Full Moon light. Even holding your face and palms up to the Moon can help. Also expose your crystals and stones to the moonlight. Don't worry if the Full Moon is not visible; indirect moonlight will work too. The Full Moon is a potent time to release intentions into the universe.

Lunar meditation

You may like to try aligning your meditation focus with the Moon's phase. Try meditating on the meaning of growth and attraction during the waxing phase, and on release, and letting go during the waning phase.

Moon water

This is a traditional practice, to capture some of the Moon's energy in water. Moon water can be used in rituals, for anointing, or for cleansing purposes. Many witches prefer a silver cup or crystal glass to hold the water (often available in charity stores), but canning jars work perfectly well. Avoid making Moon water during an eclipse of the Moon, as the water will be agitated and less useful.

To make, fill a clean container with drinking water and place it somewhere that may be exposed to the sky and moonlight. This could be on a windowsill, doorstep, roof terrace or any other location, where the Moon may be able to shine on the water. Although a bright Full Moon produces the most potent Moon water, indirect exposure to moonlight also works, so don't worry if your location does not provide a direct view of the Moon. You could also place the cup on or near some lush green Moss.

Wherever you place your water, give a nod and smile to the sky, to thank in advance for this gift. Leave the cup in position overnight and retrieve it the following morning. Thank the Moon as you collect it.

Moonwash your stones and crystals

Place stones and crystals in a shallow bowl of water and leave them all night, under the Full Moon's light. This will clear and recharge them. If leaving them outdoors is not possible, placing them on a windowsill will also work well.

Moon plants

Old herbals and grimoires often recommended harvesting plants, even different parts of the same plant, during specific lunar phases. For instance, Burdock and Dock roots are thought best harvested during the Waning Moon. And the dew on certain plants was also favoured at certain lunar phases—Lady's Mantle dew is best collected at the Full Moon closest to Beltane. Other plants are strongly associated with the Moon, often due to their silvery appearance. The Artemisias Mugwort and Wormwood are examples.

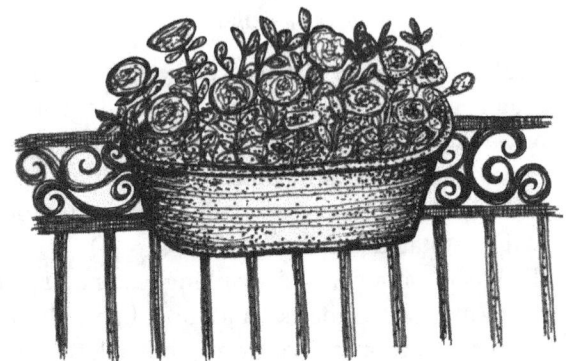

Many plants respond to the Moon's cycles, or appear playful during moonlit nights. You may notice moonlike qualities in plants such as Brugmansia, Night-scented Jasmine, or Night-scented Stock—these all release heady fragrance at night. Witch Hazel and Rowan both have a quicksilver-type energy about them. Evening Primrose opens its blooms at night, and herbs with white flowers, which can be seen last at dusk, may also be considered Moon plants.

Moon gardens

Growing Moon plants is another way to align with lunar cycles. Begin by planting a few Moon plants in a large pot or outdoors, in areas where you and neighbours may like to sit outside late into the evening. Even when tall buildings prevent you from seeing the Moon, sitting close to Moon plants can help you sense its energy. Datura is often associated with the Moon, and can make a wonderful addition to a city witch Moon garden. But, it is extremely toxic so be especially careful if you decide to cultivate it. Datura has become quite a common European city street herb, so there are plenty of seeds around.

Lunar gardening

Gardening by the Moon involves carrying out particular gardening tasks during specific phases of the Moon. The intention is to use lunar energy to provide optimal conditions for plant growth. Lunar gardeners believe that this system provides healthier plants and greater yields.

Biodynamic gardening involves lunar gardening, and is the method used by some of the highest-quality vineyards and herb farms in Europe. Detailed lunar gardening calendars are available,[34] but the following principles should help you to begin:

> Plant above-ground herbs (such as Lemon Balm and Passionflower) during the waxing phase, when the visible Moon is growing.
>
> Sow and plant herbs where the below-ground parts are valued (such as Garlic) during the third quarter, following the Full Moon.
>
> Harvest roots at New Moon, when plant energies are said to be most concentrated below ground.
>
> Harvest above-ground parts (fruit, flowers, foliage, bark) at Full Moon, when plant energies are most concentrated above ground.
>
> Weed between herbs during the Full Moon.
>
> Avoid planting and harvesting during the last quarter.

New Moon rituals

The Moon appears to grow from the New Moon until the Full Moon, 14 days later. This waxing phase is a suitable time to set intentions for the coming month. New Moon is also the optimal time to set up any potions that need about six weeks to infuse. By starting now, their magical potential will increase dramatically until the coming Full Moon, then settle and solidify, from Full Moon to New Moon. The final two weeks will allow the potion to reach its peak potential (at Full Moon).

New Moon manifestation ritual

Perform this manifestation ritual on the New Moon (Dark Moon). Ideally, start on the darkest night of the lunar month, though a night close to that will work well too. This ritual harnesses the energy of the waxing and waning phases of the Moon—the Waxing Moon to build intentions, the Full Moon for release, and the Waning Moon for transformation.

Sit comfortably, then ground and centre yourself. Calm your mind by observing your breath, then gradually lengthen your breath. Aim for a

---

[34] Such as J.R. Gower, *Gwydion's Planting Guide: The definitive Moon-planting manual* (Pan-Dimensional, 1994).

rhythm where your exhalation is slightly longer than your inhalation, perhaps inhaling for 3 counts and exhaling for 5 counts.

Light a candle, in a heatproof holder, and reflect on what you wish to manifest or develop during the coming lunar month. What do you want to grow? Visualise it as if it has already manifested, sensing it as clearly as possible with each of your senses.

Now create a short, present-tense statement that captures your intention. Phrase it as though it already exists, simply needing to become visible. Simplify your statement to keep it clear and concise, such as, "My life is balanced, abundant, and brings good to the world."

Write your statement on a small piece of paper or Birch bark. Perhaps use a natural ink such as berry juice. Snuff out the candle then fold the paper and place it under the candle holder.

Each night, from the Dark Moon to the Bright Moon, visit the candle. Light it, and for a few minutes, read the statement and visualise your intention again. Afterwards, snuff out the candle, refold the paper, and place it back under the candle.

After two weeks, at the Full Moon, perform this practice one last time. Engage all of your senses again, feeling your intention as intensely as you did at the New Moon. Feel it pulse in your chest; breathe it, see it, and let it resonate deeply within you. Read your statement aloud one last time, then release it into the universe. Visualise your intention as a starburst of light particles, spreading throughout the world to make your intent a reality.

Burn the paper using the candle flame, let it cool in a heatproof container, then bury the ashes outdoors, or bury the paper in earth.

For the remainder of the Moon cycle, trust the universe to manifest your intention. You will not need to recite the statement or light the candle again. Trust that you will be provided with precisely what you need when it is right. At the next New Moon, reflect on how the process has worked and what changes have come about as a result. You may begin the process again, either with the same intention, adjusted for what has already manifested, or with a completely different focus.

New Moon intentions are powerful so, as with any spellwork, avoid entangling others in your intentions and manifestations. Focus on the feelings and qualities you seek, rather than specific people or places, and trust the universe to sort out the details.

Blood Magic

Blood Magic uses the energy found in naturally shed natural tissues like tears, saliva, menstrual blood, hair, nail clippings, and semen. These materials, when used respectfully, carry potent life force and symbolic significance, making them suitable for various rituals and sympathetic magic. Menstrual blood, in particular, is often used for grounding, protection, and binding work. It's important to emphasise that Blood Magic does not involve harm to oneself or others.

Grounding with blood involves returning it to the earth in rituals that honour its life force. A common practice includes using menstrual blood, diluted or directly poured into the soil, especially at the base of trees. This act is both a symbolic and physical return of life force to the earth. As menstruation carries the energy and memories of the preceding weeks, women can use this process to actively release old emotions and experiences, viewing each cycle as an opportunity for renewal and transformation.

Blood Magic is not exclusive to menstruating women. Life force exists in all naturally shed materials. So anyone can work with these materials to connect with the energy present in their body.

Blood Magic is commonly used in protection, fertility, or healing work but can be woven into many spells. Feeding dried grains of blood and bone to Roses and fruit trees is a common European gardening practice, so choosing to use your own menstrual blood over animal products doesn't seem so strange. Other naturally shed materials like tree sap, bark, or resin, and a Cat's sloughed-off claws, can also be incorporated into rituals. There are many ways to do this, such as burying, burning, or adding to charm bags. All Blood Magic should be conducted with intention, respect, and an understanding of the sacredness of the materials used.

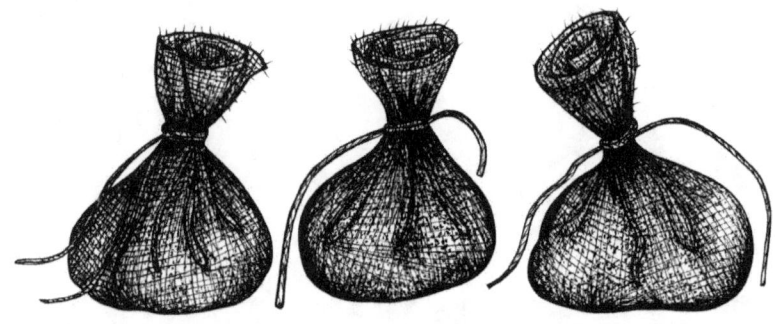

Here are two examples of how to perform Blood Magic.

Charm to banish unwanted emotions

Materials

Candle

Lighter

Small cauldron or heatproof container

Some naturally shed part of your body, perhaps a few hairs from your hair brush, or dead skin, brushed off

Tweezers.

Sit comfortably. Light the candle then ground, centre, and shield. Hold the hair or nail clippings in your hand, as you focus on the emotions or energies you wish to release. These naturally shed parts of you contain memories of events that have occurred in the past months or even years (depending on the length of your hair!). Envision any remaining heaviness or negativity, streaming into the hair or clippings, from your palms.

When ready, place the clippings into a small heatproof container, or hold them over the flame using tweezers. Watch as they burn and visualise the past negativity dissolving and drifting away with the smoke.

Say:

Be gone, what serves no more!

When complete, extinguish the candle, and bury any ashes in earth.

Binding of person to place

To bind yourself to a place, perhaps one you wish to return to, offer some naturally shed piece of yourself, such as clipped nails, hair from your brush, or diluted menstrual blood, into the soil at the base of a tree at the location. As you do so, whisper:

Through blood and root, my spirit stays,
Call me back in future days.
It is done.

The intention of this binding is to create an energetic link between you and the specific place, calling you back when the time is right. Remember to avoid binding in a way that could limit and restrict, as even ties to places can become problematic.

Shapeshifting

Temporarily adopting the characteristics of another being can help us to develop a deeper connection with them and the natural world. This can be approached at different levels, from considering how they go about their business, to actually shifting our consciousness within their body. Many myths and legends around the globe feature humans who shapeshifted into animals or plants to overcome challenges. These tales can teach us much about the skills of transformation, personal development, and the characteristics of life that are part of us all. This section shares two shapeshifting myths and explains the technique.

Ceridwen and Taliesin

Ceridwen was a witch who lived underwater, in a lake at Bala, Wales, along with her husband and twins (a boy and a girl). Her daughter was perfect but her son, Afagddu, was not so blessed and was rather an unfortunate boy. Ceridwen wanted to make him talented and attractive so she gathered herbs and began brewing a herbal potion that would magically transform Afagddu into everything that Ceridwen wished him to be.

The potion needed to be stirred for a year and a day, and after that Afagddu was to be given the first three drops, as these would provide wisdom, inspiration, and brilliance. Ceridwen was an incredible witch and her potion was potent but she had no time to stir herself, so she engaged a blind old man, Morda, to tend the fire and a young lad, Gwion Bach, to stir.

Unfortunately for Ceridwen, when the brew was just finished, three drops spat out onto the thumb of young Gwion Bach. Naturally, he sucked his thumb to ease the scorch. As he did this, the wisdom, inspiration, and brilliance intended for Ceridwen's son entered Gwion Bach. Ceridwen was livid and determined to kill the boy, but he fled. And so began a chase involving the shapeshifting of Gwion Bach, as he tries to escape the clutches of the furious witch, and the shapeshifting of Ceridwen, as she attempts to hunts him down:

Gwion transformed into a Rabbit so Ceridwen became a Dog and chased him.
Gwion became a Fish, Ceridwen chased in the form of an Otter.
Gwion became a Bird, Ceridwen chased him as a Hawk.
Gwion became a grain of Corn, Ceridwen promptly ate him, while in the form of a Hen.

Satisfied in having destroyed Gwion Bach, Ceridwen returned to the form of a woman. However, she found she was pregnant and eventually gave birth to a child, one so strikingly beautiful that she could not kill him. Knowing it was the spirit of Gwion Bach in another form, but unable to kill something so radiant, she set the baby adrift at sea, in a large leather bag. The baby in the bag was found, and raised by caring parents and became known as Taliesin, the greatest Bard of Ancient Britain.

We can learn much from the legend of Ceridwen and Taliesin, not least our need to know the special talents and characteristics of different creatures; this helps us to emulate them in times of need. The Children of Lir of Celtic mythology (who transformed into Swans) and many other well-known ancient tales likewise indicate that adopting the form of an animal can help to keep us safe.

Some of the women accused during the witch hunts of the Middle Ages described shapeshifting during their trials. Some described it as becoming "like" an animal, then described the return to their own body as "leaving" the Hare. Although these women were under cruel duress at the time, to the point of death, so we cannot take what was said as truth, it does give a strong indication that in Europe shapeshifting has been part of spiritual work for a long time. Describing the process as becoming like and then leaving the animal also indicates that shapeshifting is not as difficult to achieve as it may seem.

Daphne and the Bay tree

In the Greek metamorphosis myth of Daphne and Apollo, Daphne was a water nymph, famed for her beauty. Apollo (god of archery, music, dance, truth, prophecy, healing, and disease) had annoyed Eros (god of love) by bragging that his bow was bigger than that of Eros. Angered by the insult, Eros shot two arrows.

A golden love arrow hit Apollo, causing him to fall in love with the first person he saw, and another arrow, of lead, struck Daphne, causing her to decide to remain a virgin all her life. Apollo saw her, fell in love and wanted her. He pursued her horribly and caused her great anguish.

Apollo was like a Greyhound hunting a Hare. When finally he almost touched her, she asked her father, the river god Peneus, to protect her from Apollo's advances. Peneus agreed and promptly transformed Daphne into a Bay tree (*Laurus nobilis*). Although Apollo could no longer have Daphne as he wanted, he cast a spell on the Bay tree so its beauty would never age nor fade; to this day, it remains evergreen.

The Bay became an emblem of Apollo; Laurel leaves adorn his hair and lyre in most depictions, and the Bay became a symbol of creative achievement, music, poetry etc. However, from a shapeshifting perspective, Bay can be seen as strongly protective.

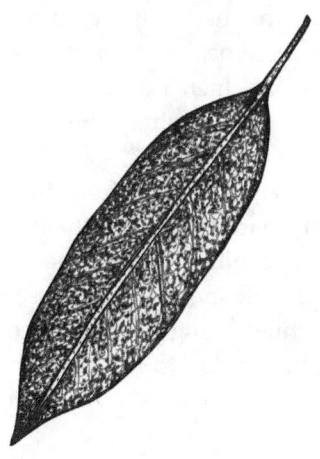

How to shapeshift

This is not suitable if you have any serious mental health illness.

You may like to have your Druid egg or anchor stone with you. Ensure you have time and space to be comfortable and uninterrupted for a while. Choose an animal or plant. You need to have observed it in some way—eventually you will be able to do this by simply thinking about the animal. Become aware of as much as you can about the animal or plant. Use your senses to build a more detailed picture of it. Mimicry comes next, so enacting some of the plant or animal's movements is a good way to begin—perhaps the movement of its branches in a light breeze, its uprightness, or how a chosen animal moves about.

If it feels right, move on to visualising that you are inside of the other being. If you sense any resistance, stop the practice and return to observing and mimicking. Ask yourself why there was resistance and see if you can work on that later. If you are able to enter, what is it like to be there? Use your powers of visualisation to feel what it is like to be seeing the world through its eyes, bark, or roots; smelling the air through its nose, skin, or pores. How does it feel to move through water, soil, or air? Which sounds are heard, what does food taste like, what looks different from inside this living being?

Travel with the being as it goes about its regular routine. Nothing is still in nature, there is always some dynamism, even in seemingly dormant times, so try to sense that.

When ready, withdraw yourself from the animal or plant, feel yourself outside of it again, separate and yet connected. Thank the being for allowing you to sense the world through it for a while. Then cut or close the connection between you; use your metaphysical scissors if needed. Become aware of how the world is through your own body, using all of your senses, one by one. Increase your awareness of sound, light, skin sensations, taste, and gut feelings. Sense the world as a human again—as you.

Observe the animal or plant again from the outside, now with an expanded awareness of what it is like to be them. Consider which aspects of this shapeshifting you could use for the good of the other being, for your personal development, and for the universe as a whole. Remember these. Relax for a while, taking deeper but comfortable breaths and taking time to thoroughly ground, centre, and shield yourself. Rubbing your Druid egg or anchor stone may help this, also clapping your hands, or standing and shaking a little, or briskly tapping your body with your fingertips.

Record any thoughts that the practice brings up for you. Return to it after having time to process the experience.

It helps to start with very short periods of shapeshifting. Let them settle and influence how you feel and work. Return later for slightly longer periods, if it feels comfortable to you.

Conclusion

Congratulations! You now have all the tools needed to weave green magic into your life. I hope you feel more confident in your practice, and that you'll return to these pages often, leaving behind traces of your own journey—leaf stains, pressed flowers, and splashes of spell ingredients. As you hold this book in your hands, take a moment to reflect on the path you've travelled. Together, we've wandered through city streets, rediscovered wild spaces, and uncovered enchantment in the everyday objects and beings that surround us.

In the *Lifestyle* section, we explored how magic can be found in every corner of the city. It doesn't matter whether your home is a shared apartment, a houseboat, or a villa—every setting is rich with possibility. Magic doesn't require special tools or grand gestures; it only asks for your presence and intention. I hope you've felt inspired to work with the turning seasons, using your practice to help shape your goals and dreams.

I imagine you'll revisit the rituals and activities in the *Wheel of the Year* chapter, adding your own personal notes and traditions. Perhaps urban foraging will become a spiritual anchor for you, as it has for many city witches, helping you forge deeper connections with your local environment. You might also find that working magic with others becomes part of your style. Just remember, each of us weaves our own path, and no path is superior to another.

Nature Lore reminded us that the wild doesn't stop at the edge of a park or garden. Urban nature is everywhere: herbs pushing through pavement cracks, houseplants with magical personalities, street trees, and Crows skilfully picking through litter. Every being is perfectly adapted to city life and has something to teach us. This knowledge deepens our love for life and strengthens our practice. Indoors or out, cities are home to countless lifeforms, and every encounter with them is an opportunity to cultivate our own strengths—strengths that can ripple out and help heal the world. Whether it's a moment spent watching rainbows in raindrops or a lunch break under a tree, our non-human neighbours are waiting to be noticed, honoured, and learned from.

In *Tools and Techniques*, we learned that your broom doesn't need to look like anyone else's. In fact, you don't need a broom at all. By choosing fair, sustainable materials (or creative alternatives) your magical toolkit becomes a true reflection of your ethics, as your tools are simply extensions of your energy and intent. We explored the relevance of symbolism, ritual, and prayer, and how to protect what matters most to you. You've begun to demystify practices like spellcasting, shapeshifting, and blood magic—rituals that were once veiled are now accessible. Magic isn't reserved for a chosen few; it's for you, me, and anyone willing to listen, learn, and explore.

The magic of the Green City Witch carries responsibility, yes, but it also brings the joy and freedom of transformation. With each step, you've been shaping a practice that is entirely your own, woven from your life, your values, and your creativity.

As you close these pages, remember that you are part of nature. You don't need perfect conditions, specific tools, star alignments, or anyone else's permission. What matters is your intent, your connection to the world, and the love you pour into your practice. Magic isn't about escaping the city; it's about working with the here and now. It's about being present, tuning in to your local environment, and knowing that you already have everything you need to create change right where you are.

No matter where you live or where you come from, you can be a Green City Witch. Whether you mutter charms in the supermarket or perform rituals in the shower, your connection to magic is real, valid, and powerful. Don't let anyone tell you otherwise. Magic is already woven into your day, your actions, and the air that connects us all.

If your fingers are itching to brew potions or explore the magic of urban herbs, you're in luck—this journey is just beginning. The next book in this series, *Recipes for the Green City Witch: Using Urban Herbs for Brews, Bites, Concoctions, and Crafts*, will take you and your local street and houseplants into the kitchen-apothecary. Together, we'll explore magical foods, potions, and remedies you can make with what's around you, enabling you to cook, heal, and enchant using sustainable, local materials.

And soon, a companion course will open its doors at www.greencitywitch.com—a guided, spiralling journey through the book, helping you grow and weave your knowledge over the cycle of thirteen moons. Visit the site to connect and be the first to know when that magic begins.

But for now, step outside. Touch the bark of a tree. Let the sap within speak to you and connect you to the circle of Green City Witches worldwide that you are a part of. You're already living your magic. You don't need a ritual to confirm it. Just take a moment to be. Breathe your city in, and send your green magic out. Acknowledge the energy around you and within.

You are a Green City Witch, and the world is ready for the magic you're about to release. May your days be enchanted, your spirit free, and your sense of wonder never fade. Weave green magic into every day. The city is yours to transform.

BIBLIOGRAPHY

@yangdawan6285. (2020). *Daylilies have a bumper harvest.* YouTube. https://www.youtube.com/watch?v=X-cVtFtPjas

Abbot, D. (2023). *20 Celtic Symbols: Ancient Irish and Druid meanings.* https://www.culturefrontier.com/celtic-symbols/

Adamatzky, A. (2022). Language of fungi derived from their electrical spiking activity. *R Soc Open Sci.* 9211926. http://doi.org/10.1098/rsos.211926

Akiyama, R., Watanabe, B., Nakayasu, M. et al. (2021). The biosynthetic pathway of potato solanidanes diverged from that of spirosolanes due to evolution of a dioxygenase. *Nat Commun* 12: 1300. https://doi.org/10.1038/s41467-021-21546-0

Al-Snafi, A.E. (2015). The pharmacological importance of *Antirrhinum majus*—a review. *Asian J Pharm Sci Tech.* 5: 313–20. Google Scholar.

Arvigo, R. & Epstein, N. (2021). *Rainforest Home Remedies: The Maya way to heal your body & replenish your soul* (Harper One).

Association of Foragers. https://foragers-association.org/

Ayres, P. (2020). Wound dressing in World War I—The kindly Sphagnum Moss. *FieldBryology* 110. https://www.britishbryologicalsociety.org.uk/wp-content/uploads/2020/12/FB110_Ayres_Sphagnum.pdf

Azab, A. (2016). Alcea: Traditional medicine, current research and future opportunities. *Eur Chem Bull.* 5: 505–14. doi: 10.17628/ECB.2016.5.505. https://www.researchgate.net/publication/313108398

Baker, M. (1996). *Discovering the Folklore of Plants* (Shire Classics).

Ball, I. (1983). *Wine Making the Natural Way* (Hunt Barnard Printing).

Bartram, T. (1998). *Bartram's Encyclopedia of Herbal Medicine: The definitive guide to the herbal treatment of diseases* (Robinson).

Beers, S-J. (2001). *Jamu: The ancient Indonesian art of herbal healing* (Tuttle).

Bendien, E., Kruijthoff, D.J., van der Kooi, C., Glas, G. & Abma, T. (2023). A Dutch study of remarkable recoveries after prayer: How to deal with uncertainties of explanation. *J Relig Health* 62(3): 1731–55. https://doi.org/10.1007/s10943-023-01750-6

Bensky, D., Clavey, S. & Stoger, E. (2015). *Chinese Herbal Medicine Materia Medica*, portable 3rd edn (Eastland Press).

Bergo, A. (2021). *The Forager Chef's Flora: Recipes and techniques for edible plants from garden, field and forest* (Chelsea Green).

Bernhardt, E. (2008). *Medicinal Plants of Costa Rica* (Zona Tropical).

Betts Ecology (2018). *Toxicotoadology*. https://www.bettsecology.co.uk/insight/toxicotoadology

Blanco-Wells, G. (2019). Ecologies of repair: A post-human approach to other-than-human natures. *Front Psychol.* 12: 633737. https://doi.org/10.3389/fpsyg.2021.633737

Bone, K. & Mills, S. (2013). *Principles and Practice of Phytotherapy: Modern herbal medicine*, 2nd edn (Elsevier).

Breverton, T. (2012). *The Physicians of Myddfai: Cures and remedies of the mediaeval world* (Llyfrau Cambria).

Brill, S. (2002). *Identifying and Harvesting Edible and Medicinal Plants in Wild (and Not So Wild) Places* (Harper).

Brockington, G., Gomes Moreira, A.P., Buso, M.S. et al. (2021). Storytelling increases oxytocin and positive emotions and decreases cortisol and pain in hospitalized children. *Proc Natl Acad Sci USA* 118(22): e2018409118. https://doi.org/10.1073/pnas.2018409118

Bruton-Seal, J. & Seal, M. (2008). *Hedgerow Medicine: Harvest and make your own herbal remedies* (Merlin Unwin Books).

Bruton-Seal, J. & Seal, M. (2012). *Make Your Own Aphrodisiacs* (Merlin Unwin Books).

Buettner, D. (2012). *Blue Zones: 9 lessons for living longer from the people who've lived the longest*, 2nd edn (National Geographic).

Buhner, S.H. (2014). *Herbal Antivirals: Natural remedies for emerging & resistant viral infections* (Storey).

Cabrol, F. (2024). Canonical Hours: Fixed portions of the Divine Office which the Church appoints to be recited at the different hours. *Catholic Answers.* https://www.catholic.com/encyclopedia/canonical-hours

Cambridge English Dictionary. https://dictionary.cambridge.org/dictionary/english/

Carr, T. (2023). *A Spell a Day: 365 easy spells, rituals and magic for every day* (Watkins).

CBI (2023). *Entering the European market for avocados*. Centre for the Promotion of Imports from Developing Countries, Netherlands Ministry for Foreign Affairs (CBI). https://www.cbi.eu/market-information/fresh-fruit-vegetables/avocados/market-entry

Chandler-Grevatt, A. (2023). Moss Safari: What lives in moss? *Science in School* 63. https://www.scienceinschool.org/article/2023/what-lives-in-moss/

Chatterjee, R. (2018). *The Stress Solution: The 4 steps to reset your body, mind, relationships & purpose* (Penguin Life).

Chen, X. (2019). A review on coffee leaves: Phytochemicals, bioactivities and applications. *Crit Rev Food Sci Nut*. 59(6): 1008–25. https://doi.org/10.1080/10408398.2018.1546667

Chevalier, G., Patel, S., Weiss, L., Chopra, D. & Mills, P.J. (2019). The effects of grounding (earthing) on bodyworkers' pain and overall quality of life: A randomized controlled trial. *Explore* (New York) 15(3): 181–90. https://doi.org/10.1016/j.explore.2018.10.001

Chevallier, A. (2023). *Encyclopedia of Herbal Medicine*, 4th edn (DK).

Collins, J.L. (2021). *The Simple Path to Wealth*.

Cooke, E. (2012). How narratives can aid memory. *The Guardian*, 15 Jan. https://www.theguardian.com/lifeandstyle/2012/jan/15/story-lines-facts

Cordoza, M., Ulrich, R.S., Manulik, B.J. et al. (2018). Impact of nurses taking daily work breaks in a hospital garden on burnout. *Am J Crit Care* 27(6): 508–12. https://doi.org/10.4037/ajcc2018131

Crawford, M. (2012). *Creating a Forest Garden: Working with nature to grow edible crops* (Green Books).

Cunningham, S. (1985). *Cunningham's Encyclopedia of Magical Herbs* (Llewellyn).

De Blécourt, W. (1994). Witch doctors, soothsayers and priests: On cunning folk in European historiography and tradition. *Soc Hist*. 19(3): 285–303. http://www.jstor.org/stable/4286217. Accessed 21 Oct. 2022.

Dhanalakshmi, U.M., Alam, T. & Khan, S.A. (2022). The folkloric uses and economic importance of some selected edible medicinal plants native to Oman: A brief overview. In: Masoodi, M.H. & Rehman, M.U. (eds). *Edible Plants in Health and Diseases* (Springer, Singapore), 1–29. https://doi.org/10.1007/978-981-16-4880-9_1

Diagne, N., Arumugam, K., Ngom, M. et al. (2013). Use of Frankia and actinorhizal plants for degraded lands reclamation. *BioMed Res Int*. 2013: 948258. https://doi.org/10.1155/2013/948258

Duggen, E. (2005). *Cottage Witchery: Natural magick for hearth and home* (Llewellyn).

Duggen, E. (2009). *Garden Witch's Herbal: Green magic and spirituality* (Llewelyn).

Elpel, T. (2013). *Botany in a Day: The patterns method of plant identification*, 6th edn (Hops Press).

Emre, G., Dogan, A., Haznedaroglu, M.Z. et al. (2021). An ethnobotanical study of medicinal plants in Mersin (Turkey). *Front Pharmacol.* 12: 664500. https://doi.org/10.3389/fphar.2021.664500

Espiritu, K. (2019). *Field Guide to Urban Gardening* (Cool Spring Press).

Fastame, M.C., Ruiu, M. & Mulas, I. (2021). Mental health and religiosity in the Sardinian Blue Zone: Life satisfaction and optimism for aging well. *J Relig Health* 60: 2450–62. https://doi.org/10.1007/s10943-021-01261-2

Fleming, M.A., Ehsan, L., Moore, S.R. & Levin, D.E. (2020). The enteric nervous system and Its emerging role as a therapeutic target. *Gastro Res Pract.* 2020: 8024171. https://doi.org/10.1155/2020/8024171

Forest, D. (2020). *Wild Magic: Celtic traditions for the solitary practitioner* (Llewellyn).

Forest Research (n.d.). Dutch Elm Disease *(Ophiostoma novo-ulmi)*. https://www.forestresearch.gov.uk/tools-and-resources/fthr/pest-and-disease-resources/dutch-elm-disease-ophiostoma-novo-ulmi/

Fowler, A. (2015). *The Thrifty Forager: Living off your local landscape* (Kyle Books).

Franklin, A. & Phillips, S. (1997). *Pagan Feasts: Seasonal food for the eight festivals* (Capall Bann).

Ganora, L. (2009). *Herbal Constituents: Foundations of phytochemistry* (Herbal Chem Press).

Gerard, J. (1994). *Gerard's Herbal: The history of plants.* Ed. M. Woodward (Senate).

Gettings, F. (1987). *Secret Symbolism in Occult Art* (Harmony Books).

González-Ball, R., Bermúdez-Rojas, T., Romero-Vargas, M. & Ceuterick, M. (2022). Medicinal plants cultivated in urban home gardens in Heredia, Costa Rica. *J Ethnobiol Ethnomed.* 18(1): 7. https://doi.org/10.1186/s13002-022-00505-z

Gower, G.R. (1994). *Gwydion's Planting Guide: The definitive Moon-planting manual* (Pan-Dimensional).

Green, J. (2000). *The Herbal Medicine Maker's Handbook: A home manual* (Crossing Press).

Green, M. (1995). *A Witch Alone: Thirteen moons to master natural magic* (Thorsons).

Grieve, M. (1971). *A Modern Herbal: The medicinal, culinary, cosmetic and economic properties, cultivation and folk-lore of herbs, grasses, fungi, shrubs & trees with their modern scientific uses* (Dover).
Griffith, F.L. & Thompson, H. (1921). *The Demotic Magical Papyrus of London and Leiden.* Oxford. https://etana.org/sites/default/files/coretexts/15139.pdf
Hamilton, A. (2024). *The First Time Forager: A complete beginner's guide to Britain's edible plants* (National Trust).
Heald, O., Fraticelli, C., Cox, S. et al. (2019). Understanding the origins of the Ring-necked Parakeet in the UK. *J Zoology* 312(1). https://doi.org/10.1111/jzo.12753
Hedley, C. & Shaw, N. (2020). *The Herbal Book of Making and Taking* (Aeon).
Hopman, E.E. (2008). *A Druid's Herbal of Sacred Tree Medicine* (Destiny Books).
Horne, R. (2023). *The Witches' Art of Incantation: Spoken charms, spells, & curses in folk magic*, 2nd edn (Moon Over Mountain Press).
Houston, T.K., Allison, J.J., Sussman, M. et al. (2011). Culturally appropriate storytelling to improve blood pressure: A randomized trial. *Ann Intern Med.* 154(2). https://doi.org/10.7326/0003-4819-154-2-201101180-00004
Inkwright, F. (2021). *Botanical Curses and Poisons: The shadow lives of plants* (Sterling Ethos).
Jakubczyk, K., Łukomska, A., Czaplicki, S. et al. (2021). Bioactive compounds in *Aegopodium podagraria* leaf extracts and their effects against fluoride-modulated oxidative stress in the THP-1 cell line. *Pharmaceuticals* (Basel) 14(12): 1334. https://doi.org/10.3390/ph14121334
Jaen, J. (1999). *Handbook of Canary Folk Medicine: The secrets of our old herbalists* (Romero).
Johnson, O. & More, D. (2004). *Collins Tree Guide: The most complete field guide to the trees of Britain and Europe* (Collins).
Jones, L. (2020). *Self-Sufficient Herbalism: A guide to growing, gathering and processing herbs for medicinal use* (Aeon).
Jones, L. (2023). *A Working Herbal Dispensary: Respecting herbs as individuals* (Aeon).
Juenong, W. & Blishem, T. (2017). *Illustrated Modern Reader of 'The Classic of Tea'* (Better Link Press).
Jupiter, K. (2020). The function of open-field farming—managing time, work and space. *Landscape Hist.* 41(1): 69–98. https://doi.org/10.1080/01433768.2020.1753984
Kanniah, J. (2020). What is coffee leaf tea? *Perfect Daily Grind.* https://perfectdailygrind.com/2020/09/what-is-coffee-leaf-tea/

Karlsson, B.G. (2022). The imperial weight of tea: On the politics of plants, plantations and science. *Geoforum* 130: 105–14. https://doi.org/10.1016/j.geoforum.2021.07.017

Kasmawati, H., Mustarichie, R., Halimah, E. et al. (2022). Unreveiling the potential of *Sansevieria trifasciata* prain fraction for the treatment of androgenetic alopecia by inhibiting androgen receptors based on LC-MS/MS analysis, and in-silico studies. *Molecules* (Basel) 27(14): 4358. https://doi.org/10.3390/molecules27144358

Kelleher, K. (2018). Scheele's Green: The color of fake foliage and death. *The Paris Review*, 2 May. https://www.theparisreview.org/blog/2018/05/02/scheeles-green-the-color-of-fake-foliage-and-death/

Kindred, G. (2006). *Herbal Healers* (Wooden Books).

Kindred, G. (2011). *Earth Wisdom: A heartwarming mixture of the spiritual, the practical and the proactive* (Hay House).

Kindred, G. (2013). *Letting in the Wild Edges* (Permanent Publications).

Kis, B., Avram, S., Pavel, I.Z. et al. (2020). Recent advances regarding the phytochemical and therapeutic uses of *Populus nigra* L. buds. *Plants* (Basel) 9(11): 1464. https://doi.org/10.3390/plants911146

Lamanna, C. (2018). A storytelling approach: Insights from the *Shambaa*. *J Med Humanit*. (39): 377–89. https://doi.org/10.1007/s10912-018-9512-6

Le Guin, U.K. (1997). *Dancing at the Edge of the World: Thoughts on words, women, places* (Tor Books).

Le Moullec, A., Juvik, O. & Fossen, T. (2015). First identification of natural products from the African medicinal plant *Zamioculcas zamiifolia*—A drought resistant survivor through millions of years. *Fitoterapia* 106: 280–5. https://doi.org/10.1016/j.fitote.2015.09.011. (https://www.sciencedirect.com/science/article/pii/S0367326X15300861)

Li, X., Jiang, S., Cui, K., Qin, X. & Zhang, G. (2022). Progress of genus *Hemerocallis* in traditional uses, phytochemistry, and pharmacology. *J Hort Sci Biotech*. 97(3): 298–314. doi: 10.1080/14620316.2021.1988728

Lin, H.Y., Tsai, J.C., Wu, L.Y. & Peng, W.H. (2020). Reveals of new candidate active components in *Hemerocallis radix* and its anti-depression action of mechanism based on network pharmacology approach. *Int J Mol Sci*. 21(5): 1868. https://doi.org/10.3390/ijms21051868. https://www.ncbi.nlm.nih.gov/pmc/articles/PMC7084327/

Liu, T., Li, Z., Li, R., Cui, Y., Zhao, Y. & Yu, Z. (2019). Composition analysis and antioxidant activities of the *Rhus typhina* L. stem. *J Pharm Anal*. 9(5): 332–8. https://doi.org/10.1016/j.jpha.2019.01.002

Mabey, R. (1989). *Food for Free* (HarperCollins).

Mac Coitir, N. (2016). *Ireland's Wild Plants Myths, Legends and Folklore* (The Collins Press).

Macdonald, G. & Penberth, J. (2007). *West Country Witchcraft* (Green Magic).
Maltman, A. (2018). *Vineyards, Rocks, & Soils: The wine lover's guide to geology* (Oxford UP).
Manniche, L. (1989). *An Ancient Egyptian Herbal* (British Museum Press).
Martin, L. & Martin, B. (2010). *Growing Tasty Tropical Plants in Any Home, Anywhere* (Storey Publishing).
Mas, F., Horner, R., Brierley, S., Harper, A. & Suckling, D.M. (2020). The scent of individual foraging bees. *J Chem Ecol*. 46(5–6): 524–33. https://doi.org/10.1007/s10886-020-01181-7
Mase, G. (2013). *The Wild Medicine Solution: Healing with aromatic, bitter, and tonic plants* (Healing Arts Press).
Mcconnochie, J. (2022). Are solar panels sustainable? *Sustainable Jungle*. https://www.sustainablejungle.com/are-solar-panels-sustainable/
McGeeney, A. (2016). *With Nature in Mind: The ecotherapy manual for mental health professionals* (JKP).
McGilchrist, I. (2009). *The Master and His Emissary: The divided brain and the making of the Western world* (Yale UP).
McGuire, W. (2018). *Long Live the Weeds* (RBG Kew). https://www.kew.org/read-and-watch/long-live-the-weeds
McVicar, J. (2009). *Jekka's Complete Herb Book* (Kyle Cathie).
Mességué, M. (1975). *Health Secrets of Plants and Herbs* (Pan).
Michalak, M. (2023). Plant extracts as skin care and therapeutic agents. *Int J Mol Sci*. 24(20): 15444. https://doi.org/10.3390/ijms242015444
Muir, L. (2018). *Wild Mocktails and Healthy Cocktails: Home-grown and foraged low-sugar recipes from the Midnight Apothecary* (CICO Books).
Norman, J. (2015). *Herbs & Spices: The cook's reference* (DK).
North Carolina Extension Gardener Plant Toolbox (2024). *Stellaria media*. https://plants.ces.ncsu.edu/plants/stellaria-media/
Nyerges, C. (2016). *Foraging Wild Edible Plants of North America: More than 150 delicious recipes using nature's edibles* (Rowman & Littlefield).
Oakeley, H. (2009). Medicines, poisons and folklore. *The Horticulturist* 18(3): 17–19. http://www.jstor.org/stable/45139670
Paine, A. (2006). *The Healing Power of Celtic Plants* (O Books).
Palumbo, J. (2022). The woman behind the world's most famous tarot deck was nearly lost in history. CNN. https://edition.cnn.com/style/article/pamela-colman-smith-tarot-art-whitney/index.html
Parry-Jones, D. (1952). *Welsh Country Characters* (Batsford).
Peterson, D. & Selsam, M. (2008). *Don't Throw it, Grow it! 68 windowsill plants from kitchen scraps* (Storey Publishing).
Peterson-Bidoshi. K. (2006). The 'Dordolec': Albanian house dolls and the evil eye. *J Am Folklore* 119(473): 337–55. https://muse.jhu.edu/article/204000

Pires Jr, E.O., Coleja, C., Garcia, C.C. et al. (2021). Current status of genus *Impatiens*: Bioactive compounds and natural pigments with health benefits. *Trends Food Sci Tech*. 117: 106–24. https://www.sciencedirect.com/science/article/pii/S0924224421000820

Podunavski, R. (2009). *Balkan Traditional Witchcraft* (Pendraig Publishing).

Pole, S. (2011). *A Pukka Life: Finding your path to perfect health: Inspired by Ayurveda* (Quadrille).

Pole, S. (2013). *Ayurvedic Medicine: The principles of traditional practice* (JKP).

Pollard, K. (2017). *Impatiens glandulifera* (Himalayan balsam). CABI Digital Library. https://doi.org/10.1079/cabicompendium.28766

Potter, C., Harwood, T., Knight, J. & Tomlinson, I. (2011). Learning from history, predicting the future: The UK Dutch Elm Disease outbreak in relation to contemporary tree disease threats. *Philos Trans R Soc Lond B Biol Sci*. 366(1573): 1966–74. https://doi.org/10.1098/rstb.2010.0395

Pseudo-Apuleius (12th century). Oxford, Bodleian Library MS. Bodl. 130. https://digital.bodleian.ox.ac.uk/objects/4ffa9d94-a1fb-495d-9deb-fcdccdec2c09/

Quinn, J., Kessell, A. & Weston, L. (2014). Secondary plant products causing photosensitization in grazing herbivores: Their structure, activity and regulation. *Int J Mol Sci*. 15(1): 1441–65. https://doi.org/10.3390/ijms15011441

Redwood, A. (2011). *The Art of Mindful Gardening* (Leaping Hare).

Ribeiro, J., Silva, V., Aires, A. et al. (2022). *Platanus hybrida*'s phenolic profile, antioxidant power, and antibacterial activity against Methicillin-Resistant *Staphylococcus aureus* (MRSA). *Horticulturae* 8(3): 243. https://doi.org/10.3390/horticulturae8030243

Rogers, V. (2000). *Your Handwriting Can Change Your Life* (Touchstone Books).

Roper, M. & Dressaire, E. (2019). Fungal biology: Bidirectional communication across fungal networks. *Curr Biol*. 29: 4. https://doi.org/10.1016/j.cub.2019.01.011.

Rose, F. (2006). *The Wild Flower Key: How to identify wild flowers trees and shrubs in Britain and Ireland* (Warne).

Roy, R. (2024). *Yoga as Pilgrimage: Sūtras for a modern age* (Sādhana Māla).

Royal Botanic Gardens Kew (2024). Plants of the World Online. https://powo.science.kew.org/taxon/urn:lsid:ipni.org:names:60021-2

Russell, S. (2004). *Manifesto* (Element).

Rzhepakovsky, I., Areshidze, D., Avanesyan, S. et al. (2022). Phytochemical characterization, antioxidant activity, and cytotoxicity of methanolic leaf extract of *Chlorophytum comosum* (green type) (Thunb.) Jacq. *Molecules* (Basel) 27(3): 762. https://doi.org/10.3390/molecules27030762

Sala, L. (2013). *Ritual: The magic perspective* (Mindlift Publishers, Hilversum).

San Jose, C. (2018). *Les Plantes Médicinales* (Artemis).

Scalise Sugiyama, M. (2001). Food, foragers, and folklore: The role of narrative in human subsistence. *Evol Hum Behav.* 22(4): 221–40. https://www.researchgate.net/publication/247233160_Food_Foragers_and_Folklore_The_Role_of_Narrative_in_Human_Subsistence/link/5f3c79eca6fdcccc43d3165a/download

Seeley, T. (2019). *The Lives of Bees: The untold story of the honey bee in the wild* (Princeton UP).

Seo, J., Lee, J., Yang, H.Y. & Ju, J. (2020). *Antirrhinum majus* L. flower extract inhibits cell growth and metastatic properties in human colon and lung cancer cell lines. *Food Sci Nutr.* 8(11): 6259–68. https://doi.org/10.1002/fsn3.1924

Sheldrake, M. (2021). *Entangled Life: How fungi make our worlds, change our minds, and shape our futures* (Vintage).

Shetty, A., Rana, M. & Preetham, S. (2012). Cactus: A medicinal food. *J Food Sci Tech.* 49(5): 530–6. doi: 10.1007/s13197-011-0462-5.

Sich, J. (2015). Healing with Herb Robert. *Julia's Edible Weeds.* https://www.juliasedibleweeds.com/general/healing-with-herb-robert/

Simmonds, M., Howes, M-J. & Irving, J. (2016). *The Gardener's Companion to Medicinal Plants: An A–Z of healing plants and home remedies* (RBG Kew).

Singh, A.K. & Khatkar, B.S. (2011). Processing, food applications and safety of *Aloe vera* products: A review. *J Food Sci Tech.* 48(5): 525–33.

Soth, A. (2018). The Toadmen, masters of equine magic. *JSTOR Daily.* https://daily.jstor.org/the-toadmen-masters-of-equine-magic/

Sowen, M. (2023). The green that poisoned Britain. *Everything is Amazing.* https://everythingisamazing.substack.com/p/the-green-that-poisoned-britain

Starhawk, Baker, D. & Hill, A. (2000). *Circle Round: Raising children in goddess traditions* (Bantam Books).

Stevenson, P. (2017). *Welsh Folk Tales* (The History Press).

Streeter, D. (2016). *Collins Wildflower Guide*, 2nd edn (Collins).

Struthers, J. (2010). *Red Sky at Night: The book of lost countryside wisdom* (Ebury).

Sultzberger, R. (2000). *Herb Gardening: Practical advice on choosing and growing herbs* (Aura Books).

Sutton, M. & Mann, N. (2022). *Druid Magic*, 2nd edn (Llewellyn).

Szewczyk, K.D.S., Zidorn, C., Biernasiuk & Komsta, L.A. (2016). Polyphenols from *Impatiens* (Balsaminaceae) and their antioxidant and antimicrobial activities. *Ind Crops Prod.* 86: 262–72. https://www.sciencedirect.com/science/article/abs/pii/S0926669016302138

Taylor, S. (2021). *The Humoral Herbal: A practical guide to the Western energetic system of health, lifestyle and herbs* (Aeon).

The Seed Sistas (2022). *Poison Prescriptions: Power plant medicine, magic & ritual* (Watkins Media).
The Witches Next Door (2017). How to use Knot Magic in your practice. *The Witches Next Door*, Patheos, 5 Dec. https://www.patheos.com/blogs/thewitchesnextdoor/2017/09/knot-magic/.
Thomsen, M. (2022). *The Phytotherapy Desk Reference*, 6th edn (Aeon).
Throop, P. (1998). *Hildegard von Bingen's Physica: The complete English translation of her classic work on health and healing* (Healing Arts Press).
Thu, Z.M., Oo, S.M., Nwe, T.M. et al. (2021). Structures and bioactivities of steroidal saponins Isolated from the genera *Dracaena* and *Sansevieria*. *Molecules* (Basel) 26(7): 1916. https://doi.org/10.3390/molecules26071916
Tilford, G. & Wulff, M. (2009). *Herbs for Pets: The natural way to enhance your pet's life* (Fox Chapel).
Tudge, C. (2005). *The Secret Life of Trees: How they live and why they matter* (Penguin).
Upenieks, L. & Thomas, P.A. (2021). Gaining faith, losing faith: How education shapes the relationship between religious transitions and later depression. *J Health Soc Behav.* 62(4): 582–98. https://doi.org/10.1177/00221465211046356
Van der Hoeven, J. (2021). *The Book of Hedge Druidry* (Llewellyn).
Vendetti, J. (n.d.). A microscopic look at snail jaws. *Natural History Museum*. https://nhm.org/stories/microscopic-look-snail-jaws
Vitimus, A. (2009). *Chaos Magic: The misunderstood path* (Llewellyn). https://www.llewellyn.com/journal/article/1799?srsltid=AfmBOor-VX-CwKXEOhaTcgQ8618Hs9jnF6L5h5xN0XWeWhP4PZpUvr7s
Wadikar, D.D. & Patki, P.E. (2016). *Coleus aromaticus*: A therapeutic herb with multiple potentials. *J Food Sci Tech.* 53(7): 2895–901. https://doi.org/10.1007/s13197-016-2292-y
Wang, Y., Hao, R., Guo, R. et al. (2023). Integrative analysis of metabolome and transcriptome reveals molecular insight into metabolomic variations during Hawthorn fruit development. *Metabolites* 13(3): 423. https://doi.org/10.3390/metabo13030423
Weed, S. (2011). *Down There: Sexual and reproductive health the wise woman way* (Ash Tree).
White, C. (2019). Some trees can change sex and are more likely to die when female. *New Scientist*, 7 June. https://www.newscientist.com/article/2205199-some-trees-can-change-sex-and-are-more-likely-to-die-when-female/
Wilde, M. (2023). *The Wilderness Cure: Ancient wisdom in a modern world* (Simon & Schuster).

Wilhelm, R. (1950). *I Ching or Book of Changes* (trans. C.F. Baynes) (Routledge & Kegan Paul).
World Birds (2024). https://worldbirds.com/
Wright, J. (2010). *Hedgerow*. River Cottage Handbook No. 7 (Bloomsbury).
Yance, D. (2013). *Adaptogens in Medical Herbalism* (Healing Arts Press).
Yosri, N., Alsharif, S.M., Xiao, J. et al. (2023). *Arctium lappa* (Burdock): Insights from ethnopharmacology potential, chemical constituents, clinical studies, pharmacological utility and nanomedicine. *Biomed Pharmacother*. 158: 114104. https://doi.org/10.1016/j.biopha.2022.114104
You, J., Wen, X., Liu, L., Yin, J. & Ji, J.S. (2023). Biophilic classroom environments on stress and cognitive performance: A randomized crossover study in virtual reality (VR). *PLOS One* 18(11): e0291355. https://doi.org/10.1371/journal.pone.0291355
Young, O. (2022). 10 Little-known facts about Abalone. *Tree Hugger*. https://www.treehugger.com/abalone-facts-5180643

INDEX

Note: Page numbers in **bold** indicate figures.

a-Maying, 58
Abalone shells, 289–290, 291–292, 360
abundance
　spells for, 59–60, 64–65
Acacia tree, 14
acorn, 13, 52, 57, 59, 66, 196, 266, 356, 390
adapting spells and charms (also see
　alternatives), 375–376
Agrimony (*Agrimonia eupatoria* L.),
　82–83, 89–90, 384
Alban Elfed, 71
alchemy, 174, 296, 394
Alder (*Alnus glutinosa* (L.) Gaertn.),
　47, 91
Aloe Vera (*Aloe vera* (L.) Burm.f),
　92–**93**, 243, 359
altars, 37, 42, 47, 51–52, 56–57, 61,
　66–67, 72, **293**–294
alternatives, 62, 291–292, 296, 299, 300,
　326, 346, 361, 374–375, 394
Amoebae, 11

Amphibians, 262–263
amulet, 327–328, 334, 364, 370, 373, 391
ancestors, 6, 36, 37, 38–39, 79, 148, 306,
　326, 332, 352
anchor stone, 39–40, 48–49, 54, 294,
　416–417
animal watching, 12
anointing, 164, 165, 195, 294, 300, 393,
　405
Ant (*Formicidae*), 273
Apollo, 98, 415
Apple (*Malus* spp.)
　foraging, 36–37, 82–83, 85, 94, 101
　uses and significance, 36–37, 38, 94,
　301, 385, 386, 396
Apple cider vinegar, 73
Ash (*Fraxinus excelsior* L.)
　foraging, 82–83, 95
　uses and significance, 73, 95–**96**,
　301, 350, 376
Association of Foragers, 80fn7

associations
- abundance, 56, 66, 118, 129, 138, 150, 164, 178, 181, 193, 210, 229, 232, 263, 271, 274, 280
- accumulation, 91
- adaptation, 12, 155, 181, 190, 265, 266, 269–270, 271, 273, 274, 275, 276, 278, 280, 281, 282
- alchemy, 174, 296
- alertness, 118, 162, 184, 267, 277, 280, 360
- ancestors, 148
- anti-enchantment, 104, 138, 204
- anti-theft, 172
- aphrodisiac, 147, 186, 193, 195, 247
- attachment, 166
- attraction, 102, 111, 142, 150, 159, 183, 230, 232, 404
- balance, 71, 99, 114, 150, 178, 273, 280
- beauty, 94, 97, 127, 155, 171, 174, 213, 272, 275, 278
- bees, 178, 180, 242
- beltane, 155, 174, 186, 195, 255, 406
- bewitchment, 174, 242
- binding, 116, 142, 167
- birds, 147, 159
- blood, 91, 100, 162
- boundaries, 106, 113, 114, 155, 159, 173, 239, 270, 273, 284
- calm, 112, 138, 140, 176, 178, 180, 190, 192, 197, 201, 215, 217, 238
- cats, 109
- change, 210, 257, 262, 263, 264, 271, 272, 273, 275, 276, 277, 282
- chastity, 98
- childbirth, 192, 271
- clairaudience, 153
- clairvoyance, 110, 153, 186, 255
- clarity, 37, 89, 140, 150, 183, 195, 215, 220, 233, 245
- cleansing, 104, 110, 116, 130, 132, 153, 165, 166, 172, 176, 213, 215, 228, 240, 242, 247, 255
- clearing, 110, 153, 165, 212
- clothing, 130
- communication, 178, 179, 206, 220, 222, 264, 265–267, 272
- community, 99, 113, 144, 150, 166, 178, 180, 184, 267, 269, 270, 271, 273, 275
- companionship, 94, 270, 279
- completion, 71
- concealing, 166
- creativity, 56, 98, 148, 169, 196, 234, 245, 253, 265, 284, 296, 323
- cycles, 127, 137, 154, 262, 276, 280, 283
- darkness, 36, 116
- death, 124, 135, 179, 199, 257, 262, 266, 276, 323
- defence, 151, 159, 162
- demons, 171, 324
- determination, 135, 151, 272, 273
- detoxifying, 100, 104, 116, 127, 172, 208, 228, 249
- dignity, 183
- divination, 89, 124, 125, 158, 187, 192, 204, 214, 217, 242, 245, 250, 253, 255, 274
- dominance, 151, 167, 230, 239, 271
- dreams, 89, 106, 192, 242
- druids, 94, 95, 187, 188, 210, 257
- elders, 148
- elegance, 183
- enchantment, 137, 164, 204
- endurance, 103, 229
- energy, 61, 106, 129, 154, 157, 184, 187, 190, 226, 230, 233, 236, 243, 259, 260
- eternity, 94, 120
- exorcism, 110, 172, 253
- fairies, 155, 159, 209, 242, 247
- fairness, 137
- family, 266, 270, 271, 276
- femininity, 162, 278, 279
- fertility, 51, 56, 92, 95, 97, 132, 144, 155, 166, 167, 169, 187, 190, 196, 197, 224, 232, 234, 236, 255, 263, 264, 271, 275, 263, 264, 271, 274, 275, 276, 277, 278, 280, 284, 339
- fidelity, 42, 113, 166, 167, 187, 279, 323

INDEX 437

fire, 138, 226, 255, 296
flexibility, 151
flow, 132
force, 160
foresight, 267
forgiveness, 165
freedom, 264, 275
fresh starts, 46, 250, 404
friendship, 120, 234
gateways, 164
goddesses, 46, 178, 192, 220, 253, 263, 278, 279
good fortune, 58, 89, 109, 140, 159, 167, 180, 188, 197, 209, 229, 249, 265, 267, 271, 272, 276, 278, 280
grace, 99, 268, 272
grief, 124
grounding, 108, 190, 195, 204, 243
growth, 116, 122, 145, 150, 154, 160, 183, 190, 224, 234, 236, 243, 249, 263, 271, 272, 282, 284, 285
happiness, 62, 127, 147, 171, 178, 180, 187, 214, 224, 228, 276
hardship, 91, 127
harmony, 89, 113, 130, 178, 197, 265, 276
healing, 46, 58, 98, 110, 122, 164, 190, 208, 210, 217, 218, 234, 242, 245, 262, 263, 264, 282, 283, 300
health, 94, 102, 104, 108, 114, 120, 133, 138, 148, 171, 178, 188, 202, 228, 238, 249
heartache, 147, 155, 159, 213, 252
hope, 68, 100, 124, 148, 275
humility, 108, 195, 284
immortality, 92, 120, 217, 275
impatience, 160
innocence, 124, 165
inspiration, 148, 296
intuition, 106, 172, 190, 278, 280, 300, 301
invisibility, 130, 144, 166, 219, 220, 240, 277
irritation, 181, 274

joy, 94, 150, 193, 265
karma, 137
language, 284
light, 61, 116, 233, 243
liminality, 112, 164, 179, 201, 289, 300
listening, 157
love, 42, 73, 92, 97, 106, 109, 113, 124, 147, 155, 180, 186, 187, 188, 197, 213, 215, 219, 224, 242, 255, 272, 276, 279
luck, 99, 102, 162, 171, 179, 192, 199, 210, 217, 234, 242, 260, 263, 266, 267, 276, 327, 328
luminescence, 162, 402
melancholy, 129, 135, 140, 215, 253
messages, 201, 206, 274, 276, 320–322
money, 72, 118, 120, 129, 135, 167, 210, 229, 259, 260
monopoly, 160
moon, 100, 166, 174, 192, 248, 250, 253, 280
nakedness, 142
negativity, 106, 110, 111, 132, 153, 190, 195, 252, 253, 284
new beginnings, 36–37, 100, 271, 280, 404
nourishment, 72, 99, 142, 195, 232, 236, 296
obstacles, 155, 186, 275, 404
old age, 148
opportunism, 125, 127, 144, 154, 169, 212, 249, 265, 266, 272, 279, 281
passion, 97, 193, 226, 369
peace, 89, 197, 201
perseverance, 150, 183, 260
persistence, 137, 159, 208, 268, 272, 273, 274, 282
poison, 130, 257, 263
positivity, 111, 116, 184, 208, 210, 230, 233, 234, 236, 265, 277
power, 151, 154, 206, 215
pride, 138, 196
productivity, 150
prosperity, 97, 111, 113, 129, 142, 144, 169, 188, 210, 224, 229, 234, 249, 263, 264, 271, 284

protection (plants), 42, 89, 92, 95, 98–99, 102–103, 106, 108, 109, 110, 111, 114, 130, 133, 140, 153, 155, 157, 159, 162, 164, 166, 169, 171, 172, 174, 176, 178, 179, 184, 187, 188, 190, 192, 193, 195, 196, 199, 201, 208, 209, 210, 213, 214, 215, 217, 218, 219, 220, 222, 228, 229, 236, 240, 242, 243, 245, 247, 252, 253, 255, 257, 260
protection (animals), 263, 267, 268, 271, 272, 276, 277, 278, 279, 282, 283
psychic powers, 215
purification, 46, 63, 73, 89, 92, 100, 103, 104, 111, 132, 140, 165, 166, 176, 193, 220, 224, 240, 242, 245, 247, 295
purity, 47, 127, 188, 234, 272, 324
rebirth, 47, 51, 94, 127, 171, 262, 263, 282, 323, 324
rejuvenation, 46, 92
relocation, 154, 259
repair, 122, 239
resilience, 42, 72, 106, 108, 125, 127, 144, 148, 155, 169, 181, 190, 195, 204, 206, 219, 260, 268, 270, 271, 273, 274, 282
return, 137, 266
samhain, 94, 155, 255
seduction, 142, 272
seizing, 116, 154, 249
sensitivity, 160
sensuality, 193
shelter, 102, 180, 236, 248, 282, 283
shielding, 130, 166
silver, 100, 166, 250
simplicity, 195
smoothing, 122
speed, 154, 269
spiciness, 98, 138, 144, 145, 154, 183, 193, 212, 243, 252
spirit realm, 91, 94, 109, 164, 176, 179, 186, 187, 192, 203, 202, 209, 243, 248, 253, 279, 282

spiritual awareness, 63, 114, 118
stability, 91, 183, 189, 190, 294
strength, 91, 95, 103, 106, 125, 138, 150, 151, 155, 162, 165, 184, 196, 202, 208, 226, 232, 234, 242, 263, 268, 273, 274
success, 89, 98, 104, 120, 130, 142, 144, 150, 151, 169, 206, 208, 229, 232, 236, 259, 262, 271
survival, 148, 273, 279, 281
sweetness, 142, 169, 230, 232, 233, 236, 274, 375
take overs, 154, 167
teamwork, 66, 91
tolerance, 155, 181, 212, 260
transformation, 98, 132, 174, 212, 262, 263, 264, 266, 267, 272, 273, 274, 275, 277, 279, 280, 281, 283, 285, 296, 301
vigour, 56, 151
vitality, 59, 97, 114, 226, 263
warmth, 56, 106, 145, 154, 172, 208, 212
water, 91, 95, 157, 187, 248, 250
wealth, 91, 108, 120, 135, 148, 150, 154, 206, 208, 212, 229, 249
whispers, 135, 201, 206, 248
wisdom, 36, 99, 108, 133, 148, 197, 206, 217, 257, 264, 268, 274, 275, 281, 283, 284, 296, 300
witches, 140, 155, 172, 209, 215, 263, 278
worries, 165
youthfulness, 151, 169, 178, 197
astrology, 304
autumn equinox (also see *herfest, mabon*), 34, 71–75, 85, 379
Avalon (see *Isle of apples*)
Avocado (*Persea americana* Mill.), 52, 97
awen, 323

banishing, 64, 106, 297, 391, 404, 410
Banyan tree, 142
Barberry (*Berberis vulgaris* L.) (also see *Mahonia*), 184–185

barefoot walking, 17, 25, 48, 59, 111, 308–309
Basil (*Ocimum basilicum*), 72, 397–**398**
Bat (*Chiroptera*), 277–278
Bat's wings, 321
Bay (*Laurus nobilis* L.)
  foraging, 81–83, 98
  uses and significance, 42, 45, 59, 63, 98, **415**
Bed Bug (*Cimex lectularius*), 273–274, 362–363
Bee (*Apis*), 16, 47, 61, 62, 64, **274**, 349, 387, 394
Beech (*Fagus sylvatica* L.), 82, 85, 99, 268
Beetroot, 52
belonging, 3–6
beltane, 33, 56–60, 82–83
binding, 42, 116, 142, 167, 299, 368, 376, **377**–378, 383, 398–399, 409, 411
Bindweed (*Convolvulus arvensis*), 74, **75**
biophilia, 7–9, 11, 130
Birch (*Betula* spp.)
  foraging, 82, 100–101
  uses and significance, 47–50, 59, 100, 295, 298, 356
birds, 12, 16, 43, 263–272, 349
Black Horehound (*Ballota nigra*), 73
Blackberry (also see *Bramble*), 66, 68, 103, 396
Blackbird (*Turdus merula*), 12, 264
bliss state, 315–316
blood magic, 409–411
Blue Tit (*Cyanistes caeruleus*), 264–265
Bluebells, 57
Bodhi tree, 142
book of hours
  for witches, 26–27
boundaries (also see *associations*), 100, 102, 110, 142, 162, 171, 201, 213, 220, 331, 357–361, 378, 382
boundary
  charm, 382
Bramble (*Rubus fruticosus* L.), 310
  uses and significance, 102, 358, 359
  foraging, 71, 80, 81–85

breathing
  balance, 72
Bright Moon (also see *Full Moon*), 408
Brigid, 46, 47, 338
broom, 103, 176, 295, 305, 360, 379
  jumping the, 100, 103
Broom (*Cytisus scoparius* (L.) Link), 103
Brownies, 337–338, 358
bug hotel, 52
Burdock (*Arctium lappa* L.)
  foraging, 67, 81–85, 104–105, 405
  uses and significance, 104–105
Butterfly, 56, 61, 104, 275

Cacti, 106–107, 359
candles, 38–39, 42, 43–45, 48, 295, 296–297, 300, 304, 327, 343, 374, 388
cards, 295–296, 341, 346
careers, 2, 22–23, 260, 372, 397–398
Carob (*Ceratonia siliqua* L.), 84–85, 108
Carr, Tree, 310
Carrion Crow (*Corvus corone*), 266, 349, 420
Cat (*Felis catus*), 12, 97, 109, 131, 278, 280
Cat claw, 328, 410
catkins, 47, 50, 52, 91, 100, 157, 206, 232, 248
Catnip (*Nepeta cataria* L.), 82–85, 109
cauldron, 183, 288, 292, 293, 296, 323
Cedar (also see *Thuja*), 386
cemeteries, 4, 6, 13, 38, 124
centring, 307, 309–310, 388
Ceridwen, 323, 413–414
Cernunnos, 51, 338
Chaffinch (*Fringilla coelebs*), 265
Chameleon Plant (*Houytuinia cordata*), 81–85, 110
Chamomile (*Matricaria chamomilla* L.; *Chamaemelum nobile* (L.) All.)
  foraging, 83–85, 112, 141
  uses and significance, 25, 52, 58, 63, 111–112, 192, 309, 314, 384
chanting, 333, 355–356, 371

chaos magic, 305, 324, 325
charging
    tools, 25, 62, 292–293, 301, 327, 405
    sigils, 335–336
charm
    boundaries, 382
    gadgets, 379
    good food, 380
    gossip, 384–385
    healing, 380
    health, 381
    love binding, 383–384
    love divination, 386
    Meadowsweet, 387
    money, 383
    negativity clearing, 381–382
    pest control, 386–387
    plant health, 380–381
    pocket, 382–383
    protection, 382
    safe travels, 379, 379–380
    seed planting, 69
    spring snow, 384–385
    wart, 385
charmers, 372–373
charms, 370–373, 379–387
    adapting, 375–376
Chickweed (*Stellaria media* (L.) Vill.)
    foraging, **60**, 81–85, 113, 250
    uses and significance, 43, 48, 113, 390
chocolate, 108, 202, 260
cider, 41
cipher wheel, 321
Circe, 137
Citrus species, 58, 108, 114–115, 226
clairaudience, 153, 342–343
claircognisance, 342–343
clairsentience, 342–343
clairvoyance, 41, 110, 153, 186, 255, 342–343
Clary Sage (*Salvia sclarea*), 299
cleansing
    tools, 21, 64, 242, 360, 292, 405
    self, 334, 360, 405
    space, 21, 331, 360, 378, 405

Cleavers (*Gallium aparine*), 46, 51, 53, 58, 82–84, 116–117
cloak, 38, 74, 166, 264, 300, 391
clouds, 10, 317, 344, 349–**350**
clutter, 20, 35, 316, 332, 360, 389
cobwebs, 142, 284, 308, 316, 360, 364, 381–382, 389
Coffee (*Coffea arabica* L.), 52, 116, 118–119, 345
Comfrey (*Symphytum* spp.), 81–85, 120–**123**, 389
communicating
    with wild beings, 16
communication
    between plants, 14
community-supported agriculture, 21
contagious magic, 305
contemplation on found objects, 18
Corn dolly, 73
Corn spirit, 73
Corvids (*Corvidae*), 265–267
covens
    activities, 30–31
    group size, 30
    safety and trust, 31–32
covens and community, 29–32
Cowslip (*Primula veris*) (see *Primrose*)
Cranesbill (see *Geranium*)
Crayfish (*Procambarus clarkii* and other species), 272–273
creativity
    spell for, 59–60
cross-quarter days, 33, 34, 36, 46, 56, 66
Crustaceans, 272–273
crystal ball, 255, 296, **343**, 345
crystals, 62, 140, **290**–291, 294, 296, 328, 330, 361, 381, 404, 405
curses, 252, 298, 364, 367–368, 372, 376–377, 378–379

Daisy (*Bellis perennis* L.)
    foraging, 81–84, 124
    uses and significance, 9, 51, 53, 57, 58, 62, 124, 372

INDEX

Dandelion (*Taraxacum officinale* F.H. Wigg.)
   foraging, 4, 81–85 125–**126**
   uses and significance, 58, 62, 104, 125, 309, 390
Daphne, 98, 415
Dark Moon (also see *New Moon*), 402, 407–408
Daylily (*Hemerocallis fulva* (L.) L.), 83–84, 127–128
Dead Nettles (*Lamium* spp.), 51, 81–85, 129
debt, 22
deity, 142, 338
Devil's Ivy (*Epipremnum aureum* (Linden & André) G.S. Bunting, 130–131
dew bathing, 17, 58
divination, 26, 38, 59, 61, 63, 73, 305, 341–350
   charm, 386
   Egyptian ritual, 327, 334
   plants and animals
     (see *associations*), 59, 63, 386
   tools for, 295–296, 298, 299, 343–344
Dock (*Rumex* species), 52, 82–85, 132, 405
Dog (*Canis lupus familiaris*), 97, 131, 278–279
dorodango, 296, 345
Dragonfly (*Anisoptera*), 275
dreams, 25, 38, 63, 89, 305, 348
dressing oil, 296–297
drinking straw, 160
druid egg, 297, 361, 416–417
Druids (also see *neo-druidry*), 94, 95, 187, 188, 210, 257, 274
drum, 333, 356

Earthworm (*Lumbricus terrestris*), 263, 270, 279, 284
egg
   magic, symbolism, 51–52, 53, 292
   staining, 52

Elder (*Sambucus nigra* L.)
   foraging, 43, 63, 81–85, 95, 133–134
   uses and significance, 41, 67, 68, 133–134, 338
elemental meditations, 18
Elm (*Ulmus* L.), 83, 135–136, 384
Enchanter's Nightshade (*Circaea lutetiana* L.; C. alpina subsp. alpina)
   foraging, 83–85, 137
   uses and significance, 137, 394–396
energy
   engaging (also see *healing*), 307, 312–313
   local, 3
enteric brain, 342–343
environmental impact
   (also see *sustainability*), 20–21, 97, 230, 289–291, 307
equinox, 33–34, 51–55, 71–75, 82, 85, 379
ethical foraging, 78–79
evil eye, 220, 276, 358, 364
Eye of Horus, 327
Eye of Newt, 321

Fennel (*Foeniculum vulgare* Mill.), 82–84, 138–**139**
fertility rites, 56, 155
festival dates (wheel of the year), 34
Feverfew (*Tanacetum parthenium* (L.) Sch. Bip.)
   foraging, 81, 83–85, 141
   uses and significance, 140, 358
Fig (*Ficus carica* L.), 85, 142–143, 359
Filbert (see *Hazel*)
finances, 20–24, 362, 368, 370, 373, 389
Fir (see *Pine family*)
fire gazing, 344
floriography, 320, 321, 322
Fly (*Diptera*), 276, 360
folk magic, 304, 305
food, 23
   charm, 380
foraging
   apps, 78 (fn6)
   as a grounding technique, 308

calendar, 80–85
    experts and teachers, 80
    guidelines, 78–79
    journal, 80
    legality, 79
    safety, 77–79
    urban, 77–85
    wheel of the year, 36, 41, 46, 51, 56, 61, 66, 71
Forsythia, 51, 53
Fox (*Vulpes vulpes*), 54, 279, 280
Foxglove (*Digitalis*), 122
Frankincense (*Boswellia*), 290–291, 298–299
Frog (*Rana* spp.), **262**–263, 321, 349
Full Moon
    rituals, 404
funeral rites, 92, 199
fungi, 13, 14, 15fn3, 17, 36–**37**, 204, 295, 369
furanocoumarins, 15

gadgets
    charm, 379
Gallant Soldiers (*Galinsoga parviflora* cav.), 81, 84–85, 144
Garlic, 68, **70**, 73, 99, 197, 212, 247, 358, 364
Garlic Mustard (*Alliaria petiolata* (M. Bieb.) cavara & Grande), 67, 81–84, 145–146, 153
geomancy, 345–346
Geranium (*Geranium sylvaticum* L.), 81–85, 147, 386
Giant Hogweed (*Heracleum mantegazzianum*), 15
Ginger (*Zingiber officinale* Roscoe), 212, 243–**244**, 381
Ginkgo (*Ginkgo biloba* L.), 81, 85, 148–**149**
gossip
    charm, 384–385
grain harvest, 66, 71
Grape Hyacinth, 52, 83
Grapevine (*Vitis vinifera* L.), 83–85, 150, **390**

graphology, 321–322, 325
gratitude, 24–25, 38, 66–68, 332, 352–354, 373
Graveyard dust, 321
graveyards, 233, 257–258, 275, 322
Great Tit (*Parus major*), 267–268
green city magic
    definition, 306
green city witchery
    guidelines, 306–307
    core techniques, 307–314
green living, 19–27
Green man, 51–52, 56–57, 61, 196, 339
greenwashing, 20
grimoire, **297**–298, 324, 374, 386, 404, 405
Ground Elder (*Aegopodium podograrium* L.), 14–15, 81–5, 151–152
Ground Ivy (*Glechoma hederacea* L.), 81–85, 146, 153
grounding (also see *associations*), 8, 11, 17, 294, 307–309, 334, 409
gut instinct (see *intuition*)
Gwion Bach (see *Taliesin*)
Gypsywort, 52

hag stone, 38, 298
hair, 10, 111, 172, 214, 238, 306, 409–411
Hairy Bittercress (*Cardamine hirsuta* L.), 81–85, 154
hamsa (see *Hand of Fatima*)
hand lens, 43, 78
Hand of Fatima, 327, 364
handwriting, 321–322
Hare, 51, 52, 53–54, 280, 415
harvest
    protection spell, 69–70
    knot, 66
    lords, 74–75
Hawthorn (*Crataegus monogyna* Jacq. and *C. laevigata* (Poir.) DC.)
    foraging, 16, 81–85, 156
    uses and significance, 17, 37, 53, 56, 58–59, 155, 310

Hazel (*Corylus* L.)
    foraging, 47, 50, 81–85, 91, 158
    uses and significance, 52, 72, 157, 164, 295
healing
    charms and spells, 377, 380, 396
healing (also see *associations, energy-engaging*), 8, 46, 58, 297, 305, 328, 332, 351, 353, 370, 372, 410, 415
health, 361–362, 381
Herb Bennet (see *Wood Avens*)
Herb Robert (*Geranium robertianum* L.), 82–85, 159, 388–389
herbs
    sustainability, 93, 184, 209, 229, 289–291, 299, 374
herbs (also see individial herbs), 4, 16, 298, 304, 305, 314, 326, 328, 330fn26, 358, 370, 374
herfest (also see *mabon*), 34, 71, 74–75, 162
Heron (*Ardea cinerea*), 147, 268, 273
hexes, 167, 172, 214, 252, 328, 368, 376–377
Hildegard von Bingen, 138, 153, 154, 172, 186, 204, 209, 381, 388
Himalayan Balsam (*Impatiens glandulifera* Royle), 83–85, 160–**161**, 349
Hinamatsuri (Doll's Festival), 171
hobby horse, 56
Holly (*Ilex aquifolium* L.)
    foraging, 81–85, 163
    uses and significance, 41, 42–43, **44–45**, 71–72, 162, 321, 360, 381
Holly King, 71, 162
Hollyhock (*Alcea rosea* L.)
    foraging, 82–85, 164
    uses and significance, 67, 164, 358
home decor and furnishings, 19
honey, 15, 49–50, 73, 103, 178, 274, **334**, 375, 396
house dolls, 364
House Sparrow (*Passer domesticus*), 268–269, 344

houseplants, 8, 19–20, 24, 35, 48, 62, 308, 380–381
Hyldemoer, 133, 338
Hyssop (*Hyssopus officinalis* L.), 83–85, 165

I Ching, 59, 320, 347
imbolc, 33, 34, 46–50, 81–82
incantation, 100, 330, 334, 355, 368–369, 370–371, 372fn32
incense, 25, 298–299, 326, 330, 331, 360, 364, 374
Indian Nettle (see *Coleus*)
ink, 38, 68, 73, 102, 237, 408
Insects, 273–277
instruments, 25, 314, 356
intention, 353, 367–368, 377, 404, 407–408, 419
intestinal worms, 95, 97, 157
intuition (also see *associations*), 26, 63, 313, 342–343
invisible ink, 237
invocation, 299–300, 332, 352–353, 367–370
Isle of Apples, 36, 37, 94
Ivy (*Hedera helix* L.)
    foraging, 81–85, 166
    uses and significance, 38, 41–43, 58, 73–74, 166, 322, 358
Ivy Arum (see *Devil's Ivy*)
Ivy Queen, 71, 73–74, 162

Jackdaw (*Corvus monedula*), 266
Japanese Knotweed (*Reynoutria japonica* Houtt.)
    foraging, 78, 82–85, 167–168
    uses and significance, 167
Japanese Plum/Loquat (*Eriobotrya japonica* (Thunb.) Lindl.), 81, 169–170
Japanese Quince (*Chaenomeles japonica* (Thunb.) Lindl. ex Spach), 82, 85, 171
Jay (*Garrulus glandarius*), 266
Jelly Ear fungus (*Auricularia auricula-judae*), 133

444 INDEX

jiva bandha, 362
journalling, 25, 38, 80, 297, 327, 348, 374, 404
Juniper (*Juniperus communis* L.), 307
    foraging, 83–84, 172–**173**
    uses and significance, 172

Kabbalah, 322
karma, 394–396
Kestrel (*Falco tinnunculus*), 269
Kimpetbrivl, 327
Kindred
    Glennie, 308
knives, 299
Kobolds, 338
Kodama, 339
Krishna, 142

Lady's Mantle (*Alchemilla* spp.)
    foraging, 81–85, 174–175
    uses and significance, 17, 174, 405
Ladybird (Coccinellidae), 276
lamen, 326–327
lammas (also see *lughnasadh*), 66
Lavender (*Lavandula angustifolia* Mill.)
    sustainability, 290–292
    foraging, 66–67, 82–84, **177**
    uses and significance, 53, 63–64, 92, 176, 295, 300, 305, 360
leaf art, 15, 237
Leiden Magical Papyrus, 327, 334–335
Lemon Balm (*Melissa officinalis* L.)
    foraging, 82–85, 178
    uses and significance, 178, 310, 311, 407
Lesser Celandine (*Ficaria verna*), 48, 53
light
    spell, 44–45
Lilac (*Syringa vulgaris* L.), 82–83, 179
Lime (*Tilia* spp.)
    foraging, 43, 81–85, 180
    uses and significance, 61–63, 64, 180, 310, 347
liminal state, 111, 164, 179, 201, 289, 300, 307, 313–314, 316, 318, 329, 332, 343

Linden (see *Lime*)
lingua magica, 320
Lizard (*Lacertidae*), 282
local
    energy, 3
    food, 4
    green connection, 4
    history and folklore, 5
local businesses, 21
London Plane (*Platanus* x *hispanica*), 181–182
Loquat (see *Japanese Plum*)
Lords and Ladies (*Arum maculatum*), 234
love
    binding, 383–384
    divination, 386
lughnasadh, 33, 34, 66–70
lunar
    gardening, 406–407
    spell casting, 404
    cycles, 401–403
    journaling, 404
    meditation, 404

mabon, 71, 85
Madder (*Rubia tinctorum*), 57, 117
magic (defining), 303–304
Magnolia (*Magnolia* L.), 43, 82–83, 183
Magpie (*Pica pica*), 12, 267
Mahonia (*Berberis aquifolium* Pursh (Mahonia)), 37, 81, 84, 184–**185**
Mallow (*Malva sylvestris* L.), 53, 81–85, 186
Mammals, 277–281
Mandrake (*Mandragora officinalis*), 290
manifesting, 24, 45, 60, 99, 170, 304, 324, 336, 338, 373, 407–408
manifesto
    personal, 24
Marigold (*Tagetes* spp.) also see *Pot Marigold*, 68, 72
mati amulet, 364
May
    bowl, 57
    day (also see *beltane*), 56
    queen, 56

INDEX   445

maypole, 56, 59
Meadowsweet
    charm, 387
Meadowsweet (*Filipendula ulmaria*
    I (L.) Maxim.)
    foraging, 63, 83–84, 90, 134, 187
    uses and significance, 67, 187
meditation, 26, 63, 292, 294, 300,
    310, 313, 315–318, 322,
    337, 362
    elementals, 18
    light, 44
    lunar, 404
    skull, 17
    snowdrop, 48–49
    tree, 17, 39
melancholy, 129
menstrual
    blood, 409–411
    cycle, 403
    leave, 22
metaphysical scissors, 377–378
Michaelmas Daisy, 72
microbes (also see *Nematodes, Amoebae*),
    8, 17, 190, 382
midsummer, 34, 83–84, 111, 180, 192,
    228, 375
midsummer's eve, 61, 63
Miner's Lettuce (see *Winter Purslane*)
Mint (*Mentha* spp.)
    foraging, 81, 83–84, 188–189
    uses and significance, 58, 72, 120,
        390, 397
misappropriation, 289, 306, 330
Mistletoe, 43
Mole (*Talpidae*), 279–280, 284
molehill soil, **67**, 68, 280
Molluscs, 281–282, 289
money
    charms, 382–383
    plants, 229, 383
Moon
    plants, 405–406
    gazing, 404
    and mind, 403
    water, 405

gardens, 406
manifestation, 407–408
Moon (also see associations)
    magic and rituals, 30, 63, 174, 250,
        292, 304, 305, 306, 330, 344,
        375, **401**–408
Morrigan, 338
Moss (Bryophytes)
    harvesting and care, 82–83, 85, 191
    uses and significance, 38, 47, 52,
        108, 308, 350, 405
    watching, 10–11, 43
motanka (see *house dolls*)
Mother-in-law's Tongue (see *Snake
    Plant*)
Mugwort (*Artemisia vulgaris* L.)
    divination, 345
    foraging, 81–85, 192, 254
    uses and significance, 63, 192,
        291–292, 299, 309, 310,
        311–312, 314, 321, 358
murmurations, 344

nail clippings, 305, 409, 410
Narcissi, 52
nasir amulet, 364
Nasturtium (*Tropaeolum majus*), 81,
    83–85, 193–**194**
natural magic
    definition, 305
nature
    -inspired symbolism, 322–323
    in magic, 306, 341–342, 343–345,
        374–376
    in spells and charms, 374–375
    signs in, 343, 349–350
    sounds in, 6, 9, 13, 314, 340, 356
    spirits, 91, 306, 324, 337–340, 342,
        352–354, 357–358, 365, 371
    urban, 2, 7–18, 420
negativity clearing
    charm, 381–382
Nematode, 11, 284–285
neo-druidry (also see *druids, OBOD*),
    305, 323, 387
NeoPagan, 33, 305, 323

Nettle (*Urtica dioica* L.), **304**
  foraging, 4, 46, 51, 81–85, 195
  uses and significance, 73, 132, 151, 195, 275, 309, 311, 326, 396
New Moon
  rituals, 407
  manifestation, 407–408
numerology, 322, 325
Nutmeg (*Myristica fragrans*), 388
nwyfre, 8, 362

Oak (*Quercus* L.)
  foraging, 81–82, 85, 196
  uses and significance, 56–57, 58, 61–62, 73, 94, 196
Oak King, 61, 71, 99, 162, 196
OBOD (see Order of Bards, Ovates, and Druids)
Ogham, 284, 347
  sticks, 299, 347–**348**
Old man (Mugwort), 321
Old woman (Wormwood), 321
Olive (*Olea europaea* L.), 83–84, 197–**198**
Onion, 52, 94, 212
oracle cards (also see *cards*), 346
Order of Bards, Ovates, and Druids (OBOD), 32, 323
ostara, 34, 51–55
oxymel, 73
Oya, 220

Pagan Federation, 32
palm stone, 309, 333
Palo Santo, 289, 292
Pansies (also see *Violets*), 48, 245–**246**, 358
Paris, 8fn2, 137
Parsley (*Petroselinum crispum* (Mill.) Fuss), 81–85, 199–**200**, 397
Passionflower (*Passiflora caerulea* L.), 83–85, 201
patterns, 16, 181, 275, 313, 317, 322–323, 343–345, 347, 404
pellars, 372–373
pentagram, 94, 320, 323–324
Peppermint (also see *Mint*), 311

perambulations, 61, 62
pest control
  charm, 386–387
petrichor, 11
photosensitivity, 151–152, 216
Pictish swirls, 323–324
Pigeon (*Columba livia domestica*), 166, 269–**270**
pilgrimage, 5–6, 46, 301
Pine family
  foraging, 78, 82–84, 203
  uses and significance, 43, 44, 68, 202–203, 390
plant communication, 14–15
plant health
  charm, 380–381
plant identification, 78
Plantain (*Plantago major*)
  foraging, 82–85, 205
  uses and significance, 186, 204
plastic, 8, 18, 21, 374
pocket stones, 25, 361
Poplar (*Populus* L.), 82–83, 206–207
Poppy, 67, 74
posessions, 20
Pot Marigold (*Calendula officinalis* L.), 24, 67, 81–85, 208
practical magic, 296, 304, 305
prana, 8, 362
prayer, 24, 36, 118, 314, 332, 351–354, 369, 375
Primrose (*Primula vulgaris* Huds.), 48, 53, 57, 82, 209
Prometheus, 138
protection
  charms, spells, rituals, 69–70, 331, 358, 376, 382, 393–394
  (also see *associations*)
  techniques, 44, 357–365, 392, 409
  tools for, 297, 299, 300, 301, 327, 361
protective herbs (also see *associations*), 358–359
Pseudo-Apuleius, 297fn20
psychic hygiene, 25, 364
Purple Dead Nettle (see *Dead Nettles*)
pyrrolizidine alkaloids (PA), 122

quarter days, 33, 41, 51, 61, 71
Quickthorn, 321

Rabbit (*Leporidae*), 51, 279, 280, 414
rain, 349–350, 356
Ramsons (see *Wild Garlic*)
Rat (*Rattus*), 12, 280–**281**, 363
rattle, 356, 360
Raven (*Corvus corax*), 267
reconnecting
  with urban nature, 7–18
Red Cabbage, 52
Red Clover (*Trifolium pratense*), 83, 210–**211**, 375–**376**, 390
Red Dead Nettle (see *Dead Nettles*), 129
renewal
  spell for, 49–50
repair cafés, 20
reptiles, 282–283
resilience (also see *associations*), 20, 22
ribbon, 59, 176, 295, 299–300, 384–385
Ribwort (*Plantago lanceolata*), 46, 66, 68, 82–85, 204–**205**
ritual
  harvesting, 63, 68, 73, 79, 218, 299
  bath or shower, 24, 48, 49, 165, 210, 334, 404
rituals, 329–336
robes (also see *cloak*), 300
Robin (*Erithacus rubecula*), 16, 159, 270
Rocket (*Diplotaxis tenuifolia*), 81–85, 212
Rook (*Corvus frugilegus*), 267
roots
  ritual harvest, 43
Rose (*Rosa* spp.)
  foraging, 81–85, 213
  uses and significance, 109, 192, 213, 310, 322, 328, 359, 372, 384, 392, 410
Rose-ringed Parakeet (*Psittacula krameri*), 270–271
Rosebay Willowherb, 295
Rosemary (*Salvia rosmarinus* Spenn.)
  foraging, 71, 81–85, 214
  uses and significance, 53, 71, 214, 301, 311, 314, 328, 348, 358–359, 360, 371, **374**, 375, 390

rosewater, 59, 98
routines, 23–27
Rubber Plant (*Ficus elastica*), 142
Rue (*Ruta graveolens*), 81–85, 199, 215–**216**, 358
runes, 27, 100, 324
Russian Sage (*Salvia yangii*), 217

Sage
  Clary (see *Clary Sage*)
  Russian (see *Russian Sage*)
  White (see *White Sage*)
Sage (*Salvia officinalis* L.)
  foraging, 81–85, 217
  uses and significance, 192, 196, 217, 299, 301, 358, 359
saining
  bundles, 63–64, 228, 240, 253, 292, 314, 331, 386–**387**
saliva, 409
Sam Webster, 14–15
samhain, 33, 34, 36–40, 81, 94
sand dunes, 58
saturnalia, 41, 98, 162
Scarab beetle, 327
scrying, 225, 296, **343**–345, 404
seasonal living
  (also see *wheel of the year*), 21
seedlings, 47, 53, 73, 115, 119, 144
seeds, 53, 54–55, 67, 69, 79, 104, 108, 115
Self-heal (*Prunella vulgaris*), 81–85, 218, 396
self-sufficiency, 20
shamanic magic, 305
Shams al-Ma'arif, 297
shapeshifting, 12, 53–54, 309, 332, 340, 413–417
shells, 18, 281–282, 289–293, 360
Shepherd's Purse (*Capsella bursa-pastoris*), 81–85, 219
shielding, 130, 166, 307, 311–312, 363
short straws, 347
sigils, 44, 230, 236, 252, 324–327, 328, 335–336, 372, 396
signs
  in nature, 343, 349
  that magic is working, 373

silk, 283, 299–300, 384
silver, 100, 289, 300, 364, 405
skin, 10, 12, 16–17, 18, 25, 39, 48, 350, 362, 364, 379–380, 404, 410
skin brushing, 25, 48, 334
skull meditation, 17–18
sky-stretch, 24–25
Slow worm, 282
Slug, 103, 140, 208, 263, 281–282
smudging, 289
Snail, 281–282
Snake (Serpentes), 283
Snake bite, 153
Snake Plant (*Dracaena trifasciata* (Prain) Mabb.), 220–221, 359
Snapdragon (*Antirrhinum majus* L.), 84–85, 222–223
snow, 350
Snowdrop, 47, 48–49
social impact, 20, 29–30, 98, 230, 307
solar panels, 20
solar plexus, 309–310, 363
solstices, 33, 34, 41, 61, 81, 83
soul nests, 38
sound, 355–356
spell
    for abundance, 64–65
    for abundance and creativity, 59–60
    for balance and growth, 54–55
    for banishing, 391–392
    for binding to prevent harm, 398–399
    for career, 397–398
    for good health, 396
    for harvest protection, 69–70
    for herfest, 74–75
    for invisibility, 391
    for karma, 394–396
    for light, 44–45
    for love, 388–389
    for prosperity, 389–390
    for protection, 393–394
    for renewal, 49–50
    for study success, 394
spells, 367–370, 373–378, 388–399
    adapting, 375–376
spellwork
    timing of, 375

Spider (*Araneae*), 142, 263, **283**–284, 360
Spider Plant (*Chlorophytum comosum* (Thunb.) Jacques), 224–**225**
spiky plants, 359
spirit flight, 264, 295, 301
spirit stopper, 214
spirits
    (also see *associations*), 38
spoons, 197, 300
spring equinox, 34, 51–55, 82
spring snow, 135, 384
Spruce (see *Pine family*)
staff, 157, 257, 300–301
Stag's Horn Sumac (*Rhus typhina* L.), 226–227
Stinging Nettle (see *Nettle*)
St John's Wort (*Hypericum perforatum*), 61, 63, 84, 228
stones, 4, 18, 25, 37, 62, 296, 298, 305, 309, 328, 331, 345–346 356, 361, 363, 370, 404, 405
Stork (*Ciconia ciconia*), 271
storytelling
    benefits of, 30fn5
Succulents, 92, 120, 229, 249, 259, 260
Sufism, 118, 314, 322
sugar, 176, 230–231, 245, 295, 236, 375
Sugarcane (*Saccharum officinarum* L.) (also see *sugar*), 230–231
summer solstice, 34, 61–65, 83–84
sustainability, 20–21, 93, 84, 209, 229, 289–291, 374–375
Swan (*Cygnus olor*), 271–272, 414
Sweet Chestnut (*Castanea sativa* Mill.), 81, 85, 232, 390
Sweet Cicely (*Myrrhis odorata* L.), 82–84, 233
Sweet Woodruff (*Gallium odoratum*), 57–58, 117
Swiss Cheese Plant (*Monstera deliciosa* Liebm.), 234–**235**
Sycamore (*Acer pseudoplatanus*), 73, 82, 181, 236–**237**, 376
symbolism (also see *associations*), 261, 292, 296, 300, 307, **319**–328, 346fn28, 347
sympathetic magic, 102, 107, 305, 409

INDEX   449

Taliesin, 323, 413–414
talisman, 274, 276, 298, 327–328, 370
Tansy (*Tanacetum vulgare*), 358, 388
Tardigrades, 11
tasseography, 345
tea leaf reading (also see *tasseography*), 38
Tea Plant (*Camellia sinensis* var. *sinensis*; *C. sinensis* var. *assamica*), 238–239
technology-free days, 34
The Herb Society UK, 80
threads, 44, 299–300, 327, 377
Thuja (Red and White cedar) (*Thuja occidentalis* L.; *Thuja plicata* L.) (also see *Cedar*), 240–241
Thyme (*Thymus vulgaris* L.)
    foraging, 81–85, 242
    uses and significance, 18, 164, 186, 242, 348, 396
timing
    magical work, 375, 403
Toad (*Bufo bufo*), 140, 217, 263
Toad men, 263
Toe of Frog, 321
toilet paper plant (see *Coleus*)
tongue scraper, 25
tools
    charging, 292, 301
    cleansing, 21, 64, 242, 360, 292, 405
    end of use, 293
    sustainable, 20–21, 289–291, 374–375
tourmaline, 290, 296, 361, 364
toxic chemicals, 19, 203, 240, 374
traditional remedies
    cardiovascular system, 97, 114, 155, 167, 238, 247, 255
    digestive system, 89, 91, 92, 98, 100, 102, 104, 108, 109, 111, 125, 132, 135, 138, 140, 142, 150, 184, 186, 187, 188, 199, 208, 215, 228, 232, 233, 238, 243, 255
    emotions, 127, 138, 140, 147, 213, 217, 252
    endocrine system, 210, 217, 224
    infections, 104, 114, 133, 150, 167, 172, 178, 226, 243, 249
    musculoskeletal, 97, 100, 122, 172, 187, 214, 224, 228, 248
    nervous system, 109, 114, 118, 148, 176, 178, 180, 183, 201, 210, 214, 228, 238
    reproductive system, 102, 140, 147, 174, 192, 199, 224, 255
    respiratory system, 99, 120, 140, 148, 153, 164, 165, 169, 180, 186, 202, 204, 209, 210, 215, 232, 242, 243, 245, 247
    skin, 89, 92, 94, 95, 97, 100, 102, 104, 110, 111, 113, 122, 132, 133, 142, 150, 151, 155, 160, 164, 166, 167, 169, 174, 176, 178, 179, 184, 186, 187, 195, 197, 204, 206, 208, 209, 210, 213, 214, 215, 218, 220, 232, 236, 238, 240, 242, 243, 245, 247, 250, 257, 260, 385
    urinary system, 116, 125, 172, 222, 226
    wound herbs, 89, 99, 124, 129, 137, 144, 159, 190, 204, 218, 219, 248, 255, 259
travel
    charms, 379–380
tree
    hugging, 18
    meditation, 17
    planting, 73
    watching, 13
treepit garden, 5
trees
    talking with, 15
triskelion, 323
Tsukumogami, 20, 293
Turmeric (*Curcuma longa* L.), 243–244
Tutsan (*Hypericum androsaemum*), 228
twilight, 10, 155, 375, 379

vagus nerve, 355–356
Violet (*Viola* spp.), 81–85, 245–246
viriditas, 8, 49, 56, 376

vital energy (also see *nwyfre, prana, viriditas*), 362
vitamin D, 16
VOCs (see *volatile organic chemicals*)
volatile organic chemicals, 8, 14, 17

walking, 3–5, 8, 43, 47, 53, 62, 72, 326, 361
   barefoot, 25, 48, 57, 308–309
walking staff (see *staff*)
Walnut, 52, 85
wand, 94, 95, 157, 197, 257, 292, 299, 301, 331, 370–371
wards, 361
wart
   charm, 385
warts, 113, 142, 160, 166, 240
wassailing, 41
Water Bears, 11
water watching, 12–13
weather
   lore, 349–350
   watching, 9–10
wells, 46, 58, 95
Wheel of the Year, 33–75
White Dead Nettle (also see *Dead Nettles*), 129
White Sage (*Salvia apiana*), 289, 291, 330, 360
Wicca, 305, 324
Wild Garlic (*Allium ursinum* L.)
   foraging, 47, 55, 82–84, 247
   uses and significance, 52, 57
Wild Rocket (also see *Rocket*), 81–85
wildlife
   refuges, 41
Willow (*Salix* L.)
   foraging, 81–85, 248
   uses and significance, 51–52, 57, 58, 61–62, 292, 295
wind, 6, 10, 18, 207, 349, 350, 356

wind chime, 356
Winter Purslane (*Claytonia perfoliata; C. sibirica*), 81–83, 85, 249
winter solstice, 34, 41–45, 81
witch balls, 328
Witch bane, 321
Witch City, 137
Witch Hazel (*Hamamelis* Gronov. ex L.), 82, 250–251, 298, 406
wood ash, 43–44, 142, 299
Wood Avens (*Geum urbanum* L.)
   foraging, 43, 81–85, 252
   uses and significance, 252, 358, 388
Woodpecker (*Picidae*), 272
Woodworm (*Anobium punctatum*), 277
work-life-nature-magic balance, 22
Wormwood (*Artemisia absinthium* L.), 83–85, 253–254, 277, 321, 347, 358, 405
worries, 17, 43, 48, 50, 165

yantras, 322
Yarrow (*Achillea millefolium*)
   foraging, 81–85, 256
   uses and significance, 38, 56, 59, 63, 188, 255, 345, 347, 358, 386, 389–390
Yellow Dead Nettle (also see *Dead Nettles*), 81–85, 129
Yew (*Taxus* L.), 203, 257–258, 300, 301, 358–359
yoga, 23, 25, 313, 315–316, 362
yule (also see *winter solstice*), 34, 38, 41–45, 100, 163, 166, 203
yule log, 41, 43

Zebra Plant (*Tradescantia zebrina* Bosse), 259
ZZ-Plant (*Zamioculcas zamiifolia* (G. Lodd.) Engl.), 260, 359

www.ingramcontent.com/pod-product-compliance
Lightning Source LLC
Chambersburg PA
CBHW051107230426
43667CB00014B/2472